DENTINAL FLUID TRANSPORT

Lifetime research of
Ralph Steinman and John Leonora
leading to a theory of hormone-axis-mediated dental cariostasis

Condensed and Edited by
Dr. Clyde Roggenkamp

Compiled by
Drs. Lin Martin, Clyde Roggenkamp
and Herbert Woodward

With Historical Foreword by John Leonora

Cover design by Richard Tinker
Educational Support Services
Loma Linda University School of Dentistry

Loma Linda University School of Dentistry
Loma Linda, CA 92350

This publication is a condensed compilation of the research work of Ralph Steinman, DDS, MS, and John Leonora, PhD. References have been edited only, with no direct authorship intended except in the Foreword, Preface and Biography of Dr. Steinman in Appendix B. Some phraseology was necessarily re-worded for succinctness without significantly altering original meanings. This publication is primarily for dental educators and others, such as students, who may be interested in reading the research involving the dentinal fluid transport (DFT) theory of dental caries resistance. Readers should refer to original sources for useful illustrations and other supporting information.

Library of Congress Catalog Card Number: 2005933671
ISBN: 1-59410-008-X

Roggenkamp, Clyde.
Dentinal fluid transport : lifetime research of Ralph Steinman and John Leonora leading to a theory of hormone-axis mediated dental cariostasis / by Clyde Roggenkamp, with historical foreword by John Leonora – Centennial edition. Loma Linda University School of Dentistry. Loma Linda, Calif. : The University, 2005, c2004.

p.. : ill. ; cm.
Annotated bibliography.
Includes index.
ISBN 1-59410-008-X
1.Steinman, Ralph—bibliography. 2. Leonora, John—bibliography. 3. Dental Caries Susceptibility. 2. Dentin Permeability--physiology. 5. Dentinal Fluid. 6. Dentistry—research. I. Loma Linda University School of Dentistry. II. Title. III. Lifetime research of Ralph Steinman and John Leonora. IV. Theory of hormone-axis mediated dental cariostasis.

WU 270 R733d 2005 2005933671

Third printing, October 2015, ECKO Publishing, Sandy, Utah, USA

FOREWORD

Historical Research Tribute to Ralph R. Steinman, DDS, MS
Written by John Leonora, Ph.D.

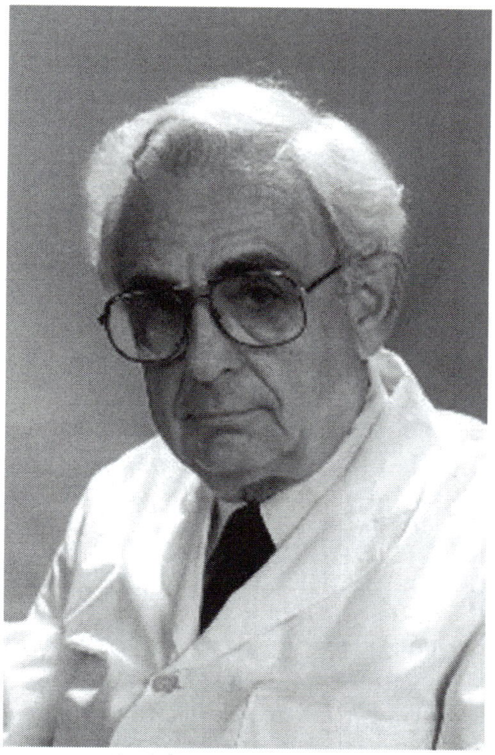

Dr. John Leonora

The purpose of this historical review of our research collaboration over several decades is to provide a stimulus to the reader to examine our published data demonstrating that systemic mechanism(s) are critical for maintaining optimal dental health. The important issue is that, in spite of a destructive oral environment, there are physiological mechanism(s) that are linked to teeth that enable them to withstand the assault of a hostile environment. Examination of the histological morphology of teeth clearly indicates that they are designed for maintaining fluid flow through the dentin and enamel; consequently, there must be a mechanism to control fluid flow. We refer to this as the dentinal fluid flow mechanism (see Figure 1). Hopefully, it should become apparent that cariogenic bacteria are opportunistic rather than deterministic. The probability that oral bacteria induce cariogenesis is greater when systemic mechanism(s) that maintain tooth vitality is/are compromised.

Over 25 years were spent in collaborative research with Dr. Ralph Steinman. It has been documented in science on numerous occasions that unforeseen events can alter the direction that one intends to follow. As an endocrine physiologist, I had planned to work in my chosen field of physiology of reproduction, until one day so long ago, when Ralph came to see me for a little help on a dental problem that took the remainder of my academic career at Loma Linda University to help, at least in part, to resolve. To put our work in perspective, I want to begin a number of years before we met because those were the years he began to question Miller's acidogenic theory as the primary cause of cariogenesis.

After graduating from Emory University, School of Dentistry, Dr. Steinman went into private practice and during WW II volunteered for the Dental Corps. During this time, his confidence in the acidogenic theory began to diminish. What he observed in patients' mouths did not always follow dogma. Also, he was strongly influenced by the writings of E.G. White on the deleterious effects of high sugar consumption. After the war, Dr. M. Webster Prince, one of the moving forces for establishing the School of Dentistry at Loma Linda, extended an invitation to Dr. Steinman to become part of the original dental faculty. To better prepare himself for academia, Ralph enrolled in the dental graduate program at the University of Michigan and obtained a master's degree in Prosthodontics. His academic experience in graduate school served as a catalyst to his thinking that the acidogenic theory was inadequate because it ignored the potential defensive role of the host. Upon his arrival at Loma Linda, he dedicated his research effort to ascertain whether the host had a role in defending its teeth against a destructive oral environment. Unfortunately, many of his faculty associates did not share his convictions and criticized him severely, even to the point of putting a sign on his laboratory door which said "searching for a systemic explanation for cariogenesis is akin to looking for the holy grail." This attitude reminds me what Dr. Albert Szent-Györgyi, 1937 Nobel Laureate in medicine, said "when everyone begins to laugh at you, then you know you are two steps ahead." Regardless of what others thought, Steinman remained undaunted in his views.

Ralph was a thorough student of dental literature relating to cariogenesis. Beginning with the literature of the late 1800s, he studied the development of dental thought as to the causal factors related to cariogenesis. Through the 1930s there were two tracks of investigations, the dominant track favored the acidogenic theory and the lesser track examined the possible role of systemic factor(s) i.e. the possible role of the host. It appears that in the 1940s, at an International Association of Dental Research meeting, Miller's acidogenic theory became the accepted dogma by committee vote, rather than science. [Larmas, M., *J Dent Res* 82:253 (2003)]. The investigators in the lesser track who emphasized the possible existence of a dentinal fluid flow system that begins at the level of the odontoblasts and extends through the dentin via cytoplasmic extensions from the odontoblasts within narrow canaliculi, were effectively ignored thereafter. The fluid in the dentinal fluid transport (DFT) system was referred to as dental lymph to distinguish it from other body fluids. [For more details see Introduction, *J Dent Res* 59: 176 (1980)].

Steinman was impressed with the possible significance of DFT, even though its regulatory mechanism was unknown. Furthermore, he concluded that the methodology developed to examine teeth microscopically was cumbersome and that the definition of the markers used to demonstrate DFT was poor because the teeth had to be demineralized before they could be sectioned. Also, the experimental approach did not provide any insight into the dynamics of DFT. His first challenge was to develop a different approach, which did not require demineralization and that could also provide some estimate of the rate of fluid flow through the dentin. He decided to work with young rats between the ages of 21-35 days old.

He found that the entire jaw could be sectioned on a microtome in the frozen state, thus averting the need for demineralization. Cutting the jaws medially through the molar teeth to a thickness of approximately 100µm provided excellent microscopic visualization of tooth structure. After trial and error, he found that the dynamics of DFT could be best visualized after an intraperitoneal injection of a fluorescent dye, acriflavine hydrochloride. His next achievement was the demonstration that the composition of a diet (cariogenic vs noncariogenic) affected the dynamics of DFT. In rats fed a noncariogenic diet, the fluorescent dye moved quickly from the pulp-dentin interface to the dentin-enamel interface within 30-45 min. In comparison, DFT occurred only to a limited extent in the teeth of rats fed the cariogenic diet. In these rats, the fluorescent dye accumulated in the pulp but did not penetrate significantly beyond the odontoblast layer. That the composition of a diet could affect DFT had never been previously observed. As with the other investigators who had observed DFT, Dr. Steinman was unable to explain the mechanism regulating DFT. However, he was convinced that the difference in the dynamics that he observed between the two groups of rats could be important. It suggested the possibility that optimal dental health required host involvement through systemic mechanism(s). He decided he needed assistance and called me for an appointment.

Our first meeting was a memorable event. His enthusiasm was compelling but because my knowledge of dentistry was deficient, I needed a quick course in Dentistry 101 to understand the significance of what he was excited about. After reflecting upon his presentation, I told him that if he was correct, a hormonal mechanism might be a plausible explanation. The question was: which of the recognized hormones at that time could be involved in the regulation of the DFT mechanism? From personal knowledge and the available literature none of them appeared to be a plausible candidate. We concluded that if a hormonal mechanism was involved it had to be discovered. This point marked the beginning of a wonderful research relationship that continued until Dr. Steinman retired July 1, 1981, and continued to a lesser degree until 1997 when he moved to Oregon to live near his son. Ralph and I had an agreement as far as our work was concerned. He would be responsible for the teeth part of our studies such as sectioning the teeth to measuring DFT and the role of DFT in cariogenesis. I would be responsible for identifying the hormonal mechanism(s) stimulating DFT, the isolation of the hormonal factor(s), and the physiological studies for characterizing the endocrine system. We developed the DFT technique into a bioassay for our physiological studies and for tracking hormonal activity during the isolation of the active fraction. It proved to be a most amiable, stimulating cooperative effort.

Our early work was devoted to identifying the hormonal factor(s) that might regulate the DFT mechanism. This work led to the discovery of a hypothalamic–parotid gland endocrine axis [see Endocrinology 83: 807 (1967) for specific details]. There is an interesting anecdote associated with our first experiment. After I conducted a literature review, looking for clues as to where we should begin our search, it seemed intuitive that the most likely first source to examine should be the hypothalamus. I prepared a crude extract from rabbit hypothalami and we assayed it for DFT activity by infusing it intravenously into 28-day-old rats. Upon completion of the assay, Ralph took the rat jaws to his laboratory to examine them for increased DFT activity. Approximately an hour later, my phone rang and it was Ralph. He was so excited that on our first experiment we had identified the source of the DFT stimulating hormone. The obvious question that arose was whether the hypothalamic factor was exercising a direct effect on the teeth or was its effect indirect, as is characteristic of other hypothalamic hormones in stimulating hormonal secretion from other endocrine glands. Our first experiment was a fortuitous small step that turned us in the right direction. We focused on the possibility that the effect of the hypothalamic factor might be mediated through one of the major salivary glands. After a series of experiments, we concluded that the effect of the hypothalamic factor was not direct on the teeth but rather was mediated through the parotid glands. The hypothalamic factor was biologically active only when administered to intact rats (parotid glands present) but was ineffective in parotidectomized animals. There was no involvement of the submandibular-sublingual gland complex. This discovery made it apparent that the DFT regulatory mechanism was more complex than a single hormone stimulating odontoblasts. The direct regulator of DFT was secreted by the parotid glands and the endocrine function of the parotid glands was controlled by the hypothalamus.

Jean-Marc Tièche, a physiology graduate student, for his Ph.D. dissertation took up the challenge to complete the isolation of parotid hormone (PH) from porcine glands. He was successful in isolating PH in pure form and he also determined its amino acid structure. Intravenous infusion of pure porcine PH stimulated the uptake of fluorescent dye by the DFT mechanism. Upon completing his Ph.D. requirements, Jean-Marc joined us and succeeded in the partial purification of the hypothalamic factor (parotid hormone releasing factor) that stimulated PH secretion. Because of insufficient funding, the isolation of this factor has not been completed. In addition, Dr. Tièche also developed an antibody against porcine PH and a radio-immunoassay and later an ELISA method (enzyme linked immunoadsorbent assay) to measure the level of PH in pig blood. These developments were essential for conducting our physiological studies. Concurrent with the hormone isolation studies, our physiological studies involved two animal models: the rat and pig.

For many decades the rat model has been the animal of choice in studies relating to cariogenesis (see Figure 2). Since we were interested in determining the role of the DFT mechanism to cariogenesis, we also did our studies in rats. Our initial studies suggested that the sucrose effect in suppressing the DFT mechanism was mediated through the suppression of PH secretion. However, further studies pin-pointed the sucrose effect as occurring at the level of the hypothalamus which inhibited the secretion of the PH-releasing factor. This inhibitory effect caused a decrease in PH hormone secretion and a concomitant decrease in DFT. At this point, our challenge was how to inhibit/ reverse the sucrose effect on the hypothalamus. We made a fortuitous discovery that the sucrose effect could be acutely reversed by either an intravenous or intra-arterial infusion of carbamoyl phosphate or carbamoyl aspartate. [Carbamoyl and carbamyl spellings are used somewhat interchangeably in the literature.] Because the dose of either compound infused through the internal carotid artery was more than ten times less than the amount infused through the subclavian vein to effectively stimulate PH secretion we concluded that the site of action was within the central nervous system. Subsequent studies indicated that the probable site of stimulation was at the level of the hypothalamus which sequentially enabled the endocrine and DFT mechanisms to function in spite of the rats ingesting a high sucrose diet. It is important to note that physiologically these two endogenous compounds are closely linked in the pyrimidine pathway leading to the synthesis of DNA.

The moment of truth had come. Could these compounds counteract the inhibitory sucrose effect on the endocrine and DFT mechanisms in rats chronically fed a cariogenic diet for three months? Dr. Steinman had shown that there was an inverse relationship between DFT activity and the incidence of dental caries. A low incidence of caries was associated with high DFT activity, and a high caries incidence with low DFT activity. With this information, we believed that if the DFT mechanism could be functionally maintained cariogenesis would be significantly reduced. We did two caries studies. With the first study, we had some trepidation because all of our studies with carbamoyl phosphate and carbamoyl aspartate had been acute studies. Each compound when infused into the circulation demonstrated essentially equal potency in stimulating DFT in sucrose suppressed rats. Unfortunately, we did not have any information as to whether these compounds could survive in the digestive system, let alone be absorbed in an effective concentration.

In our first caries study, the rats were maintained on a 62% sucrose diet for three months beginning at weaning (21 days of age). The control rats were only fed the 62% sucrose diet while the experimental animals were fed the same diet supplemented with either carbamoyl phosphate or carbamoyl aspartate. In the first study with carbamoyl phosphate, we got 89% inhibition in cariogenesis and 70% inhibition with carbamoyl aspartate. Because carbamoyl aspartate is considerably more water soluble than carbamoyl phosphate, we suspected that as a dietary supplement it might be more susceptible to degradation. In the second caries experiment we only used carbamoyl phosphate as the dietary supplement and we obtained an 82% inhibition. With carbamoyl phosphate, the average caries inhibition between the two studies approached 86%. From our perspective, the results were beyond our expectation. The degree of caries inhibition significantly exceeded that reported for fluoride. As expected, carbamoyl phosphate was ineffective in inhibiting cariogenesis in parotidectomized rats as it was in stimulating DFT. An intact hypothalamic-parotid gland endocrine axis is required for carbamoyl phosphate to be effective. The results from our acute and chronic studies with carbamoyl phosphate demonstrated that a functional endocrine mechanism had a significant role in maintaining a functional DFT mechanism and suppressing cariogenesis. Although the idea may sound foreign, in terms of contemporary thinking on the etiology of cariogenesis, it can be stated with certainty that the sucrose effect of stimulating cariogenesis actually begins at the level of the hypothalamus and ultimately leads to a failure of the DFT mechanism and an increase in the incidence of caries. [The reader is encouraged to read JDR 59: 176-185 (1980) for a more in-depth presentation].

To defuse the argument that passage of carbamoyl phosphate through the mouth may have altered the hostility of the oral environment by decreasing the acidogenic potential of the high sucrose diet, a study was done to measure the amount of acid that could be produced as a consequence of bacterial activity. Aliquots of high sucrose diet and high sucrose diet supplemented with carbamoyl phosphate were incubated for 24 hours with rat saliva. As a control, an aliquot of rat noncariogenic diet was similarly incubated with the same volume of saliva. Between the two sucrose diets, acid production was essentially equivalent. The amount of acid produced with the supplemented diet was greater but not statistically significant. Surprisingly, the acidogenic potential of the noncariogenic diet was significantly greater than both sucrose diets. We concluded that the cariostatic effect of carbamoyl phosphate was not mediated orally by decreasing the acidogenic potential of the sucrose diet but rather through the activation of a systemic mechanism, as previously described. In addition, it should be emphasized that, irrespective of the composition of the diet, the primary end product of oral bacterial metabolism is acid. Although the bacteria are programmed to produce acid, there does not appear to be a correlation between the amount of acid produced and the incidence of caries.

Another phase of our studies was to physiologically characterize the hypothalamic-parotid gland endocrine axis. Specifically, what physiological factors affected the secretion of PH? For these studies, we had to change to the pig model. Because of their large size, pigs are able to withstand the taking of numerous blood samples over extended time periods, sometimes lasting as long as 3 months, without causing hemodynamic problems. To obtain the blood samples, a catheter was introduced into the heart so that the blood samples could be obtained without stressing the animal. During the experiment the pig was not aware that blood samples were being withdrawn. Dr. Tièche had developed a radioimmunoassay for porcine PH that enabled us to easily titer the level of the hormone in the blood under various conditions. As previously indicated, our first clue of a systemic mechanism affecting the DFT mechanism was the response observed in rats to the infusion of a crude hypothalamic extract. The intravenous infusion of a highly purified preparation of porcine parotid hormone releasing factor into fasting pigs resulted, within five minutes, in a measurable increase in PH titer that peaked between 10-12 minutes post-infusion. No comparable increase in PH secretion occurred when the infusion was done in parotidectomized pigs. These findings confirmed our initial conclusion, derived from rat studies, that the stimulatory DFT mechanism was composed of a hypothalamic–parotid gland endocrine axis.

The next important issue to be addressed was the identification of the physiological stimulus responsible for stimulating PH secretion and also to determine the association between the endocrine and the neurally controlled parotid exocrine function. It is generally recognized that eating (chewing), along with visual, olfactory, and auditory cues, are effective stimulators of saliva secretion, particularly from the parotid glands. We found that these glands have the capability to simultaneously handle both functions through different mechanisms. Our data showed that feeding pigs a standard pig chow, after an overnight fast, proved to be an effective stimulus for PH secretion, along with the copious secretion of saliva. The hormone titer in the blood was quickly detectable after the onset of eating, reaching peak levels within ten and twenty minutes, and then declined slowly with time. An attempt was made to determine whether the endocrine and the neurally mediated exocrine function could be dissociated. Experiments were designed to test the effect of chewing a nonnutritive substance and the role of auditory, olfactory, and visual cues for stimulating PH secretion. Pigs that were fed crushed ice (nonnutritive substance), or were exposed to the auditory sound of rattling feed containers, to visual and olfactory cues derived from seeing and smelling containers filled with feed but deprived access to the feed salivated profusely. Blood samples taken during these experiments did not show any change in the basal level (fasting level) of PH. These experiments clearly indicated that although the endocrine and exocrine functions of the parotid glands occur concurrently they were controlled by different mechanisms. More importantly, the nutritive composition of what was eaten proved to be critical for the secretion of PH. As expected, feeding experiments done in parotidectomized pigs gave no evidence of PH secretion.

As previously explained, we were compelled to use two animal models to conduct our studies. To minimize species differences, it is best to use a single animal model for all studies. However, having identified that feeding is a powerful physiological stimulus for PH secretion in the pig, it was necessary to return to the rat model to determine whether the same stimulus activated the DFT mechanism. The results from this study were confirmatory. Rats fasted overnight and then fed for fifteen minutes reacted with a strong DFT response. The fluorescent dye in the dentin became visible twenty minutes after eating. The dye concentration peaked at twenty-eight minutes, and then began to decline by thirty-three minutes. Time-wise the appearance of the dye in the dentin appeared to parallel the rise and fall of the PH titer in pigs. Another similarity between the two species was that after parotidectomy PH secretion was not observed in pigs and neither was the activation of the DFT mechanism in the rat. Surgical removal of the other major salivary gland, the submandibular-sublingual gland complex, did not interfere with the response of the DFT mechanism to feeding. These results further confirmed the concept of an endocrine function residing in the parotid glands. The linkage of the DFT mechanism to the hormonal mechanism became more tenable.

The almost immediate secretion of PH to the feeding stimulus appears to involve recruitment of other unidentified neural and/or hormonal factors. The data suggest that neural endings in the oral mucosa and /or tongue can distinguish the difference between nutritive and nonnutritive substrates. Nutritive substrates appeared to activate neural stimuli going to the hypothalamus that ultimately activated the hypothalamic–parotid gland endocrine axis which then stimulated the DFT mechanism. The possibility exists that the PH secretory mechanism is analogous to the neural, hormonal and substrate factors that optimize the secretion of insulin in response to feeding. The secretion of both hormones responds almost simultaneously to eating.

Having gained insight into the regulatory mechanism controlling the DFT mechanism in animals fed a noncariogenic diet, we turned our attention to determine how a cariogenic diet might impede the DFT mechanism. Before beginning our collaborative work, Dr. Steinman had observed in high-sucrose fed rats that, compared to rats fed the noncariogenic diet, the uptake of fluorescent dye by the dentin appeared to be significantly suppressed. Our next study involving pigs provided the answer. With each pig serving as its own control, the PH titer secreted into the blood in response to eating a standard pig diet (noncariogenic) was measured at least two times per week over a three week period. This provided a profile of the secretion pattern for each pig. At the end of three weeks, the diet was abruptly changed to the cariogenic diet containing sixty-two percent sucrose. The pigs were maintained on this diet for sixty days. The results after the diet change demonstrated a dramatic decrease in PH secretion when compared to the secretion during the first three weeks on the noncariogenic diet. In addition to the decrease in PH secretion, a significant decrease in the PH basal blood level, the level maintained during fasting, was noted. After sixty days on the sucrose diet, the diet was abruptly changed back to the noncariogenic diet. Approximately three days after eating the noncariogenic diet there was a strong resurgence of PH secretion, indicating that the suppressive effect of the sucrose diet on the endocrine system had been overcome.

An important question that presently remains unresolved is: What is the nature of the inhibitory effect of the sucrose diet that leads to the impairment of the DFT mechanism that contributes to an increase in cariogenesis? We presently know from corroborating evidence, obtained from studies done in pigs and rats, that the chronic ingestion of sucrose blocks the feeding stimulus from stimulating the secretion of parotid hormone releasing factor which ultimately leads to a decrease in parotid hormone secretion (see Figure 1). The culprit for the inhibition is not a sustained high blood glucose level derived from the ingested sucrose. In terms of time, the clearance of blood glucose after eating, in both the rat and pig, is essentially similar to that observed when the animals are fed a noncariogenic diet. Neither is there any significant difference in the fasting blood sugar. What is evident is that maintenance of the inhibitory effect requires the daily ingestion of a high sucrose diet. If the sucrose diet is abruptly terminated, the inhibitory effect disappears and the endocrine axis becomes strongly responsive again to the feeding stimulus.

Another related question which deserves consideration is: what is (are) the mechanism(s) through which the endogenous compounds (carbamoyl phosphate and carbamoyl aspartate) inhibit the suppressive sucrose effect, presumably on the hypothalamus, that enables the endocrine system to function at a level which significantly decreases the cariogenic potency of the high sucrose diet? Since function is restored with supplementing the high sucrose diet with these compounds, it appears that, in a manner that is not understood, a high sucrose intake may cause systemic depletion of the endogenous compounds which results in the appearance of pathological changes.

In 1997 two memorable events occurred. One was anticipated, Ralph and his wife, Emily, decided to move to Oregon to be closer to family. After three decades of working together, our research collaboration was about to come to an end. Even after moving away, his interest in dental research remained strong. For several years, he would periodically go to the Oregon Health Sciences University Dental Library, in Portland, to keep abreast of the current literature. We shared our ideas by letter. The second event was an unanticipated telephone call from Dr. Leo Tjäderhane DDS, Ph.D. His call was reminiscent of Dr. Steinman's call decades before asking for help. Tjäderhane, along with other investigators in Dr. Larmas' Laboratory, at the University of Oulu Dental School, Oulu, Finland, had made what appeared to be a significant observation. Their studies showed that a high sucrose diet suppressed primary dentinogenesis in young rats. When he called, Dr. Tjäderhane was on a post-doctoral fellowship in Vancouver, Canada. He had just returned from a dental meeting in Japan where he had presented their data on the sucrose effect on dentinogenesis. Unfortunately, he had to acknowledge that he had no idea of the mechanism involved behind the sucrose effect. At the meeting, according to Tjäderhane, Dr. D.H. Pashley, School of Dentistry, Medical College of Georgia, suggested that he show his data to me for a possible mechanism. This conversation was the stimulus for his call. Dr. Steinman had not yet moved, so I invited him to meet with us.

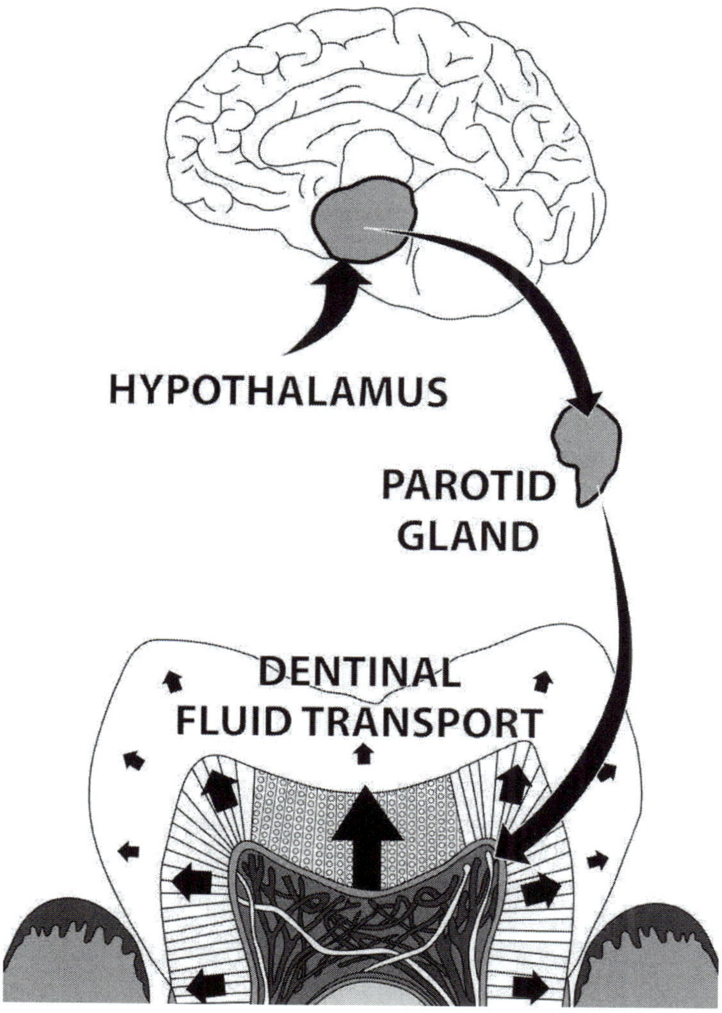

Figure 1. Diagram representing the human Hypothalamus-Parotid gland Endocrine Axis (HPEA)

The above diagram is a schematic representation of a human molar tooth illustrating that the morphology of the tooth is designed to maintain fluid flow through its structure. Dentin is composed of microscopic tubules (canaliculi) that radiate from the dentin-pulp interface to the dentin-enamel interface. At the base of the dentin, a layer of odontoblast and pre-odontoblast cells form the interface between the dentin and pulp. Functionally, odontoblasts are responsible for the secretion of dentin matrix and, because dentin is a living tissue, the maintenance of dentin vitality. Dentin, as a living tissue, should have a blood supply to maintain its physiological needs; but as the diagram shows, the blood supply terminates in the pulp chamber. To compensate for the lack of a blood supply, odontoblasts possess a dentinal fluid flow transport mechanism (DFT) that perfuses the dentin with essential nutrients derived from the blood. The capillaries in the pulp are fenestrated (have windows), allowing nutrients to diffuse out of the circulation into the pulp chamber in a lymph-like fluid which is taken up by the odontoblasts.

The uptake of nutrients appears to be parotid hormone dependent. The hormone appears to alter the permeability of the odontoblast membranes which enables the transfer of nutrient containing fluid into the odontoblasts. In addition, odontoblasts contain cytoplasmic myofibrils which enables them to function as pumps. Physiologically, the movement of dentinal fluid is in a centrifugal direction, ultimately it appears on the surface of the enamel. Fluid droplets coalesce on the surface of the enamel, forming a fluid layer. Fluid flow is greater wherever cracks occur in the enamel. Because the hydrostatic pressure within the tooth is greater than the oral pressure, diffusion of harmful bacterial products into the tooth structure is prevented and teeth remain caries free. Only when the DFT mechanism is compromised does cariogenesis occur.

After Tjäderhane's presentation, Ralph and I were impressed with the research opportunity that had been presented to us. If the mechanism(s) through which sucrose exercised its down-regulatory effect on dentinogenesis could be identified, it would be a significant achievement. We had been searching for such a tooth model where the effects of the oral environment could be separated from systemic effects on teeth. We agreed to a collaborative research approach between my laboratory and his at the University of Oulu. If successful, we were convinced that we would have irrefutable evidence on the importance of systemic mechanism(s) on teeth. Unfortunately, Dr. Steinman was not able to participate in this research because shortly thereafter he moved to Oregon. But he was with us in spirit, the studies I proposed were predicated on the research that we had done in the past.

Two major studies were done to address the sucrose effect on dentinogenesis. In our first study, we hypothesized the possibility of parotid gland involvement since a high sucrose intake, as previously discussed, is associated with a decrease in odontoblast function (↓DFT). Also, odontoblasts orchestrate the secretion of fibrillar protein matrix of the predentin and the subsequent initiation of its mineralization. We theorized that the odontoblasts, as multifunctional cells, may be responsive to PH or other presently unrecognized peptide factors secreted from the parotid glands essential for maintaining the structure and/or function in teeth. All measurements were made on first molars. The results from the first study were rewarding. First, it was necessary to confirm independently that a high sucrose intake was inhibitory on dentinogenesis, and it was.

In addition, we obtained new evidence to better understand the sucrose effect. We found that parotidectomized rats, fed a standard rat diet (a non-sucrose diet), experienced a significant reduction in dentinogenesis similar to those fed the sucrose diet, but not to the same degree. This implies, as we suspected, that the sucrose effect on dentinogenesis is not sucrose specific, but is, at least in part, parotid gland dependent through systemic mechanism(s). From an endocrine perspective, the parotids appear to be multifunctional. They contribute to the regulation of the DFT mechanism and now we had evidence that they were also involved in dentinogenesis. Conceivably, the sucrose effect in intact rats could be mediated through the impairment of the DFT mechanism and/or through a specific dentinogenic mechanism that also resided in the parotid glands. When both treatments (parotidectomy plus the sucrose diet) were combined, the inhibitory effect on dentinogenesis was significantly exacerbated over that observed with only diet. From these results, it can be inferred that the inhibitory sucrose effect mediated through the parotid glands was either incomplete and some hormonal secretion still persisted to blunt the sucrose effect or the removal of the parotids unmasked other unidentified mechanism(s) that were also susceptible to a high sucrose intake. The uniqueness of parotid involvement in dentinogenesis was further strengthened when we demonstrated that dentinogenesis was not affected by the surgical removal of the submandibular-sublingual gland complex.

Another significant observation from this study was the unique effect of diet on the weight of the parotid glands. The high sucrose diet caused these glands to significantly atrophy when compared to the weights of glands obtained from rats fed the standard diet. In comparison, the weight of the submandibular-sublingual gland complex remained essentially unaltered. We examined the possibility of whether the conversion of the pellet form of our diets (standard rat diet and high sucrose diet) into the powdered form might possibly have an effect on dentinogenesis. The data showed that changing the texture of the diet from pellet to powder did not alter the sucrose effect obtained with the pellet form. The primary determinant for inhibiting dentin apposition was the composition of the diet, the high sucrose content, and not the texture of the diet.

Since the first study demonstrated parotid involvement in dentinogenesis, our second study was to address the question: Could carbamoyl phosphate, as a dietary supplement in the high sucrose diet inhibit the sucrose effect on dentinogenesis? The results were affirmative. Carbamoyl phosphate significantly inhibited the down-regulation of dentinogenesis. The rate of dentinogenesis was essentially the same as that in rats fed the standard rat diet and the dentinal area was not statistically different from control rats. Furthermore, carbamoyl phosphate was effective only in intact rats. Parotidectomy negated the therapeutic effect of carbamoyl phosphate; therefore, the beneficial effect of the compound was mediated through the parotid glands. Another interesting effect of carbamoyl phosphate was that it prevented the atrophy of the parotid glands associated with the ingestion of the high sucrose diet. At this time, the exact mechanism through which carbamoyl phosphate exercises its beneficial effects in inhibiting cariogenesis and stimulating dentinogenesis remains unclear. However, it should be clearly evident that systemic mechanism(s), endocrine in nature, are essential for the well-being of teeth. As previously indicated, it appears that a high sucrose intake may deplete the endogenous carbamoyl phosphate.

Concurrent with our studies on dentinogenesis, Dr. Qian Zhang, beginning first as a graduate student and then continuing as a post-doctoral fellow in my laboratory, was successful in cloning the porcine cDNAs that code for the PH gene from porcine parotid glands. The amino acids encoded by the cDNAs agreed with the amino acid sequence of the hormone that we had previously isolated from porcine parotid glands. In situ hybridization and immunohistochemical staining demonstrated that the acinar calls of the parotid glands were the primary source for PH-related mRNAs. Minimal expression was found to occur in the sublingual glands and none in the submandibular glands. The expression products obtained in vitro from COS cells (kidney cells) transfected with the PH gene were assayed for biological activity using Steinman's intradentinal dye penetration assay and were biologically equivalent to the hormone isolated from porcine glands. Furthermore, the response in the rat was also equivalent to the endogenous secretion of PH due to eating.

In addition, our most recent study with a synthetic PH preparation demonstrates that the commercially synthesized protein is biologically active. Its activity is indistinguishable from either the isolated PH or the gene-expressed protein. They all stimulate the DFT mechanism (reference #100, to be published). From our perspective, the question as to whether the acinar cells in the parotid glands possess an endocrine function, in addition to their salivary function, is now a mute point.

To our knowledge, this may be the first example of a single cell type, at least among the major salivary glands, that possesses intracellular mechanism(s) that regulates two important complex functions (endocrine and exocrine). Morphologically, these cells appear well suited to regulate both functions. The apical ends of the cells open into the intercalated ducts going towards the mouth. The basal ends of the cells rest on a rich bed of capillaries well suited for hormonal transfer from the cells. If our assumption is correct that acinar cells possess dual functions, it implies that these cells have at least two transport mechanisms directing the proper distribution of molecules associated with each function, e.g., salivary proline rich proteins are directed toward the apical end of the cells and directed via the salivary ducts into the mouth. The PH is directed towards the basal portion of the acinar cells to be secreted directly into the blood to be transported to the odontoblasts and to any other responsive cells. How the molecular sorting is accomplished needs to be explored. Parotid gland proteins are unique in that they incorporate a significantly high number of proline residues into their structure. Interestingly, several studies suggest that the proline-rich domain of the proteins may have a role in sorting and regulating the secretion of parotid proteins. Ultimately, this would lead to the segregation of hormonal and salivary molecules into the appropriate pathways either to the mouth or the circulation.

SUMMARY

The foregoing is an abbreviated presentation of what Dr. Ralph Steinman and I accomplished over nearly three decades of collaborative research. Significantly more can be learned from reading our published papers. For the most part, our work was an effort of perseverance in the face of aggressive opposition, which later turned to benign denial/disinterest at both Loma Linda and the National Institute of Dental Research. In retrospect, I believe it was hoped that we might eventually disappear and the waters would no longer be troubled. However, during the past few years attitudes have begun to change. Journal editors and reviewers have looked receptively towards our work and editors have expressed their desire that we would consider submitting our papers to their respective Journals.

What began as a simple supposition on the part of Dr. Steinman that the vitality of teeth had to be dependent on unknown systemic mechanism(s) within the host led to the discovery of such mechanism(s). By recognizing the importance of a dynamic DFT mechanism and linking its functionality to these physiological mechanism(s), we believe that we have established, at least in part, a more scientifically rational approach to what is required for maintaining optimal dental health. Without a doubt the oral environment **can be** hostile to teeth but it doesn't have to be. Cariogenic bacteria are opportunistic rather than deterministic in their actions in causing cariogenesis. Epidemiological studies have clearly indicated that there isn't any correlation between the incidence of caries and the oral bacterial population, rather the correlation is with diet. The amount of sugar consumed. Our observations are in agreement with this conclusion. As previously discussed, high sugar consumption impairs systemic mechanism(s) upon which the structure (dentin) and vitality of teeth are dependent.

In the final analysis, why is DFT critical for maintaining optimal dental health? Obviously, the amount of fluid moving through the tooth structure at any moment is very small. Measurements made on the surface of the enamel of fluid volume coming through the enamel gives some idea of the volume and the rate at which the fluid flows (pig: O.4 $ul/cm^2/min$, dog/cat: 1.0 $ul/cm^2/min$, human 0.36 $ul/cm^2/min$). These measurements made by other investigators are relatively new. Prior to this, most dental researchers either denied the existence of DFT or considered it inconsequential for maintaining optimal dental health. To illustrate the point, during the 1980's I had received an NIH grant for the isolation of the parotid hormone releasing hormone from porcine hypothalamic tissue from the Endocrine and Metabolic Diseases Study Section. When the grant was up for renewal, we had a site visit and the visiting team brought a dental expert from a prestigious dental institute because, although our work was primarily endocrine in nature, the end point for following the biological activity during the isolation involved stimulation of DFT as the end point in our bioassay. Apparently, this individual was to give an assessment of our work on its significance to tooth physiology. When asked the question, his response was that he considered DFT to be inconsequential because of the minuscule amount. Obviously, with that perspective the renewal of the grant was denied. Why support something that is physiologically insignificant even though the isolation of the parotid-hormone-releasing factor was progressing, and the evidence for the already isolated PH met all of the criteria established at that time for a substance to be classified as a hormone.

To understand the significance of DFT one has to recognize three points: (1) teeth are noncompliant structures, (2) dentin is morphologically designed for fluid transport via a multitude of canaliculi that extend from the dentin-pulp interface to the dentin-enamel interface, also enamel is porous to facilitate fluid flow onto its surface, and (3) dentin, a living tissue, has no vascular supply but like all living tissues is dependent upon a transport mechanism for survival. As designed, fluid flow in teeth can be bidirectional. However, under **physiological conditions** (in healthy teeth), the direction of fluid flow is centrifugal (outward). Because teeth are noncompliant, the hydrostatic pressure within teeth is higher than in the oral cavity where the pressure is zero. The odontoblasts pump fluid from the pulp chamber through the dentin onto the surface of the enamel (see Figures 1 and 2). Under **pathological conditions** (cariogenic state), fluid flow is centripetal i.e. oral fluids can diffuse through the enamel into the dentin to cause cariogenesis. This occurs because odontoblast function is impaired. Theoretically this allows a decrease in hydrostatic pressure within the teeth which facilitates the penetration of acid and other hostile substances into the tooth structure leading to the demineralization of tooth structure. This accounts for the fact that cariogenesis always occurs in depth, even with an intact enamel over the lesion.

The fluid in the pulp chamber is derived from the blood. The capillaries in the pulp chamber are highly fenestrated (porous) which allows fluid to exit the vascular system. The composition of this fluid reflects the composition of blood minus the large protein molecules and for teeth it has been referred to as dental lymph. It contains nutrients essential for maintaining the vitality of the dentin: glucose for metabolism, amino acids for synthesizing dentinal collagen, and minerals to mineralize the dentinal collagen. To transfer all of the aforementioned from the pulp chamber into the tooth structure requires the presence of PH. This hormone appears to alter the permeability of the odontoblast cell membrane allowing the inward movement of "dental lymph" into the odontoblasts. We infer this from our studies in rats with essentially pure PH. In response to the infusion of PH dissolved in saline, the odontoblasts rapidly allowed the fluorescent dye, acriflavine hydrochloride, to penetrate into the cell body and enable the dye to move up the canaliculi. In contrast, infusion of saline

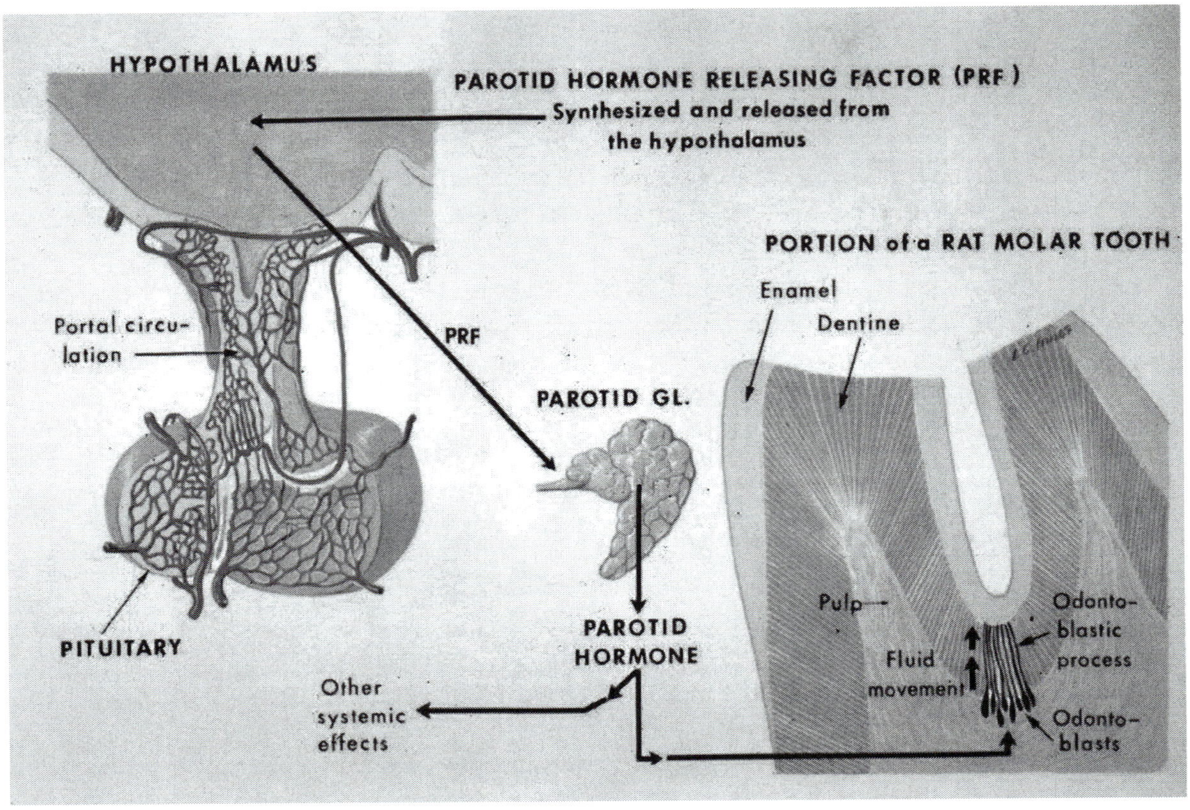

Figure 2. Diagram representing the rat model Hypothalamus-Parotid gland Endocrine Axis (HPEA)

The rat is the chosen animal model for studying cariogenesis. The above is a schematic representation of a rat molar tooth. In general, the histological morphology is similar to that of human teeth. They are designed to maintain fluid flow throughout the tooth structure beginning at the odontoblast level and terminating on the enamel surface. There are two morphological features that distinguish rat molars from human molars. The first is the lack of enamel covering the cusp tips of the molars. The second is that rat molars possess very deep occlusal grooves which are lined with enamel. It is generally accepted that enamel serves as a protective barrier against cariogenesis. Interestingly, cariogenesis is rarely observed in the cusp tips in spite of a lack of enamel. Caries occurs primarily at the bottom of the occlusal grooves which harbor the bacteria along with ample dietary substrate to produce acid. The depth of the occlusal grooves, along with the continuous impaction of diet into the grooves as a result of mastication, isolates these areas from any significant cariostatic effect that may be inherent in saliva. Therefore, any defensive mechanism against cariogenesis in these areas has to originate from within the tooth structure. We have proposed that the centrifugal movement of dentinal fluid is an essential component of the tooth's defensive mechanism against cariogenesis. See text on how cariogenesis was inhibited by approximately 90% in rats fed a cariogenic diet.

The main focus of the diagram is to illustrate the proposed mechanism that regulates dentinal fluid flow. All of our studies elucidating this mechanism were done in rats. Eating a noncariogenic diet provides sensory stimuli in the mouth that stimulates the hypothalamus to secrete the parotid hormone releasing factor (PRF) into the venous blood. Ultimately, this factor stimulates the parotid glands to secrete parotid hormone (PH). PH enters the circulation and activates the dentinal fluid flow mechanism present in odontoblasts. The result is a centrifugal movement of dentinal fluid throughout the tooth structure that is essential for maintaining the vitality of teeth and inhibiting cariogenesis. The activation of the odontoblasts creates within the tooth a higher hydrostatic pressure compared to the oral pressure. This difference in pressure prevents the ingress of cariogenic factors into the tooth. In addition, because dentinal fluid has the same pH of blood (7.4), it has a neutralizing effect on acid(s) produced by the bacteria in the occlusal grooves as it permeates though the enamel and onto its surface. When a cariogenic diet (high sugar content) is ingested, the diet has an inhibitory effect on the secretion of the parotid hormone releasing factor. The consequence is that this inhibition ultimately leads to the inhibition of PH secretion and the concomitant impairment of the dentinal fluid flow mechanism. Diminished dentinal fluid flow leads to a decrease in the hydrostatic pressure within the tooth; thereby, permitting centripetal movement (inward movement) of cariogenic factors into the tooth. The end result is destruction of tooth structure, decreased tooth vitality, and compromised dentinogenesis. The inhibition of PH secretion in response to ingesting a cariogenic diet was confirmed in our studies done in pigs.

only did not allow significant uptake of the fluorescent dye even though the dye was present in the pulp chamber. It has been reported that odontoblasts possess intracellular myofibrils and that odontoblasts, along with osteocytes, are capable of acting as pumps. If this is correct, we may infer from our studies that in addition to altering the permeability of the odontoblast cell membrane, PH may activate the pumping mechanism which accounts for the rapid movement of the dye to the dentin-enamel interface.

Lastly, another important function of dentinal fluid is that it acts as a buffer. The pH of the fluid mirrors the pH of blood, 7.4. Its buffering capacity can neutralize bacterial acids both within the tooth and on the surface of the teeth. The fluid perfuses through the enamel pores as minute droplets and coalesces on the surface of the teeth forming a possible barrier against the oral environment by acting as a buffer. The fluid flow on the surface of the teeth is exceptionally great where cracks are evident in the enamel. The latter is important because cracks provide opportunistic sites for bacterial invasion into tooth structure. The greater fluid flow at such sites is protective to prevent the ingress of bacterial products, neutralization of acids, and possible bacterial invasion. Fluid flow onto the surface of human teeth has been reported by other investigators and I have seen the process in anesthetized pigs and rats. All of these functions become impaired on a high sugar diet. The sugar suppresses the function of the hypothalamic-parotid gland endocrine axis leading to a decrease in PH secretion. In the absence of PH, the function of the DFT mechanism in the odontoblasts is compromised and DFT does not occur optimally which ultimately affects dental health.

--John Leonora, Ph.D
Professor of Physiology
LLU School of Medicine

PREFACE

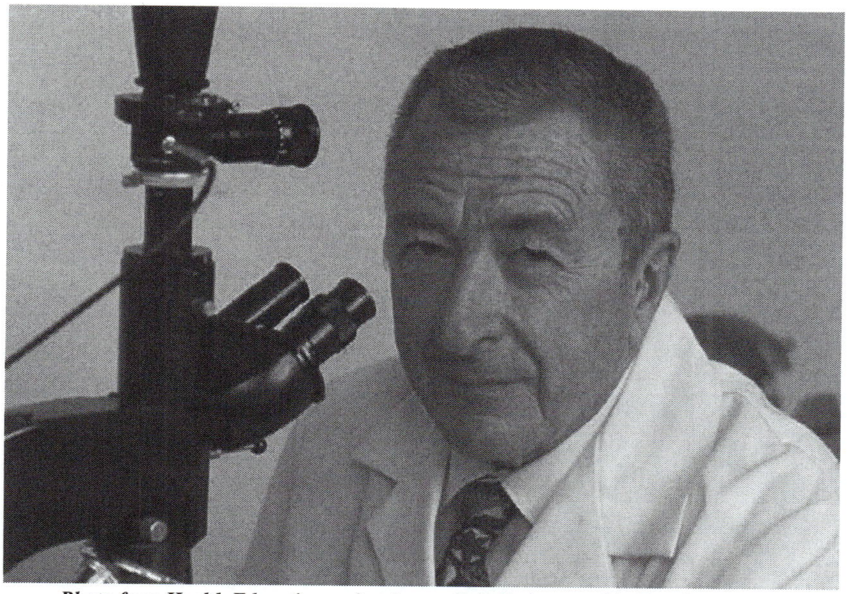

Photo from Health Education series; image digitally improved by Dr. Gary Golden
Dr. Ralph Steinman

DFT STUDIES BY DRS. STEINMAN AND LEONORA

The following condensed references were distilled from nearly 450 pages of text, and represent all of Dr. Ralph Steinman's known dentinal fluid transport (DFT) research writings. Enough details were included to understand the experimental design and credibly support the results. Documenting all 100 scientific papers side-by-side, from first to last in one document offers a chronological perspective to these investigations. In many cases, it may be important to consult tables, drawings, and photographs from the original printed articles for additional clarity. Highly significant references were mentioned by authors' names in the text. Authors' cited references that were omitted for the sake of brevity are indicated "[ref]" or "[refs]" in the text and can be obtained by checking the original articles.

Most articles were published prior to the PubMed computer search database that started in 1968. We are indebted to Drs. Lin Martin and Herbert Woodward for their valuable help in finding nearly half of these references. Some passages, worth noting for a possible later compendium article to be written, were highlighted in bold print. Much appreciation goes to the Restorative Department for continual help, particularly secretaries April, Barbara and Carol for invaluable aid in unraveling some subtler challenges of Microsoft Word as this project progressed. Richard Tinker in Educational Support Services was a steady source of computer and graphics information. We are indebted to him for the cover design and his staff including Jacob Parker, who helped with the line drawings, as well as Richard Cross, who accompanied me by private plane to Oregon to obtain an archival videotaped interview with Dr. Steinman at his Sunny Valley home. Librarian Nelia Wurangian was singularly helpful in obtaining the Library of Congress Control Number.

Many people cared to write kind words of respect and fond remembrances about Dr. Steinman. In fact, due to their great number and length, these tributes finally needed to be located in Appendix C. Be sure not to overlook reading these messages of genuine appreciation. The Restorative department has agreed to have this entire *Dentinal Fluid Transport* document made available in compact disk format.

Dr. Steinman's highly significant research, devoted specifically to previously unrecognized aspects of cariology, was accomplished on a limited budget and continued over a period spanning nearly four decades. The Loma Linda University School of Dentistry is fortunate to be the beneficiary of this sustained dedication and creative effort.

These studies involved an estimated minimum of 6,500 white rats, 108 rabbits, 17 pigs and an exhaustive array of pharmacological and biochemical agents. Today's IRB restrictions would make it more difficult to carry out such studies on animal and human tissues. Many experiments were complex and elaborate. Each was a consistent, stepwise search for truth, accomplished without money from commercial sources.

Dr. Steinman's initial inspiration came from writers including Ellen G. White on wholism and the effects of refined foods on the body, as well as by E. W. Fish in 1927 who reported the presence of "dental lymph" circulation in dentin and enamel. Dr. C. F. A. Bödecker in 1929 also had observed the controlled flow of a fluid-like substance from the pulp of the tooth to the outside through microscopically porous structures of dentin and enamel, and proposed "a new theory of the cause of dental caries." Expanding on this theme formed the basis of Dr. Steinman's research career. (Please see Article #86 for dramatic illustrations with methylene blue and acriflavine ultraviolet dyes showing fluid movement through dentinal tubules and enamel.)

Dr. John Leonora joined him in the mid-1960s. Their laboratory studies provided convincing evidence of an innate hormonal mechanism involving the hypothalamus in the lower brain, parotid salivary glands and pulpal odontoblasts. This hypothalamus-parotid gland endocrine axis (see diagrams on pp xi and xvi) is involved with generating dentinal fluid pressure out from the pulp through the natural channels and pores of the tooth structure and ultimately influences its external resistance or susceptibility to decay. Joint research with physiologist Jean-Marc Tièche in the late 1980s isolated, purified, and chemically identified the active parotid hormone believed responsible, an exacting process that can probably only be fully appreciated by reading the complete original of Article #92.

The final article by Dr. Leonora, with Dr. Qian Zhang and others, reported their successful cloning of porcine cDNAs that code for the parotid hormone (PH) gene from porcine parotid glands. The amino acids encoded by the cDNAs agreed with the amino acid sequence of the hormone that Tièche and Leonora had formerly isolated from porcine parotid glands. In situ hybridization and immunohistochemical staining demonstrated that the acinar cells of the parotid glands were the primary source for PH-related mRNAs. This laboratory-created hormone was biologically equivalent to the hormone isolated from porcine glands. Furthermore, its response in the rat was also equivalent to the endogenous secretion of PH due to eating. This research technically closes the loop on whether parotid glands possess an endocrine function in addition to salivary function.

The Foreword by Dr. Leonora is an especially important part of this book. He explains the pathway their careful and elaborate research took to arrive at what must be regarded as one of the more important breakthroughs in our understanding of dental cariological resistance. This should significantly change the way we look at the dynamics of dental caries resistance--deeper than currently being taught in any textbooks.

Please read Dr. Leonora's Foreword first to gain perspective before reading on through the rest of the material.

The concept that dental tissues are a functional part of the whole body and subject to systemic influences broadens our connections with dentistry's sister fields of anatomy, biochemistry, pharmacology, physiology, biophysics, microbiology, oral medicine, diet, and public health. Such a scope of inclusiveness is in keeping with Loma Linda University's wholistic concept of man.

--Clyde Roggenkamp, DDS, MSD
Assoc. Prof., Restorative Department
LLU School of Dentistry

TABLE OF CONTENTS

*Dr. Leonora's foreword is recommended for orientation to the nature of the research presented in this manuscript.

DRS. RALPH STEINMAN'S AND JOHN LEONORA'S SCIENTIFIC PAPERS
Listed Chronologically by Publication Dates

Compiled in collaboration with Drs. Lin Martin, Clyde Roggenkamp, Ralph Steinman, and Herbert Woodward

1. Steinman RR. Warpage produced by soldering with dental solders and gold alloys. J Prosth Dent 4(3):384-395, 1954

2. Zwemer JD [presented by Steinman RR, Haley ML]. Effect of various saccharides on the phosphate content of developing tooth buds. J Dent Res 36(2):70, Abst #182, Apr 1957

3. Steinman RR, Haley ML. The biological effect of various carbohydrates ingested during the calcification of the teeth. J Dent Child 24:211-214, 1957

4. Steinman RR, Haley ML. Effect of preweanling administration of sucrose on subsequent caries. Proc Soc Exp Biol Med 94:391-392, 1957

5. Steinman RR, Haley ML. Early administration of various carbohydrates and subsequent dental caries in the rat. J Dent Res 36(4):532-535, 1957

6. Steinman RR, Hewes CG, Hardinge MG. The systemic etiological factors of caries in white rats. J Dent Res 37(1):32, Abstr #73, Feb 1958

7. Steinman RR, Haley ML. Effect of preweanling administration of lactose on subsequent caries susceptibility. Proc Soc Exp Biol Med 97:274-275, 1958

8. Steinman RR, Haley ML, O'Day P. Intraperitoneal injections of carbohydrates to suckling rats, and subsequent dental caries. J Dental Res 37(4):719-721, 1958

9. Steinman RR, Hardinge MG, Woods RW. Experimental caries with human foods. J Dent Res 37(5):865-873, 1958

10. Steinman RR, Hardinge MG. The effect of pyridoxine and injected carbohydrate on the incidence of caries, dentinal circulation related to diet. J Dent Res 37(5):874-879, 1958

11. Steinman RR, Hewes CG, Woods RW. Histochemical analysis of caries lesions in incipient dental caries. J Dent Res 38(3):592-605, 1959

12. Wilcox A, O'Day P, Haley MI, Steinman RR. The carbohydrate content of caries-susceptible rat molars. J Dent Res 38(4):676, Abstr #59, Jul-Aug 1959

13. Steinman RR, Hewes G. Histochemical analysis of lesions in incipient dental caries. J Dent Res 38(4):687, Abstr #86, Jul-Aug 1959

14. Hewes G, Steinman RR, Woods RW. Ultrastructural changes in dentine occurring in incipient caries. J Dent Res 38(4):694, Abstr #S5, Jul-Aug 1959

15. Steinman RR, Robson B, Morrow S. The pathology of caries. J South Calif Dent Assn 27(10):339-344, 1959

16. Zwemer JD, Steinman RR. The immunohistochemical localization of plasma albumin in murine dentinal tissue. J Dent Res 38(6):1239, Abstr, Nov-Dec 1959

17. Steinman RR. The possible role of hyaluronidase in incipient carious lesions. J Dent Res 39(1):150-152, 1960

18. Steinman RR. Can dental caries susceptibility be affected by the ingestion of carbohydrates? J Indiana State Dent Assoc 39:130-134, April 1960

19. Steinman RR. The possible role of hyaluronidase in the incipient carious lesion. J South Calif Dent Assn 28(7):207-209, 1960

20. Steinman RR. The effect of weaning on the incidence of incipient carious lesions. J Dent Res 39(4):860, Jul-Aug 1960

21. Zwemer JE, Steinman RR. The endotoxic activity of a rat oral streptococcus. J Dent Res 39(5):1073, Abstr, 1960

22. Zwemer JE, Steinman RR. The endotoxic activity of human saliva. J Dent Res 39(5):1074, Abstr, 1960

23. Steinman RR. Histochemical analysis of lesions in incipient dental caries. II. Sulfhydryl and disulfide radicals. J Dent Res 39(10):1009-1013, Sep-Oct 1960

24. Steinman RR, Smith LV. The effect of stress upon the incidence of dental caries. J South Calif Dent Assn 28(11):367-369, 1960

25. Steinman RR. The in vitro changes in rat tooth structure produced by streptococcal lysate. J South Calif Dent Assn 28(12):411-412, 1960

26. Steinman RR, Brussett M, Tartaryn P. Comparison of caries incidence in exercised and immobilized rats. J Dent Res 40(1):218, Abstr, 1961

27. Steinman RR, Zwemer JD. The pathogenic role of a rat oral streptococcus in incipient dental caries. J Dent Res 40(2):378, Abstr, 1961

28. Steinman RR. Caries susceptibility as affected by electrolyte balance. J Dent Res 40(4):658, Abstr #53, 1961

29. Steinman RR. The rat molar in health and disease. J Calif. Dent Assn 37(2):103-105, Apr 1961

30. Steinman RR. The incidence of dental caries as altered by electrolyte and water balance. J South Calif Dent Assn 29(4):122-126, 1961

31. Steinman RR, Smith LV. The physiological basis for caries susceptibility and resistance. J South Calif Dent Assn 29(7):221-224, 1961

32. Steinman RR, Smith LV. Histochemical and radiographic changes observed in human teeth. J South Calif Dent Assn 29(9):294-300, 1961

33. Steinman RR, Smith LV. The effect of sucrose and 2-4 dinitrophenol upon odontoblastic function. J South Calif Dent Assn 29(10):315-317, 1961

34. Steinman RR. The possible presence of sulfhydryl, disulfide radicals and adenosine triphosphate in human teeth. J South Calif Dent Assn 29(11):360-364, 1961

35. Steinman RR. The possible presence of adenosine triphosphatase and choline esterase in human teeth. J South Calif Dent Assn 29(12):400-404, 1961

36. Steinman RR. The role of an enzyme in caries production. Dental Progess 2(2) 45/109-47/111, Jan 1962

37. Steinman RR. Molecular changes observed in dental caries and their possible nutritional implications. J Applied Nutr 15 (nos. 3 & 4):188-191, 1962

38. Steinman RR. Caries and cellular nutrition. Dental Progress 2(3):64/208-66/210, April 1962

39. Steinman RR. The histochemical distribution of magnesium in dentinal tissues. J South Calif Dent Assn 30(4):124-127, 1962

40. Steinman RR. The cellular physiology of caries susceptibility. J Calif. Dent Assn 38(5):403-404, Oct 1962

41. Steinman RR, DeVincenzo J, Voth E. The physiology of the dental pulp. Part 1. J South Calif Dent Assn 30(10):336-340, 1962

42. Steinman RR. The possible role of acetylcholine esterase in resistance to dental caries. J South Calif Dent Assn 30(11):365-367, Nov 1962

43. Steinman RR. The presence and distribution of succinic dehydrogenase and monoamine oxidase in the pulp of adult human teeth. J South Calif Dent Assn 30(12):388-391, 1962

44. Rathbun WE, Bond DE, Steinman RR. The effect of cows milk, soy milk, and chocolate milk upon the incidence of caries in the rat. J South Calif Dent Assn 31(9):299-301, 1963

45. DeVincenzo JP, Steinman RR. The physiology of the dental pulp. Part 2. A perfusion method for maintaining the viability of the intact pulp tissue of human teeth in vitro as determined by adenosine triphosphate concentrations. J South Calif Dent Assn 3(10):323-328, 1963

46. Steinman RR, Gilliland Y, Saunders M, Holub V, Tague C. A demonstration of the effect of human food combinations upon dental caries in rats. J South Calif Dent Assn 31(12):400-402, 1963

47. Steinman RR, Woods RW. Heredity, environment, diet and caries. J South Calif Dent Assn 32(5):163-166, 1964

48. Steinman RR. The possible hydrolysis of enamel protein. J South Calif Dent Assn 32(7):192-198, 1964

49. Kijak E, Foust G, Steinman RR. Relationship of blood sugar level and leukocytic phagocytosis. J South Calif Dent Assn 32(9):349-351, 1964

50. Steinman RR. Calcium and phosphorus release from intact human enamel under anaerobic conditions. J South Calif Dent Assn 32(10):384-387, 1964

51. Steinman RR. The possible role of carbon dioxide in initiating dental caries. J South Calif Dent Assn 33(1):28-31, 1965

52. Steinman RR. The chemical control of the release of calcium, phosphorus and amino acids from human dental enamel. J South Calif Dent Assn 33(5):230-234, 1965

53. Steinman RR. The possible chemical reactions between human enamel and carbon dioxide. J South Calif Dent Assn 33(9)434-436, Sep 1965

54. Steinman RR. Some chemical characteristics of the loosely bound amino acids of human enamel. J South Calif Dent Assn 33(10):462-467, Oct 1965

55. Steinman RR. A possible physiological mechanism of resistance to dental caries. J South Calif Dent Assn 33(11):514-516, Nov 1965

56. Steinman RR. The possible character of the protein-mineral bond on dental enamel and how it may be stabilized. J South Calif Dent Assn 34(4):67-72, Feb 1966

57. Steinman RR. The inherent chemical instability of dental care. J South Calif Dent Assn 34(5):247-249, May 1966

58. Steinman RR. Movement of acriflavine HCl through rat molars in health and disease. J Dent Res 46:162, Abstr #493, 1967

59. Steinman RR. The movement of acriflavine hydrochloride through molars of rats on a cariogenic and noncariogenic diet. J South Calif Dent Assn 35(4):151-157, 1967

60. Steinman RR. The pharmacologic control of dental caries in the rat. J Dent Res 47:196, Abstr #634, 1968

61. Steinman RR. Pharmacologic control of dentinal fluid movement and dental caries in rats. J Dent Res 47(5):720-724, 1968

62. Leonora J, Steinman RR. Evidence suggesting the existence of a hypothalamic parotid gland endocrine axis. Endocrinology 83:807-815, 1968

63. Steinman RR, Leonora J. Suppression of dental caries by chemical activation of the hypothalamic-parotid endocrine axis. J Dent Res 48:S207, Abstr #666, 1969

64. Sanchez A, Steinman RR, Leonora J. Effect of diet on dentinal fluid movement in germfree and nongermfree rats. Am J Clin Nutr 23:686-690, 1970

65. Steinman RR, Leonora J. Relation between early changes in dentin and later dental caries. J Dent Res 50:247, Abstr #780, Mar 1971

66. Steinman RR, Leonora J. Relationship of fluid transport through the dentin to the incidence of dental caries. J Dent Res 50(6) Part 2:1536-1543, 1971

67. Steinman RR. Studies of the parotid hormone in the pig. Personal notes, ca 1971

68. Steinman RR, Leonora J, Shiroma E, Dwyer T. Lactic acid concentration in various tooth structures in rats maintained on either a cariogenic or noncariogenic diet. J Dent Res 54(2):419, Abstr, 1975

69. Steinman RR, Leonora J. Effect of infusing selected chemical compounds on dentinal fluid movement in the rat. J Dent Res 54(3):567-569, 1975

70. Steinman RR, Leonora J. Effect of selected dietary additives on the incidence of dental caries in the rat. J Dent Res 54(3):570-577, 1975

71. Steinman RR, Leonora J. Acidogenic potential of cariogenic and noncariogenic diets in the rat. J Dent Res 54(3):578-580, 1975

72. Steinman RR. Physiological basis for resistance to dental caries – a new look. Texas Dent J 93(12):6-8, 1975

73. Steinman RR, Leonora J. Physiologic resistance to dental caries. J Missouri Dent Assn. 57(3):14-21, 1977

74. Steinman RR. The control of dental caries by manipulating dentinal fluid movement. J Missouri Dent Assn. 57(5):14-20, 1977

75. Steinman RR. The clinical significance of the physiologic approach to the control of dental caries. J Missouri Dent Assn. 57(7):15-18, 1977

76. Steinman RR. Is caries susceptibility an internal problem of the tooth? Quintessence Int 10:95-99, 1978

77. Steinman RR, Leonora J, Tièche JM. Susceptibility to dental caries. Austral Dent J 24:222-224, 1979

78. Steinman RR. The biological approach to the health and disease of teeth. What about carbohydrates and dental caries? What about cereals and dental caries? Unpublished teaching syllabus, 1979

79. Steinman RR, Leonora J, Singh RJ. The effect of desalivation upon pulpal function and dental caries in rats. J Dent Res 59(2):176-185, 1980

80. Tièche JM, Leonora J, Steinman RR. Isolation and partial characterization of a porcine parotid hormone that stimulates dentinal fluid transport. Endocrinology 106:1994-2005, 1980

81. Tièche JM, Leonora J, Berk LS, Steinman RR. A radioimmunoassay procedure for quantitating parotid hormone. Biochem Biophys Res Comm 98:154-162, 1981

82. Leonora J, Steinman, RR. DFT, its cariostatic effect. Teaching syllabus, ca 1981

83. Steinman RR. The physiologic nature of caries susceptibility. Part I. J Alabama Dent Assn. 66:20-23, 1982

84. Steinman RR. The physiologic nature of caries susceptibility. Part II. Interactions between plaque, bacteria and the tooth. . J Alabama Dent Assn 67:51-53, 1983

85. Steinman RR. The physiologic nature of caries susceptibility. Part III. Physiologic aspects of resistance to dental caries. J Alabama Dent Assn 67:46-49, 1983

86. Steinman RR. Biologic activity in the tooth in health and disease. Comp Contin Educ Dent 9:722-728, 1984

87. Steinman RR. The carious process. Class syllabus, 1984

88. Steinman RR. Physiologic activity of the pulp-dentin complex. Quintessence Int 10:723-726, 1985

89. Steinman RR. Nutrition of the teeth and dental caries. J Appl Nutr 39(1):42-50, 1987

90. Leonora J, Tièche JM, Celestin, J. Physiological factors affecting secretion of parotid hormone. Am J Physiol 252 (Endocrinol. Metab. 15):E477-E484, 1987

91. Leonora J, Tièche JM, Cook, DS. Evidence for insulinotropic effect from rat parotid glands. Diabetes (April) 37:441-445, 1988

92. Tièche JM, Leonora J. Biological and chemical evidence for the existence of a porcine hypothalamic parotid hormone-releasing factor. Biochem Biophys Res Commun. March 159(3):899-906, 1989

93. Leonora J, Tièche JM, Steinman RR. The effect of dietary factors on intradentinal dye penetration in the rat. Arch Oral Biol 37:733-741, 1992

94. Leonora J, Tièche JM, Steinman RR. Stimulation of intradentinal dye penetration by feeding in the rat. Arch Oral Biol 38:763-767, 1993

95. Leonora J, Tièche JM, Steinman RR. Further evidence for a hypothalamus-parotid gland endocrine axis in the rat. Arch Oral Biol 38:911-916, 1993

96. Tièche JM, Leonora J, Steinman RR. High-sucrose diet inhibits basal secretion of intradentinal dye penetration-stimulating parotid hormone in pigs. J Appl Physiol 76:218-222, 1994

97. Tièche JM, Leonora J. Acute secretion of immunoreactive parotid hormone in response to different diets in the pig. Arch Oral Biol 40(6):559-565, 1995

98. Leonora J, Tjäderhane L, Tièche JM. Parotid gland function and dentin apposition in rat molars J Dent Res 81(4):259-264, 2002

99. Leonora J, Tjäderhane L, Tièche JM. Effect of dietary carbamyl phosphate on dentine apposition in rat molars. Arch Oral Biol 47:147-153, 2002

100. Zhang Q, Szalay AA, Tièche JM, Kyeyune-Nyombi Eru, Sands JF, Oberg KC, Leonora J. Cloning and functional study of porcine parotid hormone, a novel proline-rich protein. J Biol Chem 250(23):22233-22244, 2005

CONDENSED NOTES OF STEINMAN'S AND LEONORA'S STUDIES

Article #1

Warpage Produced by Soldering with Dental Solders and Gold Alloys

Steinman RR. J Prosth Dent 4(3):384-395, May 1954

This article was Dr. Steinman's first publication following graduate training at the University of Michigan from his master's research on avoiding dimensional changes produced by soldering dental gold bridges. Since this was prior to his work dealing with dentinal fluid transport (DFT), it has not been condensed and transcribed here.

Article (abstract) #2

Effect of Various Saccharides on the Phosphate Content of Developing Tooth Buds

Zwemer JD [presented by Steinman RR, Haley ML]. J Dent Res 36(2):70, Abst #182, Apr 1957

Exposure of suckling rats to only 6 days of various saccharides produced significantly greater caries susceptibility, not attributable to local factors since the molars were unerupted. Decreased blood glucose 3 hours after the administration of sucrose, glucose, or fructose was accompanied by a 20-30% decrease in serum Pi, probably needed for the phosphorylation of glucose. This compensation came at the expense of the developing 16-day first molar buds, which showed a 10% reduced total phosphate content than normal.

Article #3

The Biological Effect of Various Carbohydrates Ingested During the Calcification of the Teeth

Steinman RR, Haley ML. J Dent Child 24:211-214, 1957

STUDY 1: To determine if various carbohydrates may affect molars from early calcification to eruption, 60 albino rats were divided into 4 groups and fed 3x/day with the following solutions from the first day after birth until the 21st day: (1) 20% sucrose, (2) 20% lactose, (3) 20% glucose, and (4) 20% equal mix of glucose and fructose. At weaning, they were placed on a high-caries solid diet containing 65% sucrose. Carious lesions were analyzed after 13 weeks. Sucrose Group– 53, Lactose Group– 35, Glucose Group– 37, Glucose/Fructose Group– 41, Control Group– 20.

STUDY 2: To determine what time during the suckling period is most vulnerable. 36 new-born caries-susceptible rats were divided into 4 equal groups and fed 3x/day with 20% sucrose solution as follows: (1) birth to 6th day, (2) 7th to 13th day, (3) 14th to 21st day, and (4) no sucrose but only maternal milk as a control. When weaned at 21 days, all were placed on the cariogenic diet. Animals were examined for caries scores at 13 weeks. Group 1– 38, Group 2– 42, Group 3– 46, Control Group– 20.

STUDY 3: To determine amount of added carbohydrate necessary to produce an increase in caries. At 14 days 60 animals were divided into 4 groups and fed 3% carbohydrate formula to which additional carbohydrates were added as follows: Group 1– 1.85% lactose, Group 2– 1.85% sucrose, Group 3– 5.35% lactose, Group 4– 5.35% sucrose. At 14 days the animals were weaned and placed on a cariogenic diet. At 14 weeks molar caries scores were obtained: Group 1– 5, Group 2– 10, Group 3– 15, Group 4– 25.

Greatest caries increase was from sucrose, least from lactose. **Sucrose administered by eye dropper showed 100% increase in caries over littermates compared to only 10%**

for lactose. The addition of only 1.85% sucrose was sufficient to ↑ caries. Average U.S. diet = 18% added sucrose. Teeth developing and erupting in this environment may have ↑ caries susceptibility. Implications apply to infant formulas containing sucrose.

Summary: Carbohydrates during calcification increased caries susceptibility. Sucrose showed greater caries-producing ability than lactose.

Article #4

Effect of Preweanling Administration of Sucrose on Subsequent Caries

Steinman RR, Haley ML. Proc Soc Exp Biol Med 94:391-392, 1957

To test if increased sucrose during calcification of teeth affects later caries, 36 newborn caries-prone rats were divided into 4 groups and fed 20% sucrose solution orally 3x/day in sequences as follows: (1) birth through 6th day, (2) 7th through 13th day, (3) 14th through 21st day, and (4) no sucrose but only maternal milk as a control. Carious lesions were analyzed after 13 weeks. Group 1– 38 caries, Group 2– 42 caries, Group 3- 46 caries, Group 4– 20 caries. **Over 100% increase in Groups 1, 2, and 3. Results imply changes are systemic in nature and irreversible. Clearly separates systemic from purely local factors.**

Article #5

Early administration of various carbohydrates and subsequent dental caries in the rat

Steinman RR, Haley ML. J Dent Res 36(4):532-535, 1957

Sognnaes found ↑ sucrose diet through the formative period in several rat generations increased caries susceptibility through pre-weaning changes in maternal milk as well as by the post-weaning high-sugar diet. Similar results were found with Rhesus monkeys whereas teeth formed prior to high sucrose exposure were immune to decay. Scandinavian children during and after WWII tended to reflect a similar contrast.

This study was to determine effects of various carbohydrates on molars from early calcification to eruption. Suckling NIDR caries-susceptible rats were divided into 8 groups:

Group 1– 20% sucrose, Group 2– 20% lactose, Group 3– 20% raw cornstarch suspension, Group 4– 20% glucose, Group 5– 20% equal glucose/fructose mixture, and Group 6– tap water.

Young from 2 other litters were exchanged 3 days post-birth, with one group receiving 20% sucrose and the other an equal amount of water till weaned. The sucrose group had 33 carious lesions compared to 13 for the water group.

Young from 2 other litters were exchanged 3 days post-birth, with one group receiving 20% lactose and the other 20% raw cornstarch suspension. After weaning, all rats received a high sucrose diet for 14 weeks. The lactose group had 8 carious lesions and the raw starch 53.

In a further experiment 62 pre-weaned rats were divided into the following groups: Group 1– 20% sucrose, Group 2– 20% lactose, Group 3– 20% glucose, Group 4– 20% glucose/fructose mixture. After weaning, all were placed on a high-sucrose diet for 13 weeks, then examined for caries with the following results: Sucrose group– 53, Lactose group– 35, Glucose group– 37, Glucose/fructose mixture group– 41.

Summary/Conclusions: **Numbers of cavities in each group were fairly uniform except for the lactose group which was considerably lower. Milk formulas may be of considerable importance regarding amount and kind of carbohydrates they contain. It was obvious that animals receiving carbohydrate solutions the day after birth had the highest caries scores. The earlier sugar was ingested the greater the number of teeth totally destroyed. Sucrose consistently increased later caries greater than the other carbohydrates tested.**

Article (abstract) #6

The systemic etiological factors of caries in white rats

Steinman RR, Hewes CG, Hardinge MG. J Dent Res 37(1):32, Abstr #73, Feb 1958

This study was to determine if sugar has a systemic effect in producing dental caries besides the accepted local effect, 21 post-weanling rats were fed a typical American diet for 13 weeks

STUDY 1: American diet without desserts

Group 1– 10 received injections of glucose/fructose intraperitoneally (i.p.) t.i.d.

Group 2– Controls on American diet alone

STUDY 2: American diet with desserts

Group 1– 16 mg/kg vit. B_6 was added

Group 2– Controls on American diet alone

STUDY 3: 2% Trypan blue was injected intraperitoneally (i.p.) weekly for 3 weeks

Group 1– High sucrose diet

Group 2– Purina chow diet control

STUDY 4: 0.5 ml 4% trypan blue injected on the 35th day, then observed at various time intervals

Results:

STUDY 1: i.p. Glu/fru group had molars scoring 10.9 on Shaw caries scale, control littermates scored 3.18

STUDY 2: i.p. B_6 group scored only 4.0 whereas score on diet alone was 8.8 (i.e. caries was reduced by addition of vitamin)

STUDY 3: Teeth of Purina group were visibly bluer than high sucrose diet group after 12 wks

STUDY 4: Tooth structure became visibly discolored in 10 min's, then blue in 24 hrs

Conclusion:

Results may indicate that a metabolic disturbance is integrally associated with dental caries.

Article #7

Effect of preweanling administration of lactose on subsequent caries susceptibility

Steinman RR, Haley ML. Proc Soc Exp Biol Med 97:274-275, 1958

The last study showed that pre-eruption ingestion of sucrose increased post-eruption caries potential. This study is to determine if lactose can also produce later significant caries potential.

58 rats were divided into Group 1– 20% lactose and Group 2– controls given only maternal milk from their 3rd through 21st day. From the 22nd day all were fed a cariogenic diet and molars examined after 13 weeks. **Results between groups were not statistically different, which was in contrast to the previously studied sucrose group**

which showed 100% increase. Explanation may be that GI absorption of sucrose is much more rapid than for lactose and may cause a temporary mineral imbalance during the suckling period, which coincides with the dental calcification stage, translating to a later significant post-eruption caries increase.

Article #8

Intraperitoneal injections of carbohydreates to suckling rats, and subsequent dental caries

Steinman RR, Haley ML, O'Day P. J Dental Res 37(4):719-721, 1958

This study was to determine if caries increase with carbohydrate ingestion during the suckling period is due to digestive disturbance or mainly systemic in nature.

STUDY 1: 19 rats were divided into 2 groups: Group 1– 20% glucose via intraperitoneal injection and Group 2– 20% glucose fed orally. This occurred for both groups from days 1 through 4 with normal maternal nursing through the 21st day then weaning to a synthetic cariogenic diet. Carious lesions were examined after 13 weeks. Group 1 = 16 carious lesions, Group 2 = 9 carious lesions.

STUDY 2: 34 rats were divided into 3 groups: Group 1– 20% glucose/fructose mixture via i.p. injection, Group 2– 20% glucose/fructose mixture taken orally, and Group 3– cariogenic diet after weaning. This occurred for all groups from days 3 through 21. All were examined for caries after 13 weeks. Resulting caries scores were: Group 1 = 23, Group 2 = 22, Group 3 = 15.

STUDY 3: To determine if vitamins B_6 and C added to injected solution would affect subsequent caries.

47 rats were divided into 3 groups. Group 1– 20% glucose/fructose via i.p. injection, Group 2– 20% glucose/fructose via i.p. injection + 0.1 mg vit C/10 g body wt, Group 3 20% glucose/fructose via i.p. injection + 0.1 mg vit B/10 g body wt. This occurred 3x/d from the third through 21st days. All animals were then weaned and placed on a synthetic cariogenic diet. Molars were examined for caries after 13 weeks. Caries scores were: Group 1 = 16, Group 2 = 8, Group 3 = 7.

Apparently i.p. monosaccharide injections during calcification caused a subsequent molar caries increase compared to controls. This was comparable to oral administration groups, and was consistent with another study [ref] **showing a corresponding increase in caries when carbohydrates were increased during the last third of the suckling period. Decreased caries in the vitamin-supplemented groups may indicate mere dilution of the carbohydrate ingredients, however vit. C has been shown necessary during calcification of the teeth.**

Article #9

Experimental caries with human foods

Steinman RR, Hardinge MG, Woods RW. J Dent Res 37(5):865-873, 1958

This study was to determine the effect of various diets on caries score and nutritional status through successive generations. 8 diets were employed representing variations on the theme of the "average American diet" with servings of each item proportioned according to popularity. Diets were isocaloric and with nearly equal amounts of carbohydrate and protein. The mean lengths of mandibles of each group were statistically compared. For purposes of comparison of dietary differences, a caries index

"C" and a nutritional index "N" were formulated and a coefficient of correlation was calculated to be 0.78.

If the nutritional index is known, the caries index can be calculated from the following formula: I_c = Mean Caries Index + most probable deviation from the mean ± probable error of the Index

$$I_c = 68.8 - 0.65\,(I_n - 57.1) \pm 11.5$$
$$= 0.965\,I_n + 13.7 \pm 11.5$$

A deteriorated physical condition was associated with an increase in caries. The nutritional status and physical well-being of all animals showed an inverse correlation with caries incidence.

Article #10

The effect of pyridoxine and injected carbohydrate on the incidence of caries, dentinal circulation related to diet

Steinman RR, Hardinge MG. J Dent Res 37(5):874-879, 1958

Need for a fermentable carbohydrate as a substrate for bacterial activity was shown by Kite, Shaw and Sognnaes. **But there appears to be no consistent correlation between the amount of carbohydrates passing through the oral cavity and the degree of caries present—caries appears dependent on some additional etiological factors. It is reasonable to suspect that interference with the metabolic cycle contributes to this group of additional etiological factors.**

Accepted for publication March, 1958, this is Steinman's first allusion to "circulation" in the dentin. Ability to concentrate **trypan blue** was employed to determine its extent of activity. 0.5 ml of 4% trypan blue was injected intraperitoneally and the amount of blue stain uptake was measured in the dentin. Slight gray-blue staining occurred within 10 minutes and became heavy blue by 48 hours. It was noted that younger animals demonstrated more efficient color deposition.

STUDY 1: Weaned littermates were divided into 2 groups: Group 1– Purina chow, Group 2– Cariogenic diet. All rats were injected weekly with 2% trypan blue intraperitoneally for 3 weeks. At 25 days of age, gold crowns were placed on the lower right first molars of 3 rats in each group. After 12 weeks all teeth were examined for their relative dye concentrations. Group 1 teeth were found to be significantly darker than Group 2 teeth. No color difference was observed between crowned and uncrowned teeth. Microscopic observation revealed wavy concentric lines in the secondary dentin only in the cariogenic group, confirmed with another group on the same diets but not receiving trypan blue.

STUDY 2: To evaluate the effect of specific nutrients on caries production. 21-day-old rats were divided into 2 equal groups: Group 1– Diet I (average US diet), Group 2– Diet I plus pyridoxine (vit. B_6) at 16 mg/kg of rations. Molars were scored for caries after 13 weeks: Group 1= 9, Group 2 = 4.

STUDY 3: 21-day-old rats were divided into 2 equal groups: Group 1– Diet VII (average US diet minus desserts), Group 2– Diet VII (average US diet minus desserts) plus intraperitoneal glucose/fructose mixture at 1 mg/g body wt. injected 3x/day. This 20% of total calories sugar level parallels American adolescent intake. Molars were scored for caries after 13 weeks: Group 1 = 4, Group 2 = 11.

Results in Group 2 of Study 2 confirm Rinehart and Greenberg's study demonstrating caries reduction with pyridoxine.

Bypassing the oral route of intake indicates cariogenic effect of sugar results from systemic action. It follows that the carbohydrate-related caries increase is related to both the well-established local action and the currently demonstrated systemic effect.

The previously published study showed that teeth which remained caries-free through 3 rat generations were found to be also in uniformly good physical condition. Conversely, caries-ridden teeth were associated with rats in poorer health. A review of the literature clearly indicates post-eruptive caries production is affected by factors influencing circulation, nutrition, and metabolism. Examples are vessel ligation (restricted circulation) ↑ caries, chewing hard substances (stimulated circulation) ↓ caries, increased dietary pyridoxine (nutrition) ↓ caries, reduced L-lysine (nutrition) ↑ caries, x-ray therapy (circulation) ↑ caries, increased androgens (metabolism) ↑ caries, increased thyroxin (metabolism) ↓ caries, increased acetazoleamide (metabolism) ↑ caries.

Circulation
- **Vascular ligation ↑ caries**
- **Chewing hard substances ↓ caries**
- **X-ray therapy ↑ caries**

Nutrition
- **Dietary pyridoxine ↓ caries**
- **Reduced L-lysine ↑ caries**

Metabolism
- **X-ray therapy ↑ caries**
- **Increased thyroxin ↓ caries**
- **Increased androgens ↑ caries**
- **Increased acetazoleamide ↑ caries**

From this it is reasonable to assume that the currently established theory that caries is exclusively a local phenomenon is no longer tenable. Published findings favor the concept that host metabolic disturbance precedes and predisposes dental caries by systemically lowering the tooth's resistance.

Article #11

Histochemical analysis of caries lesions in incipient dental caries

Steinman RR, Hewes CG, Woods RW. Dent Res 38(3):592-605, 1959

The purpose of this paper was to describe an innovation in tissue preparation, the application of histochemical methods, and the emerging picture of the premonitory lesion in experimental caries.

Induction of caries – Thin ground or decalcified tissue sections have commonly been employed for microscopic studies. Drawbacks are that tubular protoplasm is dehydrated, the pulp is macerated, and the heat of grinding the sections can inactivate any enzymes present. Therefore another technique was devised to preserve food present in the grooves of the teeth, bacterial plaque, enamel, dentin, pulp, and supporting structures. Animals were decapitated and the major portion of flesh was removed from the jaws which were immediately frozen. They were mounted in ice and sectioned with a microtome in the deep freeze. 8 μ sections were made till half the tooth was shaved away.

Tests used for various aspects:

Protein – ninhydrin-Schiff method
Polysaccharides – Hotchkiss periodic acid method
Sulfur – Macallum method
Reducing agents – Eränkö $AgNO_3$ microstaining method
Oxidation-reduction systems – modified Semenoff technique
Enamel diffusion – methylene blue powder bags were placed in the Rats mouths
Caries progress – contact microradiography

Findings: **The presence of an oxidation-reduction system was found uniformly throughout the dentin at all ages studied. As rats became older the evidence of diffusion decreased. Observations made in this study are consistent with the suggestion that the increased availability of carbohydrate and protein is the result of mineral loss. Properly prepared tissues reveal striking changes which precede the classical picture of the carious lesion. These changes include a cessation of oxidation-reduction, an increased stainability of carbohydrate and protein, the presence of a reducing agent, and loss of mineral.**

Article (abstract) #12

The carbohydrate content of caries-susceptible rat molars

Wilcox A, O'Day P, Haley MI, Steinman RR. J Dent Res 38(4):676, Abstr #59, Jul-Aug 1959

Purpose: To compare the CHO content of molars of rats on high sucrose vs. regular Purina chow diets.

STUDY: 18 litters of post-weanling white rats were divided, half on Purina ration and the other half on a 65% sucrose cariogenic diet. CHO content was determined using a modified colorimetric anthrone technique on 1st and 2nd molars weekly from 29 to 49 days.

Results: At 28 days, after the rats had been on the diet for 1 week ($p = 0.001$)
Purina fed group – mean CHO content was 325 μg/100 mg
Sucrose fed group – mean CHO content was 247 μg/100 mg
No further differences were noted at subsequent 35-, 42-, and 49-day intervals

Conclusion: **Significantly greater CHO was contained in regular-fed rats indicating a possible metabolic inhibition of uptake by the high-sucrose-diet rat molars.**

Article (abstract) #13

Histochemical analysis of lesions in incipient dental caries

Steinman RR, Hewes G. J Dent Res 38(4):687, Abstr #86, Jul-Aug 1959

STUDY: 600 post-weanling caries-susceptible rats were placed half on a high-sucrose cariogenic diet and the other half on Purina lab chow. Jaw sections were analyzed serially at 21 to 50 days of age. The following tests were employed: Ninhydrin-Schiff protein, Hotchkiss polysaccharide, Macallum sulfur, Ëränko vitamin C, Semenoff succinic dehydrogenase, Villamil and Mancini cytochrome oxidase, and the Quincke iron test.

Results: **By 28 days in the depth of many of the major grooves of cariogenic diet teeth, there was ↑ reactive protein, CHO, and ↓ mineral; cessation of oxidation reduction, absence of cytochrome oxidase and ↑ of Fe.**

Article (abstract) # 14

Ultrastructural changes in dentine occurring in incipient caries

Hewes G, Steinman RR, Woods RW. J Dent Res 38(4):694, Abstr #S5, Jul-Aug 1959

STUDY 1: Teeth of weanling rats injected i.p. with trypan blue **exhibited incipient caries within 7 days on a high sucrose diet**. Dentin of high-sucrose diet teeth appeared less discolored than Purina chow controls.

STUDY 2: Electron microscopic analysis of teeth from animals not given trypan blue demonstrated that the **odontoblastic processes of molar teeth of sucrose-fed rats appeared as patent tube-like structures compared to the nearly closed or solid protoplasmic processes in dentine of Purina chow controls.**

Article #15

The pathology of caries

Steinman RR, Robson B, Morrow S. J South Calif Dent Assn 27(10):339-344, 1959

This paper discusses some pathological dental tissue changes preceding actual cavitation of the teeth and relates these to certain embryological and histological features.

Skin tissue is histologically related to teeth by origin, metabolism and function. Enamel and dentin are respectively of ectodermal and mesodermal origins which also correspond with the protective outer epithelium and its deeper underlying supportive corium.

Disturbances in the balance of the component internal tissues through systemic and nutritional factors can influence the overlying external tissues. The host's systemic health status affects resistance or susceptibility to dental caries as reported in previous studies. **Besides heredity, nutrition can affect incidence of caries: L-lysine, vitamin B_6, parenteral carbohydrates, nutritional status, dibasic sodium phosphate. Other systemically induced factors are thyroxin blood levels, castration, administration of diamox, dental vessel ligation, and x-ray therapy.**

Bacteria are essential to dental caries in fissures or proximal surfaces. If diffusible material from bacterial action finds host dental tissues pre-conditioned by minor changes, the initiation of caries can occur.

Histopathology involves (1) permeability, (2) enzyme breakdown, (3) tissue changes, and (4) enamel integrity.

Permeability – **Pits, fissures, and interproximal gingival areas of newly-erupted teeth are immature and permeable** to diffusible material as evidenced experimentally by oral introduction of **methylene blue dye**. In another study, systemic injection of **trypan blue in white rats showed a definite outward flow mechanism. By the time the tooth reaches maturity, it has organized a structure that allows flow of diffusible material largely in an outward direction. This maintains nutrition and support for the overlying enamel which shields and protects the deeper structures from injurious agents. When nutritional, hereditary and systemic host factors are in good order, the entrance of bacterial products is prevented.**

Enzyme breakdown – **Enzyme systems were stable in rats fed a noncariogenic diet, but there was breakdown in the cariogenic group**. Methylene blue stain turns

colorless when oxidized. Under anaerobic conditions sodium succinate acts as a substrate for succinic dehydrogenase, which is essential for oxidation-reduction processes. **Persistence of methylene blue stain indicated absence of oxidation in the dentinoenamel junction areas** shown in Fig. 1. **Tissue cannot maintain its continuity in the absence of normal enzyme activity, and subsequent pathological changes occur.**
Tissue changes – The actual clinical appearance of the carious lesion did not occur until around 50 days of age, 22 days after the histological evidence appeared. Fig. 5 shows caries after 65 days.
Sloughing – As underlying dentin is destroyed by decay, the enamel can eventually no longer maintain its integrity.
The earliest pathological change noted in the hard tissues is an alteration in metabolism or enzyme activity. A breakdown of affected tissues results. These changes were not found in the teeth of animals on a noncariogenic diet. **It is suggested that the resistance of the host is the key to caries control**.

Article (abstract) #16

The immunohistochemical localization of plasma albumin in murine dentinal tissue

Zwemer JD, Steinman RR. J Dent Res 38(6):1239, Abstr, Nov-Dec 1959

Although fluorescent-labeled antibodies have been used to localize plasma proteins in cells and interstitial spaces, there are no studies for bone or dentinal tissues. **The purpose of this study was to investigate possible plasma albumin in albino rat dentin.**
STUDY: Fluorescein isothiocyanate-labeled anti-rabbit γ-globulin sheep globulin was employed on frozen hemi-mandibular sections of Osborne-Mendel albino rats 19 to 42 days of age. Controls followed the protocol of White (Ft. Detrick, Frederick, MD).
Results: Specific fluorescence referable to plasma albumin was readily demonstrable in the dentinal tubules of the experimental group for at least the proximal half of their course and in the pulpal margin of the dentinal matrix. Staining was more pronounced in younger animals. Controls did not exhibit the characteristic fluorescence.
Significance: **Plasma albumin was shown present in at least the pulpal half of the lengths of the dentinal tubules**.

Article #17

The possible role of hyaluronidase in incipient carious lesions

Steinman RR. J Dent Res 39(1):150-152, 1960

The purpose of this study was to investigate the possible role of bacterial hyaluronidase in incipient caries pathogenesis.
STUDY: Half of a group of 70 18-day-old Osborne-Mendel rats were given a cariogenic diet and the other half the same plus 1% antihyaluronidase, which acts by competing with natural substrate for hyaluronidase. Teeth were histochemically analyzed when rats were 18 days old.
Results: 9 rats died in the antihyaluronidase group. The average of the 31 remaining was 0.8 incipient lesion per animal compared with 4.09 incipient lesions per animal in the group not receiving antihyaluronidase.
Streptococci are capable of producing a variety of enzymes, toxins, and acids. The incipient lesion showed marked increase in permeability, reducing agents, and possible

mucopolysaccharide breakdown suggesting the possible presence of bacterial hyaluronidase.

Conclusions:

· **Dietary antihyaluronidase in experimental animals appears capable of significant caries reduction**

· **Suggests possible role bacterial hyaluronidase may play in initiating caries**

Article #18

Can dental caries susceptibility be affected by the ingestion of carbohydrates?

Steinman RR. J Indiana State Dent Assoc 39:130-134, April 1960

Three pre-conditions for caries must occur—bacteria, fermentable CHO, and susceptibility of the tooth [plus time]. Dentistry must utilize all known means of reducing dental susceptibility. The systemic environment during tooth formation is becoming recognized. Genetic make-up is a contributor. Availability of nutrients and their proper assimilation can also control susceptibility. Vitamins A, C, D as well as minerals Ca and P are essential for formation and calcification of enamel. Trace elements like F reduce caries susceptibility. The health and welfare of the forming tooth is intimately associated with the health and welfare of the individual as a whole.

Absorption of Ca and P depends on an acid environment to maintain salts in solution and is also favored by vitamins C and D and by the presence of lactose. An excess of fat may interfere by forming insoluble calcium soaps. Excess salts of Fe, Al, and Mg may form insoluble salts with P and prevent its absorption. Proper foods must be present and in the right proportions.

Nutritional diseases can be induced by excesses as well as by stark deficiencies. Excess protein can cause nephrosis, excess fat is related to cardiovascular diseases. Even known essential elements when taken in excess can become toxic, such as iodine and sodium. Is it possible some nutritional problems facing dentistry in this country are directly related to excesses rather than to deficiencies?

Sognnaes observed that maternal rats on a purified ration complete in known essentials except that all CHO was supplied as sucrose produced offspring with a significantly higher caries rate than offspring of mothers on natural diets.

Monkey studies also showed that teeth forming when the animals were placed on a high-sucrose ration were more caries-susceptible. Was it due to excess dietary sugar or to some unknown essential ingredient?

Calcification of the developing 1st and 2nd molars until their oral eruption coincides with the suckling period. The 3rd molar involves the last ¼ of the suckling period plus ca 14 days beyond weaning. This is the window of time that the amount or type of CHO can influence caries susceptibility by affecting developmental calcification.

Work by Haley & Steinman with sucrose administered via eye dropper t.i.d. to suckling rats showed that compared to littermates receiving only water instead, there was a subsequent increase in caries from sugar given for only 1/3rd of the suckling period. Lactose was the sugar least likely to produce subsequent caries.

In another study by Steinman et al, subsequent caries was found proportional to the amount of CHO in the synthetic formula of weaned baby rats. Sucrose, Karo refined corn syrup, and dextromaltose, caused greatest increases in subsequent dental caries.

Caries susceptibility of World War children in Europe was reduced due to enforcement of fewer refined foods in general and less sugar in particular. In countries such as India and China with high CHO consumption but low caries incidence, it is notable that their CHO is largely in the form of starch. Experimental animals given CHO by injection after the teeth erupted developed significantly more caries than their litter mates did on the same human food diet but without the sugar injections.

It is known that lactose causes the smallest increase in subsequent caries compared with other simple sugars, even though metabolism is similar for all simple sugars. The difference may be that lactose favors the absorption of minerals such as Ca and P. Also, lactose absorption into the blood is much slower than other sugars, so might cause less change in the blood glucose level.

A rapid rise in the BSL is accompanied by a decrease in serum inorganic phosphate, which could affect availability for the developing tooth buds in suckling rats. In fact, a 10% decrease in total phosphate content of molar buds has been reported. It may be that this altered phosphate content causes teeth to be more susceptible to caries. Sobel found a relationship of reduced dietary phosphate to increased caries susceptibility. The slower absorption of lactose compared to other simple sugars appears associated with both the least blood phosphate level changes and caries susceptibility effects.

When the ↑ sugar content of synthetic diets is replaced by a polysaccharide such as starch, there is a marked decrease in caries. Conversely, when sugar was ingested intraperitoneally, there was an increase in caries. It could be that rapidly absorbed sugar produces a systemic effect in addition to the well-known effect. From this it would seem advisable to include more slowly-absorbed sugars in the diet.

Physiologic effects of dietary carbohydrates depend on (1) the amount of CHO in the diet, (2) the speed of absorption, (3) availability of phosphate for phosphorylation, (4) endocrine balance, and (5) presence of the nutrients necessary for metabolism. Although this balance may be otherwise well maintained, it can still be disturbed by a rapid physiologic excess of CHO producing a sudden bloodstream influx. If this concept is valid, nutrients are needed in the correct amounts for an optimally healthy metabolism.

If breast feeding is impossible, the formula that is used should be one in which lactose is incorporated as the CHO.

Between-meal snacks high in sugar and very low in all other nutrients should be eliminated from the diet, especially for children, in order to benefit both existing and yet-developing teeth.

Since CHOs are needed as a source of energy, the bulk should be obtained from starch, which is found in abundance in whole grains and vegetables.

<u>Conclusions:</u>

· The effect a CHO may have on caries susceptibility may depend on its rapidity of absorption into the bloodstream

· Caries reduction, therefore, would be favored by:

- Mothers nursing their infants as much as possible
- Choosing baby formulas containing lactose as the available CHO instead of other simple sugars
- Eliminating between-meal snacks
- Replacing rich desserts with fruits or vegetables

Article #19

The possible role of hyaluronidase in the incipient carious lesion

Steinman RR. J South Calif Dent Assn 28(7):207-209, 1960

Histochemical changes are summarized as follows [see Fig. 1, original article,]:

- Changes in Enamel (1-4 days)
  - Permeability
  - Reactive to $AgNO_3$ (reducing agents)
- Changes in Dentin (within 1 week)
  - Sulfhydryl depleted from tubules
  - Cessation of oxidation-reduction
  - Depolymerization of mucopolysaccharide
  - Partial demineralization of dentin
- Changes in Dentin (3+ weeks later)
  - Necrosis of overlying enamel
  - Bacterial invasion
  - Sloughing

Purpose of this study was to investigate the possible role of bacterial hyaluronidase in the pathogenesis of the incipient carious lesion.

Conclusion: Without going into the experimental details on this study, **it was found that antihyaluronidase administered to animals on a cariogenic diet significantly reduced the number of incipient carious lesions. Bacterial hyaluronidase may play a role in the carious process.**

Article (abstract) #20

The effect of weaning on the incidence of incipient carious lesions

Steinman RR. J Dent Res 39(4):860, Jul-Aug 1960

The weaning process as brought about naturally by the maternal rat is gradual and would normally extend a number of days past the weaning dates superimposed by experimental laboratory protocol. **This study was to determine the effect of sudden weaning upon incidence of incipient carious lesions in young rats.**

STUDY: 60 weaned Osborne-Mendel rats were placed on cariogenic diets. 30 animals in each litter were weaned at 20 days of age. The other 30 remained with the dams. Jaws were sectioned and examined at 30 days of age. Presence of incipient lesions was analyzed histochemically using the ninhydrin reaction.

Results: No significant difference in weight was noticed between the groups. Subjects weaned at 20 days of age had an average of 8.3 incipient lesions whereas their unweaned littermates had an average of 3.6 incipient lesions.

No. Days on Cariogenic Diet	Age Weaned	No. Rats	No. Lesions	Average
0-30	20	30	249	8.3
0-30	(not weaned)	30	108	3.6

Reduction of caries by mothers milk was to be expected from a report by Shaw et al, J. Nutrition 67:253, 1959. The cariogenic diet may be suspected of being inadequate for optimal development of rat teeth at this stage of their development. Further studies may be needed to elucidate whether other factors such as bacterial or emotional may be contributory.

Article (abstract) #21

The endotoxic activity of a rat oral streptococcus

Zwemer JE, Steinman RR. J Dent Res 39(5):1073, Abstr, 1960

It is now known that reactions induced by endotoxins such as the delayed skin response, local and generalized Shwartzman phenomena, febrile response, and the potentiation of epinephrine are also elicited by lysates of Group A β-hemolytic streptococci [ref]. Streptococcal species have been shown to produce dental caries in gnotobiotic rats [ref]. **The purpose of this study was to establish the possible endotoxic activity of a streptoccal microorganism**.

STUDY: Oral streptococcus strain FA-1, which induces dental caries in gnotobiotic rats was obtained from NIDR. Streptococcal lysate was prepared. 28 normal albino rabbits were maintained on Wayne rabbit diet and tested for delayed skin reactions, local and generalized Shwartzman, febrile responses, and endotoxin potentiation of epinephrine. Each reaction was typically observable as a 1-3 cm skin lesion.

Results:

·Delayed local inflammatory reaction – Intradermal lysate injection produced characteristic erythema, induration, and edema at 24 hrs. Saline-injected controls were non-reactive.

·Local Shwartzman – i.v. *E. coli* endotoxin injection caused severe hemorrhagic necrosis at initially reactive sites from previous skin reactions

·Generalized Shwartzman – i.m. cortisone injections for 3 days developed cortical necrosis following provocation by i.v. 2 ml strep lysate in 1 out of 5 rabbits

·Febrile response – i.v. injection of either 2 ml lysate or washed cell suspension showed significant body temperature elevation compared with controls injected with saline

·Epinephrine potentiation – i.v. injection of 2 ml lysate then intradermally 2 ml saline at one site and 2 ml epinephrine at a second site uniformly developed severe hemorrhagic necrosis at the epinephrine site within 24 hrs. These reactions were identical with those in rabbits tested with 200 μg *E. coli* lipopolysaccharide.

Significance:

Strep lysate toxicity was shown strongly as delayed local inflammatory reactions; strongly in the generalized Shwartzman, slightly in the generalized Shwartzman reaction, significantly as febrile response, and strongly in the epinephrine potentiation test.

Article (abstract) #22

The endotoxic activity of human saliva

Zwemer JE, Steinman RR. J Dent Res 39(5):1074, Abstr, 1960

Lipopolysaccharide somatic antigens of gram-negative bacteria are called "endotoxins". It has been suggested that endotoxins play a role in the pathogenesis of gingival and periodontal disease. **This study is to confirm the presence of endotoxins in the mouth and oral fluids by a uniquely identifiable and sensitive means.**

Endotoxin specifically potentiates the necrotizing action of epinephrine ≤1000x, producing extraordinary hemorrhagic necrosis in rabbits receiving I.V. injections of endotoxin within previous 4 hrs.

STUDY: 53 albino rabbits were used to test individual human saliva samples from 5 subjects in good oral health and 2 with moderate to advanced periodontal disease. After

I.V. injection with 1 ml of individual human saliva specimens, all rabbits were injected intradermally with 0.2 ml saline at one site and 0.2 ml epinephrine at a second site. 5 control animals received 200 μg *E. coli* lipopolysaccharide. 5 additional control rabbits were not given any I.V. injections. All rabbits were examined for local lesions 24 hours after intradermal injection. Lesion size variabilities were disregarded.

Preparative Controls		Saliva of Healthy Subjects					Saliva/Perio Patients	
Non-injected	Endotoxin	1	2	3	4	5	6	
0/5	5/5	1/10	2/5	4/5	2/5	3/5	2/8	5/5

Results: **Clearly all specimens of saliva exhibited some endotoxic activity. Saliva from the advanced perio patient induced hemorrhagic necrosis in all 5 tested animals**

Article #23

Histochemical analysis of lesions in incipient dental caries. II. Sulfhydryl and disulfide radicals

Steinman RR. J Dent Res 39(10):1009-1013, Sep-Oct 1960

Reported previously, histochemical changes in the dentin preceding caries include cessation of oxidation reduction, increased stainability of CHO and protein, presence of silver nitrate reducing agent, and some loss of mineral. The purpose of this paper was to find whether sulfhydryl and disulfide radicals exist in dentinal tubules normally and under pathological conditions.

STUDY: 100 Osborne-Mendel caries-susceptible rats were divided into two groups at 20 days of age. Group 1 was given the cariogenic diet while Group 2 was on a noncariogenic diet. Jaw sections were examined using the lead acetate method for sulfhydryl and disulfide groups at various times between 20 and 30 days.

Results: Lead sulfide was visible as a black precipitate in dentinal tubules (fig. 1). Fig. 4 is a section showing dentin from the noncariogenic diet until 30 days of age, compared with that of a littermate on the cariogenic diet in fig. 5. The area of pathosis showing no tubular precipitate was found as early as 26 days of age in cariogenic diet subjects. A sharp line of demarcation between affected and unaffected dentin is usually present at 28 days of age.

Discussion: **Sulfhydryl groups are essential in a number of enzyme systems [ref]. Failure of the oxidation-reduction system fails within the area of early pathology [ref]. Diminution of reactive sulfhydryl groups in incipient carious lesions further implicates the organic phase of the tooth in early caries pathogenesis.**

Summary:

· **A sensitive method for possible demonstration of sulfhydryl radicals within dentinal tubules was presented**

· **Evidence that sulfhydryl groups disappear during incipient caries pathogenesis was shown**

[Note: Histochemical techniques often require an acid medium, unsuitable because of decalcification and other invalidating alterations to dental tissues. The options were limited. Dr. S. tried the ditetrazolium chloride method but the color was weak and definition poor. Through trial and error he found that the lead acetate method worked.]

Article #24

The effect of stress upon the incidence of dental caries

Steinman RR, Smith LV. J South Calif Dent Assn 28(11):367-369, 1960

All white rats in this study were littermates placed on a cariogenic diet *ad libitum.* Rats confined to wire cages allowing no freedom of movement had a poor general appearance and weighed about 22% less than unconfined animals that had been allowed to exercise in a rotating cage. In the experimentally confined group there was an average of 14.9 lesions compared with 5.9 for the exercised controls.

Stress may be a significant factor in increasing caries susceptibility, at least in young animals. Caries susceptibility was not overcome by allowing exercise to the confined young rats.

Article #25

The in vitro changes in rat tooth structure produced by streptococcal lysate

Steinman RR. J South Calif Dent Assn 28(12):411-412, 1960

The purpose was to determine the effect of a streptococcal lysate upon rat tooth structure and find the active agent involved.

STUDY: A lysate of rat oral streptococci strain FA-1 was prepared and frozen until use. Finely divided tooth particles were washed twice in water and the precipitate centrifuged, 300 mg of which was placed in test tubes divided into three groups. Group 1– 1 ml of water was added, Group 2– 1 ml of lysate, Group 3– 1 ml of lysate inactivated by 10 min's at 60ºC. These were incubated at 37ºC for 4 hrs. The mixtures were centrifuged and 1 ml of 0.5% ninhydrin solution was added to the supernatant. Rapidity of reaction was considered proportional to concentration of reactive proteins present.

Group 1– Slight reaction, very slow, Group 2- Reacted rapidly and markedly, Group 3- Slight reaction, very slow.

Therefore, something in the lysate released proteins and the substance is heat-labile.

In vivo studies show incipient lesions have a marked increase in reactive proteins to ninhydrin. This in vitro experiment would tend to support this view. Streptococci produce many noxious agents including enzymes.

Agents other than acid may be involved. Studies report caries occurring in neutral medium, and in an alkaline environment. Also, streptoccal enzyme hyaluronidase has been shown to decalcify teeth. It appears that in the incipient lesion there is an uncoupling of all components—collagen, mucopolysaccharides and mineral. Certainly acid plays a part in the sloughing process of caries, however the incipient, early pathology may be initiated by enzyme activity.

Article #26

Comparison of caries incidence in exercised and immobilized rats

Steinman RR, Brussett M, Tartaryn P. J Dent Res 40(1):218, Abstr, 1961

Resistance of rats to caries may be related to their physical status including diet. **The present study of immobilized vs exercised rats shows that physical status *exclusive of diet* may have a profound effect upon decay resistance.** ([See also "Effect of stress…" in article #24 above].

Article #27

The pathogenic role of a rat oral streptococcus in incipient dental caries

Steinman RR, Zwemer JD. J Dent Res 40(2):378, Abstr, 1961

Streptococcus in gnotobiotic rats has shown causal relationship to dental caries. It can produce acids, enzymes, toxins, and delayed hypersensitive response.

STUDY: Incipient lesions from Osborne-Mendel rats 20 to 50 days old and fed either Purina chow or the cariogenic diet, were analyzed by ninhydrin-reactive protein, dehydrogenase activity, and availability of sulfhydryl radicals.

Fluorescein isothiocyanate conjugated with rabbit anti-streptococcal globulin was used to stain sectioned tooth samples. High fluorescence, corresponding to bacterial concentration, showed mostly in the debris found in the grooves. There was little in the surface enamel in the grooves, and none in the underlying dentin. Streptococcal-lysate-exposed tooth sections from more than 100 rats consistently indicated a specific, marked diminution in dehydrogenase activity and reduced availability of sulfhydryl radicals. Efforts are now being made to characterize the streptococcal component involved and its effects on the dental substrate.

Article (abstract) #28

Caries susceptibility as affected by electrolyte balance

Steinman RR. J Dent Res 40(4):658, Abstr #53, 1961

Recent experiments [refs] have shown that stress in young rats significantly increased caries. Prominent among various physiological changes induced by stress is change in electrolyte balance potentially affecting the water-transport system and nutritive state of all body cells [ref]. Ligating dental arteries also increased caries rates [ref]. Poor nutritional state was related to increased caries [ref]. **The purpose of this study was to determine whether altered electrolyte balance could be a factor in caries susceptibility.**

STUDY: 182 Osborne-Mendel rats were placed on a cariogenic diet at weaning (21 days). At 31 days of age the teeth were analyzed histochemically and caries scores determined.

	Caries scores
Group 1– 44 Controls were given water ad lib	7.0
Group 2– 41 were given 0.9% saline ad lib	10.44
Group 3– 26 Controls on water alone	6.72
Group 4– 30 were given 1 mg/gm **Diuril** in their ration	3.68
Group 5– 21 Controls on water	6.08
Group 6– 20 were given 0.1 ml/35 gm wt **Percorten (DOCA)** at 21 days of age, .05 ml at 28 days	9.88

Significance: **Chi-square analysis was valid (p = 0.001) that an electrolyte imbalance could be one systemic factor affecting caries susceptibility under chemically-induced stress conditions.**

Article #29

The rat molar in health and disease*

Steinman RR. J Calif. Dent Assn 37(2):103-105, Apr 1961

Rats are probably the most universally used experimental animal due to their economy, adjustability to lab conditions, and abundance of published data as reference material. Fortunately, they are also subject to one of man's most prevalent diseases, dental caries. Histologically, rat molars are similar to human molars. Odontoblasts lay down secondary dentin throughout the lifetime of the rat. Incidence of disease in rats appears altered by many of the well-known conditions similar in man.

The tooth, a functioning entity. Enamel, dentin, and pulp cannot exist alone but each contributes to the welfare of the whole. Vital staining [refs], isotopes [ref] and fluorescent-labeled technique [ref] all indicate existence of a vital connection between circulation within the pulp and the outer hard structures of the tooth. There would appear to exist a "circulation" within the dentin [ref] and that the enamel matures from within out [refs] which is dependent on a vital pulp [ref].

By what means can the dependence of an interchange between these various tissues be mediated? They are two embryologically different tissues necessitating metabolic interaction separated by a considerable distance. If it is similar to other body tissues, communication is dependent on an electron transfer system probably involving a sulfhydryl configuration [ref]. Any interaction would depend upon the odontoblast and its protoplasmic process which reaches to the DEJ. Histochemically, the presence of an oxidation reduction system in the dentin and the possible presence of sulfhydryl in dentinal tubules have been demonstrated.

A number of important pathological changes occur in rat molars by 28 days of age: (1) a marked increase in permeability beneath the food in the enamel, (2) a cessation of oxidation reduction in the dentin, and (3) a possible depletion of sulfhydryl within the dentinal tubules just beneath the affected enamel. These are important changes involving function of the tissues.

About this time changes in structure may be observed, characterized by a marked increase in reactive protein [ref], a marked increase in reactive carbohydrate, and partial demineralization of the dentin. After 3 or 4 more weeks bacterial invasion and sloughing occur leading to typical cavity formation. As typical of disease processes in other tissues, caries appears to occur in a sequence of events terminating in necrosis, bacterial invasion, and sloughing (dissolution). It is of interest that many of the changes observed *in vivo* can be duplicated *in vitro* using streptococcal lysate.

Resistance of the host. A number of nutritional factors [refs] and non-nutritional factors [refs] have been shown to affect the incidence of caries in the posteruptive period. Immobilization stress in young rats was found to increase incipient caries incidence nearly 3 times. Prominent among the changes induced by stress is increased secretion of ACTH, which will primarily induce ↑ secretion of N, K, P and secondarily retain Na and Cl with consequent water retention. Through such a mechanism it would be possible for stress to alter the electrolyte and water balance. Since all nutrients carried to the cells and waste material carried from the cells depend on the water transport system, this could affect the functional status of every cell in the body.

It was reported that administration of desoxycorticosterone trimethylacetate (DOCA) to weaned rats caused a significant ↑ in caries. This hormone produces marked cellular retention of Na and Cl. Administration of chlorothiazide (Diuril) diuretic increases excretion of Na and Cl which reduced the incipient caries rate. Manipulation of the electrolyte balance appears to produce a marked effect on caries susceptibility.

Cellular changes. It is known that all cells have a polarized membrane inside of which is located the machinery necessary for certain functions. This cellular machinery is activated by depolymerization of the membrane to perform specific functions. The qualities of this reaction are dependent upon the intracellular ionic atmosphere which is controlled by the rate at which ions enter and leave the cell. This ionic concentration can be altered by stress or by administration of DOCA. This change in permeability is accompanied by entrance of plasma proteins and Na into the cell along with the exit of potassium ions into the extracellular fluid space. This tends to equalize the intracellular and extracellular fluids away from optimal balance and could adversely affect the flow of nutrients into the hard structures as well as alter the osmotic relationship of the tooth to its external environment.

Metabolic energy is required to pump sodium outside the cell. The higher the concentration of sodium outside, the faster this metabolic pump must work to maintain the gradient. This may place an added load upon the cell and CHO metabolism. The degree of hydration also influences the rate of cell membrane ion exchange.

Discussion**:** It is generally thought that the increase in caries following removal of the salivary glands is the result of local action on the tooth. It is well to note that removal of major salivary glands is also accompanied by increased adrenocortical activity. It has been noticed that these animals grew more slowly than normal rats. Possibly salivary glands produce a hormone which may account for the slower growth of animals when absent. It is known that some sex hormones cause increased serum sodium concentrations. Could this explain caries reduction observed following castration of young animals?

It is possible that the higher Na and Cl within the pulp and the tooth could affect caries resistance in 2 ways. By altering osmosis and water transport, it could influence the nutritive state of the tooth and affect maturation and resistance to disease. Any change in osmotic balance could alter its relationship to the external environment. It is possible under certain circumstances that normal osmotic pressure would repel noxious bacterial agents, whereas under circumstances induced by abnormal osmotic pressure it would encourage ingress of noxious materials into the tooth. Thus the electrolyte balance of the tooth may play a vital role in susceptibility or resistance to disease.

The caries problem apparently is as complex as life itself. Perhaps the best answer is an improved way of life including heredity, correct nutrition, freedom from over-stress, fresh air, and appropriate intake of water for optimum host resistance against caries.

Summary:

- **The tooth is a group of dissimilar, interdependent tissues**
- **Optimal health depends on harmonious interactive function with each of its component tissues**
- **Disease is the result of disturbance of optimal function, in whole or in part**
- **The ultimate control of infectious disease rests on effective host resistance**

[*Ed. note: This seems to be Steinman's best over-all functional summary and descriptive literature review to date]

Article #30

The incidence of dental caries as altered by electrolyte and water balance

Steinman RR. J South Calif Dent Assn 29(4):122-126, 1961

Nonspecific stress will cause an increased secretion of corticotropin. It is known that corticotropin in normal animals will cause sodium retention. This alters the water transport system and influences the nutritive state of every cell in the body. Sodium and chloride are the major electrolytes in the extracellular fluid, controlling osmotic pressure and water balance. **The purpose of this study was to determine if sodium chloride retention could be one of the systemic factors involved in the increase of incipient carious lesions under stress conditions.**

STUDY 1: 85 Osborn-Mendel rats fed a cariogenic diet were divided into groups at 21 days of age.

Group 1– drank water only, Group 2– drank 0.9% saline only. Teeth were examined histochemically after **32 days of age** to determine occlusal and interproximal incipient lesions

Results: **The saline caused significant increase in incipient carious lesions.** Caries score for the control group was **6.77** compared to **10.34** for the saline group.

STUDY 2: 30 Osborn-Mendel rats fed a cariogenic diet were divided into groups at 21 days of age and at age 35 days were divided into 2 groups of litter mates.

Group 1– Drank 0.9% saline only, Group 2– Drank water only. At **56 days of age** all teeth were examined histochemically for lesions.

Results: **Drinking 0.9% saline had no affect.**

STUDY 3: 41 Osborn-Mendel rats fed a cariogenic diet were divided into groups at 21 days of age.

Group 1– Received 0.4% DOCA (desoxycorticosterone trimethylacetate) and at 28 days of age another 0.05 ml DOCA., Group 2– Received the cariogenic diet. At 31 days of age all teeth were examined histochemically.

Results: **DOCA produced significant increase in caries.** Caries score for the control was 5.81 compared to 9.40 for the DOCA group.

STUDY 4: 56 Osborn-Mendel rats fed a cariogenic diet were divided into groups at 21 days of age.

Group 1– Controls on the cariogenic diet, Group 2 – Cariogenic diet plus 1 mg Chlorthiazide (Diuril) per gram of rations. *Water for all animals was ad libitum and not otherwise controlled.* All teeth were examined for incipient lesions at 30 days of age.

Results: **Diuril decreased the incidence of caries.** Control animals had a score of 6.46 whereas the Diuril group had only 3.60.

STUDY 5: 30 Osborn-Mendel rats fed a cariogenic diet were divided into groups at 21 days of age.

Group 1- Controls on the cariogenic diet, Group 2 – Cariogenic diet plus 1 mg Chlorthiazide (Diuril) per gram of rations. *Water for all animals was controlled to be equal.* All teeth were examined for incipient lesions at 30 days of age.

Results: **Diuril under controlled water intake conditions had no effect.**

In 1933 Moore suggested that large amounts of NaCl could be a contributing factor in the large amount of dental caries among civilized groups. A recent report indicated ↑ chloride ion was associated with ↑ caries incidence. It was thought to act at the local level, however it is needed for amylase activity and our diet contained no starch. Therefore, the ↑ chloride ion might be a reflection of a plasma ↑ in chloride ion. The younger animals placed on 0.9% saline were more affected which could suggest interference with the normal metabolism and maturation of the teeth.

Discussion**: It is generally thought that the increase in caries accompanying the removal of the major salivary glands of the rat is the result of a local action upon the surface of the teeth. In this connection it is well to note that the removal of the**

major salivary glands is accompanied by ↑ adrenocortical activity. The adrenal cortex plays a major role in electrolyte balance. It has further been noted that these animals grow more slowly than do normal rats [ref's]. There is the possibility that the salivary glands produce a hormone, which may account for the slower growth of animals with the salivary glands removed [ref]. It is also known that some sex hormones cause a rise in the concentration of serum sodium. Could this explain the reduction in caries following the castration of young animals? [ref]

When water availability is limited, more systemic sodium is retained and may explain the lack of caries reduction in rats given Diuril. Sodium and chloride electrolytes affect water transport through osmotic balance. **Interference with normal balance can affect the nutritive state within the tooth and alter its maturation and disease resistance. Abnormal osmotic pressure can also influence the tooth's ability to discourage the ingress of noxious material from its external environment. The electrolyte balance of the dental pulp may play an important role in susceptibility or resistance to disease.**

Beyond changes in digestion, alteration of intestinal function and accompanying loss of appetite, a change in the water transport system potentially affects every cell and fiber of the system. Perhaps the basic answer to dental caries prevention is a total way of life including sound nutrition, freedom from undue stress, regular exercise, fresh air, sunlight, and water intake. **The physiological state of hydration may be more significant to dental health than commonly recognized.**

Article #31

The physiological basis for caries susceptibility and resistance

Steinman RR, Smith LV. J South Calif Dent Assn 29(7):221-224, 1961

Although the first line of tooth defense is the outer enamel, its properties of hardness or density alone do not confer total immunity to carious attack. In fact, clinically it is observed that even hypoplastic areas do not necessarily decay. Studies have shown that stress and systemic electrolyte imbalance can ↑ caries susceptibility. When NaCl retention was artificially induced experimentally with DOCA, caries incidence increased. Conversely, experimental induction of NaCl excretion in rats using Diuril resulted in caries reduction. These findings would suggest dental susceptibility to caries ingress is influenced by a balance of osmotic flow within the tooth. **The purpose of this study was to determine more about the nature of this osmotic defense.** [Was H_2O_2 employed as an agent to produce atypical destruction of the tooth surface and possibly physiologically induce inward flow using methylene blue dye as a visible tracking agent?]

STUDY: Osborn-Mendel caries-suceptible rats weaned at 21 days of age were placed on either the cariogenic diet or on Purina lab chow. At various ages from 17 to 35 days of age, a filter-paper bag of 25 mg methylene blue dye was placed in the rats' mouths for 6 to 8 hours, after which the subjects' teeth were sectioned for assessment of dye penetration.

Group 1– given cariogenic diet and plain water to drink

Group 2– given cariogenic diet and 1% hydrogen peroxide by mouth, stomach tube, and intraperitoneally.

Group 3– given noncariogenic diet and plain water to drink

Group 4– given noncariogenic diet and 1% hydrogen peroxide by mouth, stomach tube,

and intraperitoneally.
Group 5– Some animals received hydrogen peroxide from 21 to 26 days of age and then were placed on plain water.
Group 6– Whole removed mandibles were also placed in methylene blue dye for 3 to 12 hours as dye penetration controls.
Results: Methylene blue showed no penetration through any molar cusp tips from 17 days of age onward, Fig. 2. The most susceptible areas were the depths of grooves where food accumulated. Animals age > 40 days failed to show penetration even in these areas. The mandibles of animals sacrificed at 26 days old and soaked in dye solution 2.5 hours showed significant dye penetration, the average shown in Fig. 1 with penetration through cusp tip and enamel.
Group 1– exhibited marked penetration of dye opposite food in grooves (Fig. 4)
Group 4– showed very marked cusp tip and enamel dye penetration beginning after 48 hours of peroxide ingestion (Fig. 5). There was also uniform penetration of the enamel of these teeth. Some rats receiving hydrogen peroxide from only 21 to 26 days of age, then placed on water, showed a marked reversal with no dye penetration.
Group 5– One section (Fig. 6) had one tooth in which no recovery occurred with its adjacent tooth showing almost complete recovery
Group 6– Dye penetrated typically through cusp tips and enamel (Fig. 1)
Discussion:

- **Failure of in vivo penetration of dye at 17 days of age contrasted with marked penetration of dye-soaked post-mortem mandibles suggest that prevention of penetration was associated with its living function.**
- **Marked penetration of dye in teeth of hydrogen-peroxide-fed animals, whether by mouth, stomach tube, or intraperitoneal injection, indicates that this vital process is likely systemic in nature.**
- **Isotope studies show tracer molecules on the tooth surface can be picked up internally and vice versa [ref]. Patients receiving silver salts were found to have marked deposition throughout the dentin and deeper enamel layers [ref]. These studies suggest 2-way transfer through dentin.**
- **Pathology does not appear to occur when the transport system is functioning normally. Hydrogen peroxide reverses this transport and produces very rapid pathology.**
- **See diagram of directions of flow through dentin. External flow is preventive of material from entering the tooth. A net inward flow would draw noxious material from the surface into the tooth. Conceivably this could reach the odontoblast and reduce its ability to function.**
- **Stepwise, there is first an altered function of involved tissue. This altered transport system is largely controlled *systemically.***
- **External factors having systemic effects are electrolyte balance and undue stress, which have been shown to ↑ caries.**
- **Where there was penetration of methylene blue, there apparently was an area of abnormal transport.**
- **Oral streptococci produce hydrogen peroxide. Something like hydrogen peroxide may be involved in the early pathosis of caries.**

· Change of function in the active transport system of teeth is followed by cessation of oxidation reduction, depletion of sulfhydryls, marked increase in reactive protein and carbohydrate, and partial demineralization of the dentin at the DEJ.

Summary: **An active transport system appears to operate within the teeth. This normally prevents ingress of external noxious material to maintain health of the tooth. An abbnormal transport system might allow or encourage external noxious materials into the tooth leading to irreversible pathology.**

Article #32

Histochemical and radiographic changes observed in human teeth

Steinman RR, Smith LV. J South Calif Dent Assn 29(9):294-300, 1961

Purpose of this study was to see if histological changes induced by streptococcal microorganisms in rats' teeth such as alterations in oxidation-reduction or ↑ stainability of dental carbohydrate and protein components can be also demonstrated in human teeth.

STUDY: 175 teeth from 11-45 year old humans were frozen immediately upon extraction. Half of each tooth was removed, then while still frozen, the other halves were removed leaving thin mid-tooth sections only 50 to 150 μ thick. These specimens were incubated in 0.5% ninhydrin 24 hrs to demonstrate presence of reactive proteins, then re-frozen to preserve color. Presence of polysaccharides was demonstrated with the Hotchkiss periodic acid method. The presence of an oxidation-reduction system was demonstrated with the Semenoff technique. Testing for the presence of reducing agent (vit. C) employed the Eränko method. Radiographs were made to correlate radiolucent areas and distinguish various histochemical changes.

Tooth sections tested positive for presence of reducing agents (Semenoff technique) except when first heated to 90° C for 10 minutes. Areas in dentin associated with deep grooves and opposite interproximal contacts where no demineralization was observed showed greatest methylene blue decolorization. Where demineralization was detected radiographically, the dentin beneath it no longer decolorized methylene blue.

Ninhydrin samples indicated no demineralization associated with incipient caries at the DEJ. It appears that the reaction followed the odontoblastic processes and covered a far more extensive area than had been decalcified.

Silver nitrate appeared to follow the direction of the enamel rods.

Early incipient changes in enamel reacted markedly to mucopolysaccharide tests. A marked increase in the dentin for mucopolysaccharides usually did not occur until the lesions became more extensive.

Discussion: Histochemical changes in human enamel seemed to follow the enamel rods, quite noticeably when treated with silver nitrate. Ninhydrin followed odontoblastic processes toward the pulp of the tooth. Dentin mucopolysaccharide changes occurred later and were less circumscribed. Once pathology reached the dentin, histochemical changes proceeded far in advance of radiographically determined demineralization. Oxidation-reduction appeared to occur faster in areas where there was no pathology present. No oxidation-reduction occurred in the dentin for 1 mm around pathology but was surrounded by an area of increased activity—evidence of a resistance phenomenon? Evidence from these histochemical reactions indicated that human teeth were also affected by streptococci like rats and hamsters. In all probability the early pathology is initiated by agents other than acid, then acid plays a part in cavitation/sloughing once started. A parallel observation from other body tissues is that infection by organisms is resistance-related. If host resistance is great enough, no infection will occur. From what is now known, there probably is an active transport system in the dental hard structures. It is reasonable to suspect that one of the first alterations in normal physiology may involve this transport system–stepwise with first susceptibility in the depths of the grooves and interproximally, then facial and lingual surfaces, and finally the whole tooth breaks down.

Conclusions:

- **Histochemical changes in human teeth were similar to rat teeth.**
- **Changes appeared to follow organic pathways far in advance of radiographic evidence.**
- **Evidence shows that caries in humans is initiated by *streptococci* rather than *lactobacilli.***

Article #33

<u>The effect of sucrose and 2-4 dinitro phenol upon odontoblastic function</u>

Steinman RR, Smith LV. J South Calif Dent Assn 29(10):315-317, 1961

Hydrogen peroxide produced marked systemic effects upon the normal transport system of the tooth, probably by affecting odontoblastic function to reverse its normal flow from outward to inward. Likewise, injected sugar systemically increased caries susceptibility. The purpose of this study was more specifically to determine this mechanism by comparing odontoblastic functions relative to induced transport system alterations.

STUDY: 21-day-old weaned caries-susceptible rats were placed on a cariogenic diet. Group 1- At 24 days their teeth were exposed to methylene blue for 8 hrs and observed for extent of dye penetration. Group 2– received 0.5% 2-4 dinitrophenol (2-4 DNP) in their diet before 24th day dye penetration observation. Group 3– received injections of a 20% mixture of glucose and fructose 4x/day before 24th day dye penetration observation.

<u>Findings</u>: Group 1– No penetration through cusp tips on cariogenic diet alone. Group 2– Marked penetration through cusp tips. Group 3– Marked penetration through cusp tips.

<u>Discussion</u>: The first line of dental defense is ability to prevent ingress of noxious material into the substance of the tooth. 2-4 DNP blocks this ability. Odontoblasts act as miniature pumps to control this active transport system and require energy from glucose. Glucose utilization requires phosphate. Both 2-4 DNP and excess glucose effectively reversed the normal transport flow of the tooth probably by interfering with oxidative phosphorylation. 2-4 DNP uncouples the oxidative phosphorylation while an excess of sugar probably reduces the amount of phosphate available for energy production. To support this concept, it was found that adding phosphate to the diet reduced caries [ref]. Control of caries is a biological problem affected by heredity, nutrition, endocrine balance, stress, and other factors. It is possible for material to enter the tooth and be transported to the odontoblast. If this material is of a noxious nature, the efficiency of the odontoblast could be reduced. Animals on a noncariogenic diet overcame this invasion evidenced by absence of dye penetration or pathogenesis.

<u>Conclusions:</u>

- **Sugar and/or 2-4 DNP may reverse the active transport system.**
- **Excess sugar may cause caries systemically as well as from its local effect.**

Article #34

<u>The possible presence of sulfhydryl, disulfide radicals and adenosine triphosphate in human teeth</u>

Steinman RR. J South Calif Dent Assn 29(11):360-364, 1961

The purpose of this study was to determine the presence or absence of sulfhydryl radicals and ATP that may be associated with dentinal active transport metabolism.

STUDY: 100 vital teeth from 12-50 year old patients were sectioned and tested for sulfhydryl and disulfide radicals using the BT method of Barrnett and Seligmon. ATP was measured as a function of exposure reaction to luciferase as recorded on photographic film for 10 minutes. Film darkness was proportional to amount of ATP present.

Findings: Early incipient caries showed presence of sulfhydryl or disulfide radicals in enamel but much less in dentinal tubules from the DEJ extending towards the pulp. Ninhydrin-treated sample showed a flame-shaped area devoid of pigment below the lesion pointing toward the pulp chamber. Luciferase autoradiographs with no luminescence in the DEJ just beneath a groove lesion suggested an area of ATP depletion from there towards the pulp. This was typical in areas with larger lesions.

Discussion: Ninhydrin coloration in the enamel may be due to breakdown of the organic portion making demonstration of the sulfhydryl and disulfide radicals possible. Presence of sulfhydryl radicals and presence of ATP, along with methylene blue decoloration [ref] suggests that an active metabolism exists particularly in the dentin. Failure of certain areas to decolorize methylene blue along with a decrease in sulfhydryl radicals and absence of ATP suggest pathologic metabolic changes preceding changes in normal mineral content. High ATP concentration adjacent to the pulp suggests this is an area of greater metabolic activity. Odontoblasts are suggested as osmotic pumps controlling an active hard-structure transport system. Hydrogen peroxide [ref], 2-4 DNP [ref], and mersalyl (mercurial compound) [ref], changes in electrolyte and water balance [ref], and stress factors [ref] can alter this normal function. Mersalyl was found to alter metabolism and cell permeability to water by tying up sulfhydryl groups [ref]. The tooth must be considered an active functioning organ not merely left to the mercy of an unfavorable environment. It would appear that hope for control of caries rests upon the condition of the internal metabolism of the tooth, as is true for any host against diseases of bacterial origin. Nutrition at the cellular level is critical for resistance.

Conclusions:

- **Sulfhydryl and disulfide radical presence or absence suggests relationship to pathology in human teeth.**
- **ATP presence or absence suggests relationship to pathology in human teeth.**
- **Resistance of teeth to caries may be related to these factors.**

Article #35

<u>The possible presence of adenosine triphosphatase and choline esterase in the human teeth</u>

Steinman RR. J South Calif Dent Assn 29(12):400-404, 1961

Absence of sulfhydryl radicals and ATP to a considerable depth in tooth structures beneath the location of first evidence of demineralization in the enamel has been reported suggesting an active hard-structure metabolism. Movement of the liquid

phase of a tissue is affected by electrolyte balance influenced by selective biological membrane permeability, which depends on the integrity of the sulfhydryl groups [Belkin & Hardy]. One of the enzymes involved in this vital process is acetylcholine esterase. Another possible enzyme in this system is ATPase. **This study was to determine distribution of ATPase and cholinesterase in dentinal structures in relation to any pathological changes that may be present.**
STUDY: 100 human teeth with incipient carious lesions were frozen and sectioned. Presence of ATPase was tested by the method of Wachstein and Meisel, and cholinesterase presence by the method of Gomori.
Results: ATPase appeared largely confined to the tubules, greater towards the pulp. Dimunition of reaction was noted in dentin beneath the occlusal groove. Depletion of enzyme was evident to the pulp in fig's 1-6. Cholinesterase seemed to follow the same general pattern as the ATPase.
Discussion: Essential metabolites and enzymes necessary to perform normal selective permeability have been demonstrated in dentinal tubules of normal teeth and absent or markedly reduced in dentinal tubules immediately beneath enamel showing first evidence of pathological change. It appears from animal experimentation that failure of this system allows noxious material on the surface to penetrate deeply into the tooth. Electrolyte balance affects osmosis and influences the flow of liquid phase through tissue. This lends support to the vital concept of functional resistance. With rats it was found that salt retention following DOCA administration caused significant ↑ in caries whereas Diuril which causes NaCl excretion resulted in ↓ caries incidence. Deleterious agents on tooth surfaces alone do not cause disease until allowed to penetrate. This is paralleled by other host-disease interactions. In this case it appears to occur as a result of failure of the transport system. Evidence indicates streptococci are the external causative agents for caries. Dental resistance to streptocci appears to be related to the less easily defined factors of correct nutrition, harmonious function of the endocrines, physical state of not being overly stressed or fatigued, all of which collectively affect incidence of caries but individually do not completely control the disease.
Conclusions:
- **Possible presence of ATPase and cholinesterase has been demonstrated in dentinal tubules from the pulp to the DEJ.**
- **These enzymes appear to be absent in dentinal tubules adjacent to the pulp beneath the first evidence of demineralization of the enamel.**
- **Roles of these enzymes in other tissues are known and are suggested in dentinal tissue resistance as well.**

Article #36
Role of an enzyme in caries production

Steinman RR. Dental Progess 2(2) 45/109-47/111, Jan 1962

Streptococci as the causative organism of dental caries has been demonstrated in gnotobiotic animals by Orland and Fitzgerald. This leads to examination of the histochemical processes that may be involved.

Hyaluronidase experimentally acts as a catalytic agent of hydrolysis. Similarities have been noted in other body tissues when this enzyme hydrolyzes the intercellular cement [ref], including a marked ↑ in reducing agents, ↑ in permeability, as well as some evidence of simplification of mucopolysaccharide chemical structure [ref]. Adding antihyaluronidase experimentally to otherwise cariogenic diets of rats reduced caries production sharply [ref].

The purpose of this study was to determine the relative presence of hyaluronidase in rat oral streptococci as a potential link in the mechanism of action for caries production.

STUDY: Rat oral streptococci were cultured and lysated by the Stetson method, then frozen ready for testing. Hyaluronidase was colorimetrically determined with respect to a solution of known hyaluronidase concentration and compared with a strep sample control which had its potential enzyme action heat-destroyed at 60ºC for 10 min's. Turbidity was proportional to hyaluronidase transmittance corresponding to the unheated lysate.

Results: **A striking parallel was seen (Fig. 2) between the rising percentage of transmittance of the unknown lysate and the known hyaluronidase shown in Fig. 1. This seems to indicate the presence of hyaluronidase in the unknown lysate. In contrast, the control was represented by a horizontal line indicating complete absence of transmittance.**

Discussion: This raises several questions. **Is hyaluronidase a single enzyme or a number of yet undetermined biochemical constituents? Is this enzyme actually present in the area of oral pathology?** There is evidence to support this assumption but the actual enzyme's presence in the lesion is yet to be found. **How does hyaluronidase enter the tooth?** It seems there is an active metabolic defense mechanism to prevent external foreign material from entering and the defense cell is believed to be the odontoblast. Evidence for this is when the cell's metabolism is altered by chemical or nutritional means, the tooth loses ability to repel surface invasive agents. Heavy atomic weight agents such as methylene blue (mol. wt. 285) and fast green (mol. wt. 762) enter the tooth readily when metabolism is altered. **How large a molecule may enter a tooth under circumstances of altered dental defense?** If hyaluronidase is present in incipient carious lesions, studies should be employed to trace this to its streptococcal pathway of pathology.

Significance: **Colorimetric testing provides circumstantial evidence for the presence of hyaluronidase in streptococcal lysate which might be potentially assumed to aid in penetration of the deleterious bacterial products leading to dental caries.**

Article #37

Molecular changes observed in dental caries and their possible nutritional implications

Steinman RR. J Applied Nutr 15 (nos. 3 & 4):188-191, 1962

Claude Bernard once stated, "The organism is an entity, a whole from which no single part can be isolated." Can teeth logically be considered apart from the whole body? We often see what we are looking for. Perhaps I have looked too intently for the biological processes which may or may not be present in the teeth to correctly evaluate certain observations. About 25 years ago biologists began studying cellular changes at the molecular level. It is this approach that gives us added insight into the importance of nutrition.

The cell membrane and selective permeability. Normally there is 4 times the amount of sodium outside the cell as found inside, and there is about 18 times the amount of potassium inside the cell as found outside. This essential differential in sodium and potassium concentrations is maintained by the "sodium pump." It is a process which requires energy and the functional, healthy physiological balance of the cells is very much dependent on it. Among the various necessary factors are (1) integrity of the sulfhydryl (SH) groups, (2) presence of ATP, and (3) formation and breakdown of acetylcholinesterase. If any one of these factors fails, the system itself fails and normal cellular function and metabolism are altered.

There are a number of important ways this system may be altered. (1) Undue stress in experimental animals has been shown to cause the intracellular fluid to become more nearly like the extracellular fluid and adversely affect normal metabolism. (2) Excess retention of NaCl can overload this system and impede its efficiency. (3) The system may be blocked by chemicals such as mersalyl diamox. (4) Deficiency of certain metabolites and associated factors such as phosphate, pyridoxine, pantothenic acid, or protein can conceivably alter the cells' normal selective permeability.

Let us note that in animals under stress, in animals with excess systemic NaCl, in animals given diamox, and in animals with a deficiency of phosphate, pyridoxine, pantothenic acid or of protein, their caries rate increases.

Histochemical limitations in human teeth. Histochemical difficulties encountered with laboratory research include unsuitability of normal means of tissue preparation such as formaldehyde fixation, decalcification, and paraffin impregnation and sectioning. Even heat normally produced by grinding tissue sections would inactivate many enzymes present. This necessitated rapid freezing immediately following dental extractions then mounting in ice blocks and sectioning in a deep freeze on a small metal lathe. Only techniques suitable on frozen sections could be used. One other limitation is that techniques requiring a low pH are unsuitable due to decalcification of the histological sections.

Histochemical and radiographic findings summarized. Beneath the first radiographic evidence of demineralization in the enamel, there appears a depletion or marked diminution of cholinesterase, ATPase, ATP, SH, disulfide, and Mg in the underlying dentin extending in a confined band practically the full length of the dentinal tubules almost to the pulp. Dentin immediately adjacent to the enamel in this band exhibits the first evidence of demineralization and shows a marked ninhydrin reaction indicating possible breakdown of protein matrix in this area. It appears that caries occurs to a considerable depth rather than being just a surface phenomenon. Deeper changes are associated with altered enzyme patterns and metabolites associated with possible organic dentinal breakdown extending not quite to the pulp of the tooth. Fig. 1 is a line drawing summarizing the histochemical findings and various factors significantly influencing dental caries:

Chemicals – DOCA, Diuril
Heredity
Hormones – Thyroxin, insulin, sex
Nutrition – Ca, P, protein, CHO, F, vit A, vit C, vit D, pyridoxine, pantothenic acid
Saliva – Fluid cleansing, lysozyme, phagocytosis
Streptococci – Toxins, acids, enzymes
Stress – Electrolyte imbalance, water balance

[Note: Mg, SH, SS, ATP, ATPase, and cholinesterase, present in surrounding dentin and supported by nutrition and hormones, are absent in the reactionary dentinal tubular path or tract to incipient enamel caries fed by deleterious streptococcal agents.]

The importance of a substrate or food to supply the building blocks for the various enzymes and associated metabolites becomes apparent. Also this explains why various investigators have found such diverse molecules as pantothenic acid, pyridoxine, phosphate, and protein to have an effect upon the incidence of caries under varying conditions.

One must admit that the answer to this multifactorial problem is an improved way of life including good genes, proper lifetime nutrition, freedom from undue stress, adequate water, sunlight, fresh air, exercise and control of other environmental factors. A program of prevention based upon sound principles is the answer to man's physical problems. It is unpopular because man desires to eat his cake (and between-meal snacks) and have his teeth, too, which isn't likely to happen any time soon!

[Ed. note: This address was delivered at the International College of Applied Nutrition convention, Pasadena, CA, March 23, 1962]

Article #38

Caries and cellular nutrition

Steinman RR. Dental Progress 2(3):64/208-66/210, April 1962

To produce caries, more than the presence of bacteria is necessary; an important factor is host resistance, which is effected by nutrition.

Whether the microorganism penetrates the tooth depends in part on that tooth's metabolism. As in any infectious disease, the resistance of the host is a vital factor. If this resistance is high, large numbers of bacteria can be present and there will be no disease. If resistance is low, disease follows.

Noxious agents involved: Streptococci are among the most versatile organisms known and produce a variety of toxins, enzymes, and acids. Acid alone cannot initiate dental disease but may hasten destruction of dental tissues once metabolism has been altered. Then noxious agents such as such as H_2O_2 [ref], hyaluronidase [ref], and other enzymes produced by organisms can enter.

Similarity of metabolism with other organs: Many of the metabolic processes observed in teeth are similar to those of other organs. The chemical composition of the liquid parts of dentin is similar to interstitial fluid, contains amino acids, glucose, Mn, Fe, Ca, P, Cu, and Na [ref]. There is a rapid exchange between this fluid and other body fluids [refs], and this exchange rate varies [ref].

Means of resistance: The first line of defense of the body in general and of the teeth specifically is a physical barrier to external noxious materials. Both teeth and skin provide a mechanical barrier, but the tooth depends upon additional metabolic "shields" as well. Some of these are ATP, ADP, acetylcholine, coenzyme A, ATPase, cholinesterase, and sulfhydryl radicals [refs]. It has been shown that some metabolic shields were absent in dentin adjacent to pulp at the first evidence of pathology [ref].

Impediments to normal resistance: Animal studies [refs] have shown that when some of these protective factors are blocked, methylene blue, for example, can penetrate through both enamel and dentin—and an excess of sugar has the same effect as a deficiency of P in this regard [ref].

Stress can also alter electrolyte balance through changes in cell membrane selective permeability.

Other metabolic factors. Hamsters contracting spontaneous diabetes also developed rampant caries, even on a noncariogenic diet [ref]. Thyroxin deficiency has been reported with higher caries incidence [ref]. Pyridoxine defiency in rats, hamsters, and monkeys was associated with increased decay compared to controls [ref]. Castration decreased caries incidence [ref] perhaps via lowered serum Na level [ref]. Heredity apparently plays an important part [ref]. Nutritional elements also have been shown to affect caries incidence [refs].

Earliest changes. Caries first changes local metabolism and enzyme activity immediately beneath earliest evidence of demineralization of the enamel, then follows the dentinal tubules as organic pathways extending all the way to the pulp. The 2nd change is in the organic portion of the tooth involving probable depolymerization of the dentinal protein and mucopolysaccharides. The 3rd change is demineralization of dental hard structures, but by the time the DEJ is reached histochemical changes can already be observed extending to the pulp.

Caries characterized. Caries is a fairly typical disease process. It is not a mere surface phenomenon but occurs in depth as a consequence of events leading up to cavitation or necrosis and sloughing. Development proceeds from early metabolic alteration, through changes in enzyme activity and organic structure, to final demineralization and/or cavitation.

Systemic etiology. The important foundation of resistance to caries appears to rest upon the nutritional state of the host at the cellular level. Logically, then, caries control is an improved life style including sound nutrition and freedom from over-stress, and there is much evidence to support this preventive approach.

Article #39

The histochemical distribution of magnesium in dentinal tissues

Steinman RR. J South Calif Dent Assn 30(4):124-127, 1962

Sulfhydryl, ATP, ATPase, and a cholinesterase have been demonstrated histochemically in human dentinal tubules, but absent or markedly diminished in tubules between the pulp and first evidence of enamel demineralization. Phosphate and magnesium are an integral part of dental structures and are associated with various metabolic processes. Mg is an activator of many glycolic system enzymes, which tooth integrity, health, and function depend upon. **This study was to determine the presence and distribution of magnesium in dentinal structures.**

STUDY: 60 human teeth were frozen and sectioned. **Titan yellow was used to demonstrate Mg.**

Findings: **Mg was shown present throughout the length of the dentinal tubules, mostly adjacent to the pulp except when beneath demineralized outer enamel. Areas of depletion correspond to carious lesions and directly follow dentinal tubules.**

Discussion: **The Mg revealed by this method is apparently free Mg available for metabolism since it was found to be confined to the dentinal tubules. It followed the same distribution for sulfhydryl, ATP, ATPase and a cholinesterase in normal functioning dentin. This is one more link in the chain of evidence which suggests that the first change in dentinal tissues to occur in the development of caries is a**

change in metabolism. The decalcification associated with caries is not the same pattern observed in patients who suck a lemon or take other acids. Fitzgerald showed that acid from lactobacillus is unable to initiate caries in a germfree environment which suggests other bacterial products are needed first. Drawing (fig. 4) shows all the factors, including nutrition, shown in scientific literature to influence caries in teeth.*

Conclusions:

- **Histochemically magnesium has been demonstrated in dentinal tissues.**
- **Magnesium was observed throughout dentinal tubules especially adjacent to the pulp.**
- **Areas of presence or absence of Mg share a similar pattern with other molecules of metabolic importance, suggesting metabolic significance.**

Article #40

The cellular physiology of caries susceptibility

Steinman RR. J Calif. Dent Assn 38(5):403-404, Oct 1962

It is generally accepted that three conditions must exist for dental caries, (1) microorganisms, (2) a food supply, and (3) the deciding factor is dental susceptibility to caries.

Cell physiology controlled by selective permeability: Intracellular distribution of various molecules in optimum amounts determines the health, integrity and function of all body tissues. Necessary concentration of these molecules is controlled and maintained by selective permeability. This vital process requires energy. A well-known example is the sodium pump which regulates intracellular concentrations of sodium and potassium vastly different from that found outside the cells. Essential factors for this function are sulfhydryl (SH) radicals, ATP and acetylcholinesterase.

Marked histochemical changes occur in the dentin just beneath first evidence of enamel demineralization including ↓ ATP, ATPase, cholinesterase, SH disulfide and magnesium. These suggest failure of the metabolic system supporting selective permeability.

Outside factors affecting the selective permeability system are nonspecific psychological stress and certain sulfonamides which (-) carbonic anhydrase. Factors that (+) caries in hamsters are diamox, desoxycorticosterone trimethyl acetate (DOCA), and excess dietary NaCl. Bacterial toxins, blockage of SH radicals, chemotherapeutic radiation, and presence of H_2O_2 (-) the function of this system. **These can produce caries in animals on noncariogenic diets which suggests interference with the selective permeability system as a possible mechanism.**

A suitable substrate is necessary, which may explain why such diverse deficiencies as pyridoxine, pantothenic acid, phosphate, and protein can cause an increase in caries rate. Diabetes also produces failure of the transport system resulting in a cellular glucose deficiency. Thus, even the increase of caries in hamsters which had spontaneously developed diabetes might be related to inadequate substrate.

Experimental evidence also shows that this system is involved with caries resistance. Experimentally blocking the selective permeability system using H_2O_2 and 2,4-dinitrophenol was associated with marked penetration of dyes such as methylene blue into the tooth structure.

The mere external presence of noxious agents on teeth does not necessarily produce caries. Evidence suggests that failure of selective permeability is the primary mechanism of caries susceptibility, and is what appears to occur in dentinal areas beneath enamel with high concentrations of certain bacteria. First there is blockage in the local dentinal pathway leading to the pulp allowing initial entrance of noxious material beyond the tooth surface. As the process continues, cavitation results.

As unpopular as it might seem, the control of caries may rest upon a way of life which would include sound nutrition, freedom from undue stress, sunlight, exercise, and water. Having cake plus between-meal snacks and healthy teeth, too, has so far eluded science.

Article #41

The physiology of the dental pulp – Part 1

Steinman RR, DeVincenzo J, Voth E. J South Calif Dent Assn 30(10):336-340, 1962

Fish [ref] may have been the first to demonstrate a connection between body fluids and dentinal structures. He suggested there is a movement of fluid throughout the tooth structure. This was extended by Bodecker and Lefkowitz with dyes showing actual 2-way movement through the dentin. Steinman and Hardinge suggested this fluid movement may be altered by dietary means. Sognnaes, Shaw, and Bogoroch confirmed 2-way transfer of dentinal fluid. Yen, Bogoroch, Sognnaes, and Shaw in a radiophosphorus and radiosodium uptake study showed greater turnover of molecules in dentin than in enamel and greater in teeth of younger animals than older ones. **No studies to date outline how the fluid movement occurs or the exact route it follows. The effect of various chemicals, nutrients, bacterial products, or physical conditions upon this transport system needs to be studied.**

STUDY: Freshly extracted teeth were perfused with Eagle's nutritive medium under 20" hydrostatic pressure at 37° C through tubing joined near the cervical junction and exiting at the roots. The occlusal enamel was removed flat with a diamond bur. Masking tape was used to form a wall around the top of the tooth and sealed with sticky wax. 0.5% methylene blue was placed on the cut surface contained by the tape. Following the experiments, teeth were removed, frozen, sectioned, immediately wrapped in absorbent facial tissue paper to prevent spread of the dye, then examined microscopically.

Findings: Dye did move into the pulp chamber without need of hydrostatic pressure, but not when the pressure was applied. Dye moved into dentin toward the pulp against the hydrostatic pressure if at the correct temperature. The longer teeth were allowed to sit on the lab bench beforehand, the less dye penetrated. Only slight penetration occurred when teeth sat for 6 hrs beforehand. Dye did not penetrate against the hydrostatic pressure when temperature was chilled to 4° C. Marked penetration occurred in tubules of normal dentin at 37° C for 3 hrs, but none in exposed carious dentin.

Discussion: The movement of dye through freshly extracted teeth is evidence of an active transport system within dentin. Failure of flow in teeth chilled to 4° C indicates immobilization of the active system. Failure of dye penetration of carious dentin but its ability to penetrate adjacent normal dentin against hydrostatic pressure suggests a physiological reason. Histochemical findings show a depletion of necessary molecules to operate selective permeability in dentin beneath first evidence of enamel pathology. Many conditions inducing caries also inhibit selective permeability in other tissues [ref's]. Odontoblasts in the crown of a rat molar opposite the occlusal surface vary in length from short to long. Could it be that the odontoblasts are caught at the time of sacrifice in various stages of function (fig. 4). It would appear that one tubule at a time is having dye pulled into it towards the pulp of the tooth. Perhaps other odontoblasts are moving fluid in the other direction out the dentinal tubules towards the enamel. This is a passive process but probably under the influence of selective permeability. One would suspect it is not a purely physical process but under biological influences not yet fully understood—generally by endocrine, hereditary, or nutritional factors. Noxious bacterial products are permitted entry and inhibit normal transport. Or detoxification of noxious material is reduced in an area of reduced metabolism, usually opposite the concentration of bacteria (grooves and interproximal contacts). The first change in caries initiation is altered metabolic activity (selective permeability) in the odontoblastic processes almost to the pulp, leaving this area to the mercy of invading bacteria. The perfusion technique herein described has many possibilities for further studies of this and related types of problems.

Conclusions:

· A simple, effective technique for study of physiological function in freshly extracted human teeth is described.

· Certain observations concerning the movement of dentinal fluid through the dentin have been reported.

Article #42

The possible role of acetylcholine esterase in resistance to dental caries

Steinman RR. J South Calif Dent Assn 30(11):365-367, Nov 1962

Choline esterase, prominent among enzymes present, is markedly reduced in dentinal tubules where caries is starting in the overlying enamel. It is a chemical mediator of nerve activity in the formation and breakdown of acetylcholine. Also, it may be related to selective permeability of cells, which possibly plays a role in caries resistance. **The purpose of this study was to inhibit normal acetylcholine esterase to see if it will produce caries in rats on a noncariogenic diet.**

STUDY: 30 experimental rats 21 days old were divided into 3 equal groups and placed on noncariogenic Purina Lab Chow. Group 1– received intraperitoneal injections of diethyl p-nitrophenyl phosphate (paraoxon) 3x/day. Group 2– received intraperitoneal injections of paraoxon plus pyridine-2-aldoxime methiodide (2 PAM). Group 3– received intraperitoneal injections of an equivalent amount of water 3x/day. Teeth were examined histochemically at 42 days of age.

Results: Teeth receiving antiacetylcholine esterase were found to have significant decay. No other significant difference was found between the other two experimental groups.

Discussion: Paraoxon is a known specific irreversible inhibitor of acetylcholine esterase. 2-PAM also acts as a reversible competitive inhibitor. It would appear that the process of decay is similar in the choline-esterase-fed rats on the noncariogenic diet and the ones on the cariogenic diet, and confirms its suggested role in decay resistance. Factors linked to the metabolic chain necessary for selective permeability have been demonstrated in teeth and absent in dentinal areas immediately associated with beginning enamel caries. Conditions known to affect this process are deficiencies in necessary substrates such as pyridoxine, pantothenic acid, phosphorus, and protein [ref's]. Acetylcholine esterase is one of the factors involved and relates to caries resistance when this system is altered. **It may not be what is upon the surface of the tooth that determines caries susceptibility but rather what is allowed to penetrate into the tooth due to altered selective permeability, which in this case appeared to include acetylcholine esterase.**

Conclusions:
· Administration of anti-acetylcholine esterase to animals on a noncariogenic diet produced significant dental decay compared to controls.
· Acetylcholine esterase is therefore thought to play an important role in resistance to decay.

Article #43

The presence and distribution of succinic dehydrogenase and monoamine oxidase in the pulp of adult human teeth

Steinman RR. J South Calif Dent Assn 30(12):388-391, 1962

Using histochemical techniques developed in this laboratory it is possible to preserve enzymes, compounds, and elements of histochemical and metabolic importance in the mature tooth. Dehydrogenases are the first members of a chain of enzymes which transfer H atoms or electrons from substrates to molecular oxygen. Succinic dehydrogenase (SDase) is an iron-containing flavoprotein found in mitochondria. Its concentration in tissue depends upon the oxidative capacity of the tissue. Monoamine oxidases (MAO) occur in animal tissues in small concentrations, but higher in heart, brain, liver and kidneys; probably for detoxification. **The purpose of this study was to determine the presence and distribution of SDase and MAO in the human tooth.**
STUDY: Teeth must be kept below the freezing point throughout section preparation and satisfactory sections must be from the center of the tooth and no thicker than 100 μ. The method of Nachlas et al was used with tetranitro BT to demonstrate SDase in human pulp tissue. The method of Glenner et al with the newer tetranitro BT was used to demonstrate the presence and distribution of MAO in the tissues.
Findings: In single-rooted teeth the greatest concentration of SDase was observed in odontoblasts whose processes extended to the enamel, and less concentration in the root portion of the pulp chamber. Odontoblasts on the floor of the pulp chamber of multi-rooted teeth showed significantly less succinic dehydrogenase activity, contrasted with considerable SDase activity in odontoblasts that reached to the enamel. Fig. 3 shows diminished SDase activity in odontoblasts opposite the carious lesion. The distribution of MAO in the odontoblastic layer of the pulp chamber follows a pattern similar to SDase. MAO appears more sensitive to pathosis than SD (fig.4) with marked reduction in the odontoblastic layer opposite an incipient carious lesion by the central groove, also in the odontoblastic layer opposite two amalgam fillings (fig.5).
Discussion: Concentration of SD in the odontoblastic layer of the pulp opposite the enamel suggests that this area has a rather high oxidative capacity. A previous study demonstrated ATP in dentinal tissues. Evidently considerable energy is being expended in the pulp of adult human teeth. This provides considerable evidence for the presence of an energy-requiring transport system. The eye is an example of a fluid and ion transport system mediated over a considerable distance and operates between two histologically different tissues, the stroma and the epithelium. There is considerable dehydrogenase activity in the stroma providing an oxidizing potential. The other tissue, the epithelium, has a reducing potential. This difference in potential maintains an ionic current to direct water and ions from the stroma to the epithelium. A similar condition may be present in teeth. The surface of rat teeth carries a reducing potential which attracted deposits of silver when rats were given 1.5 parts per 1000 to drink for several months [ref]. Previous reports [ref's] showed dyes would penetrate into teeth when the animals' metabolisms

were inhibited with certain antimetabolites, but would not penetrate when animals were on a noncariogenic diet. Thus it appears energy is required to prevent ingress of noxious material into the tooth. Three conditions must exist in the mouth for decay to occur—susceptible teeth, bacteria, and food for the microorganisms. **This present paper suggests resistance is not only a mechanical feature of the tooth but that it is metabolic also. The purpose of this transport system is probably two-fold. It prevents ingress of noxious material into the tooth and plays a role in the maintenance of the tooth. One suggested function of MAO is detoxification of certain noxious materials. It seems to be depleted in areas of overlying enamel pathology.**

Conclusions:

· **Significant SD is present in the odontoblastic layer of the pulps of adult human teeth, associated with ↑ oxidative capacity.**

· **Significant MAO is present in the odontoblastic layer of the pulps of human teeth, possibly associated with some role in detoxification of noxious material which may penetrate into the tooth.**

[This basically was a histochemical exploratory demonstration study]

Article #44

The effect of cow's milk, soy milk, and chocolate milk upon the incidence of caries in the rat

Rathbun WE, Bond DE, Steinman RR. J South Calif Dent Assn 31(9):299-301, 1963

The purpose of this study was to obtain quantitative information regarding the effects of cow's milk, soy milk, chocolate milk and a high sugar diet on the growth rate and caries incidence in rats teeth.

STUDY 1: 44 15-day-old rats were divided into groups. Group 1– 11 controls were left with their mothers with the high sugar diet available as a supplement until 21 days of age when they were switched totally to the high sugar diet. Group 2– 11 were fed cow's milk twice daily. Group 3– 11 were fed soy milk twice daily. Group 4– 11 were fed chocolate milk twice daily. At 45 days the jaw segments were dissected, quick frozen and sectioned. Reactive proteins associated with carious lesions were demonstrated using the Ninhydrin-Schiff method.

Finding: The chocolate milk produced nearly three times the incidence of decay as any other group.

STUDY 2: 72 15-day-old rats were divided into groups. Group 1– 17 controls were left with their mothers with the high sugar diet available as a supplement until 21 days of age when they were switched totally to the high sugar diet. Group 2– 18 were fed cow's milk twice daily. Group 3– 18 were fed soy milk twice daily. Group 4– 18 were fed chocolate milk twice daily. At 45 days the jaw segments were dissected, quickly frozen and sectioned. Reactive proteins associated with carious lesions were demonstrated using the Ninhydrin-Schiff method.

Findings: Growth rates of the 3 experimental groups were substantially less than the control group on a high sugar diet. Differences in growth rates between the 3 groups were not significant. The chocolate milk group developed significantly more carious lesions than any other group. The cow's milk group developed a similar number of carious lesions as those on the high sugar diet.

Discussion: Chocolate milk contains 11% carbohydrate and the control diet 63% sucrose. Another study [ref] under similar experimental conditions, except that the milk was fortified with iron, copper and manganese, developed no caries. It is poor nutritional practice to depend upon only one food. Why should milk with almost no fermentable CHO produce decay? Why should a liquid diet produce decay equal to that produced by solid foods?

Conclusions:

· Growth rates were similar among all experimental groups but substantially less than high-sugar group.

· The number of lesions in the chocolate milk group was much larger than in other groups.

· Soy milk and cow's milk groups developed similar numbers to those on a high-sugar diet.

[Note: The control high-sugar diet also contained more nutritious casein, corn oil, salts, whole liver, vitamins, and choline ingredients which might seem to explain the paradoxical results compared with the less wholesome milk-only diets]

Article #45

The physiology of the dental pulp. Part 2

DeVincenzo JP, Steinman RR. J South Calif Dent Assn 3(10):323-328, 1963

This report describes a perfusion procedure which appears to be capable of maintaining the pulp in a physiologically functioning condition without necrosis for an extended period. ATP levels were monitored as indicator of viability. Microdetermination of ATP was demonstrated by an autophotographic technique of the pulp and immediately adjacent dentin.

STUDY: Dental pulp tissue was perfused with tissue culture medium via 30 ga. needles threaded through root apices up to the coronal pulp horns. A cotton gauze cylinder functioned as an absorbent wick for escaping perfused fluid from the apices and bathed the outside of the teeth in the perfusion medium. Temperature was maintained at 36° C with 100% humidity. A 97% O_2 and 3% CO_2 mixture was bubbled through the medium. Medium pH was 7.3. A 95% O_2 and 5% CO_2 mixture was passed through the incubator. Up to 50 mm Hg head of pressure was maintained to achieve the minimum critical tissue O_2 supply. Penicillin and streptomycin were added to the medium as antibiotics. ATP analysis was possible to $\pm$ 0.02 μg using a luciferin-luciferase complex from firefly tails with luminescence measured by a Turner fluorometer.

Discussion: Considerable variations in ATP concentrations were found, not correlating with age, sex, or caries activity. **Table 2 suggests that without perfusion the ATP levels are negligible after 30-60 minutes. This indicates the procedure used is capable of maintaining pulp tissue ATP levels within the range of ATP of freshly extracted teeth for a minimum of 24 hrs. Thus it is likely that the procedure maintains viable pulp tissue in vitro within the intact calcified tooth.**

Conclusions:

· A perfusion technique is described capable of maintaining ATP concentration of intact pulp tissue in vitro.

· ATP levels were determined and compared in freshly extracted teeth, perfused teeth, and unperfused.

· All pulp tissue from freshly extracted teeth contains ATP but is destroyed or utilized in 30-60 min's.
· Pulp tissue of perfused teeth contains high amounts of ATP for a minimum of 24 hours.

Article #46

A demonstration of the effect of human food combinations upon dental caries in rats

Steinman RR, Gilliland Y, Saunders M, Holub V, Tague C. J South Calif Dent Assn 31(12):400-402, 1963

The purpose of this study was to demonstrate the effect that certain common food combinations may have upon the incidence of dental caries.

STUDY: 44 weaned caries-susceptible rats were fed special diets for 5 weeks as follows:
Group I – Wheat germ, cottage cheese, eggs, whole wheat bread, potatoes, navy beans, and milk
Group II – Wheat germ, cottage cheese, eggs, enriched white bread, potatoes, navy beans, cherry pie, soft drink
Group III – corn flakes, enriched white bread, potatoes, spaghetti, ice cream, cherry pie, soft drink

Combination I –	Cariogenic diet	200 g
	Whole wheat flour	400 g
Combination II –	Cariogenic diet	200 g
	Unenriched white flour	400 g

Results:

Diet Group	#	1^0 Wt	End Wt.	Gain	Aver. Caries
Group I	10	47	170	123	1.16
Group II	10	46	148	102	3.64
Group III	10	45	51	6	9.08
Combo I	7		181		4.14
Combo II	7		177		11.14

Animals no doubt would have benefited from some fresh green foods. Addition of refined foods to the diet is suggested to have ↑ decay rate. It may be well to give more importance to whole grain cereals daily. Primitive peoples subsisting upon natural foods usually are quite decay-free whereas same racial stocks eating more "civilized" foods have significant decay. So much major attention is given to sugar content that little mention is made of refined cereal products consumed.

Conclusions:
· Various food combinations produced marked differences in caries rates.
· Increased refined food intake was generally associated with increased caries.
· More value needs to be placed on unrefined foods in the diet.

Article #47

Heredity, environment, diet, and caries in children

Steinman RR, Woods RW. J South Calif Dent Assn 32(5):163-166, 1964

A lengthy questionnaire was circulated to dental alumni and other dentists from California to Massachusetts. Dental exams were conducted by the fathers. Questions about children's habits were answered by the father or mother. **The present study was designed to assess the relative value of several factors which may influence the incidence of dental caries in children.**

STUDY: 278 children ages 4-20 were questioned regarding eating habits, heredity, frequency of brushing, fluoride exposure, and incidence of dental caries. 164/278 reported no caries, 114/278 had some caries.

Habit	No Decay	Decay	Stat. Diff.
Brushing teeth	161	111	-
White bread	**153**	**105**	**99%**
Whole wheat bread	159	106	-
Pie, ice cream, cake, etc.	161	112	-
Between-meal snack	**160**	**110**	**90%**
Whole grain cereal	**165**	**110**	**90%**
Packaged cold cereal	**152**	**109**	**90%**
Mouth breathing	151	93	-
Meat/flesh food	156	113	-

DMF 1-2 = **13% snacked**, DMF 3-5 = **35% snacked**, DMF 6+ = **67% snacked between meals.**

More of those who had decay ate between meals more frequently than those who had no decay.

Refined cereals might be a factor in caries production.

Conclusions:

· **Children with decay used white bread and packaged cold cereals more than those with no decay.**

· **The caries rose proportionately with frequency of between-meal snacks.**

· Community water is the choice of delivery for F.

Article #48

The possible hydrolysis of enamel protein

Steinman RR. J South Calif Dent Assn 32(7):192-198, 1964

The earliest change in enamel from decay is loss of soluble organic matrix. How this matrix becomes soluble is of prime importance. Enzyme molecules are probably too large to pass through enamel. Testing pH 3 lactic acid on ground tooth structure for 24 hrs failed to show protein hydrolysis. Cellular activity is known to influence the redox potential of the environment by reducing the oxygen tension and shifting the potential more negatively. Cultures of hemolytic streptococci have been reported as going gradually negative in anaerobic environments (with the lids on). Dental plaque in deeper grooves is in an anaerobic environment. **This study was to determine what effect a change in oxygen tension or potential might have upon enamel proteins.**

STUDY 1: **Oxygen Tension vs. Enamel Release of Amino Acids.** Freshly extracted teeth were preserved frozen until sectioned into 2 or 4 equal parts. Exposed dentin, cut enamel, and root surfaces were covered with wax. These pieces were incubated at 37 C in 0.5 ml water for 48 hours. Then 0.5 ml 95% ethanol was added under agitation for several minutes. The fluid was placed on chromatographic paper. Amino acids were shown by spraying 0.2% ninhydrin in N-butanol.

Series I – odd numbers **aerobic** while even numbers anaerobic **with Hydrogen**

Series J – repeated series I with **all pieces run aerobically**

Series K – repeated series I except with **odd numbers anaerobic**

Series M – all **anaerobic with odd numbers at 2 C and even at 37 C**

Series N – odd numbers were **aerobic** while even numbers were anaerobic **with Argon**

Series O – **all anaerobic** with odd numbers in **water** while even numbers were **in 60% ethanol**
Series Q – **all anaerobic** with odd numbers incubated **with water** and even numbers **without water**
Results:
Series I, J, and K – all anaerobic atmosphere samples with evident streaks compared with very faint to nonexistent streaks for aerobic samples
Series M – comparing near-freezing with body temperature specimens showed all equally distinct. Series N showed fairly distinct streaks for Argon anaerobic but almost nonexistent for aerobic.
Series O – some water-incubated streaks showed more strongly than any ethanol-incubated ones
Series Q – only some water-incubated streaks showed, some vividly, the dry didn't show at all
STUDY 2: **Electrical Potential vs. Release of Enamel Amino Acids.** Orthodontic extractions with roots excised and pulps removed had remaining crown portions fitted into plastic tubing 3" long with edges sealed by tacky wax. The enamel crown portion inside the tubing received 1 ml 09% saline. This was placed into a test tube also containing 1 ml 0.9% saline. One electrode was connected to the crown inside the tubing and the other to the solution outside in the test tube with 1 milliamp potential. Testing was done with positive polarity, no electricity, and negative polarity to potentially induce enamel protein dissolution or hydrolysis.
Results: Table 1 indicates protein present in solution when the enamel electrode was negative but not when positive or zero. Table 2 showed some reductions in transmittance for zero and even greater reductions for negative polarity.
[Difficult to compare the saliva specimen with the plain water specimen because of variables introduced by salivary proteins which may have been spun down and lost during the centrifugation step. This could have influenced the suggestion that since there was no supernatant protein it "passed into the enamel of the tooth"]
STUDY 3: **Recording Normal Electrical Potentials of the Human Tooth.** A polygraph recorded differences in electrical potential between various surface features of the tooth relative to the pulp. Freshly extracted human teeth were immediately perfused with nutrient medium to maintain metabolic function during testing. The pulp was found negative compared with enamel surfaces. The potential dropped when cold was applied and rose with heat (fig. 5). [Temperatures used were not explained.] Marked potential existed between the enamel and the cementum on the same tooth (fig. 6). Pits and fissures were found with negative polarity compared with the surrounding enamel surface (fig. 7).
STUDY 4: **Macroscopic Enamel Changes under Anaerobic Conditions.** All except the tips of canine cusps were covered with wax and the teeth anaerobically incubated 72 hrs at room temperature in 0.5 ml water. 0.5 ml 95% ethanol was added and the teeth examined.
Results: An opaque area developed where exposed to the anaerobic environment (fig. 8). The control incubated aerobically showed no change in surface enamel (fig. 9). [Not the same quality photo. It appears over-exposed and difficult to tell for sure.]

STUDY 5: **Porosity Reversal Controlled by Electrical Potential.** Painting the opaque area with methylene blue penetrated and could not be washed off.
Results: Placing the specimen in saliva and subjecting the enamel to 1 ma current positive electrode for 5-8 hrs reversed the porosity so methylene blue did not penetrate. [May not be controlled well in comparison with the tooth in plain water alone due to influences from salivary constituents and osmotic differences.]
Discussion: Change in oxygen tension was accompanied by a marked removal of protein from intact enamel. This protein with transmittance values at 440 mμ suggests significant amounts of proline and hydroxyproline were being removed and needs further study. The change in the enamel surface under anaerobic conditions resulted in an opaque appearance with porosity that could be reversed by a positive current applied to the enamel. This is consistent with the normal potential of the tooth maintained by metabolism and would encourage movement of salivary protein into the enamel. There appears to be a change from positive to negative in grooves and pits along with being the first tooth locations to initiate caries. Electric potential is associated with normal metabolism since this falls at temperatures that would inhibit metabolism. **It is possible that microbes causing caries are capable of producing an anaerobic environment deep in the developmental grooves and beneath plaque, which simultaneously changes it to a negative electrical potential and reduces oxygen tension. In this way it would hasten release of amino acids from enamel and make it more permeable to noxious materials.**
Conclusions:
· **Amino acid release from dental enamel was induced by anaerobic conditions and by a change in electrical potential.**
· **This hydrolysis is probably of a chemical and/or electrical nature and not the result of an enzyme.**
· **Hydrolysis may be the method of protein removal from human enamel suggested by Darling.**
· **Protein possibly moves into enamel under certain biological conditions.**

Article #49

Relationship of blood sugar level and leukocytic phagocytosis

Kijak E, Foust G, Steinman RR. J South Calif Dent Assn 32(9):349-351, 1964

Engulfment by leukocytes is the first line of defense for the body. The average number of microbes engulfed per leukocyte is the phagocytic index, and can be affected negatively by abnormal systemic nutritional conditions. Normal fasting blood glucose levels are 60-100 mg %. This is frequently tested with oral administration of 100 gm glucose in 500 ml water. The degree of subsequent rise or fall of blood sugar concentration aids in diagnosis of certain pathological conditions. **The purpose of this study was to determine the phagocytic index at different blood glucose levels.**
STUDY 1: 45 diabetic patients were tested after fasting 6-12 hours. A 10-cc blood sample was drawn before and after glucose administration. 5 cc were mixed with *Staphylococcus albus* and incubated at 37 C for 30 min's. After 30 minutes, blood smears were made and treated with Miles stain for microscopic analysis. The phagocytic indexes (PI) were ascertained by sampling 100 leukocytes per subject and counting the average number of phagocytized foreign particles. The remaining 5 cc of blood were tested to determine reference blood glucose levels in mg glucose/100 cc (i.e. mg %).

Results: Table I shows decreasing PI with increasing BSL.
STUDY 2: Nine "pseudo-diabetic" patients were given 100-, 75-, 50- and 25-gram portions of glucose orally and blood samples were drawn after 45 min's.
Results: The PI also tended to decrease as the BSL increased. Could this represent part of the reduced microbial resistance of the diabetic patient?

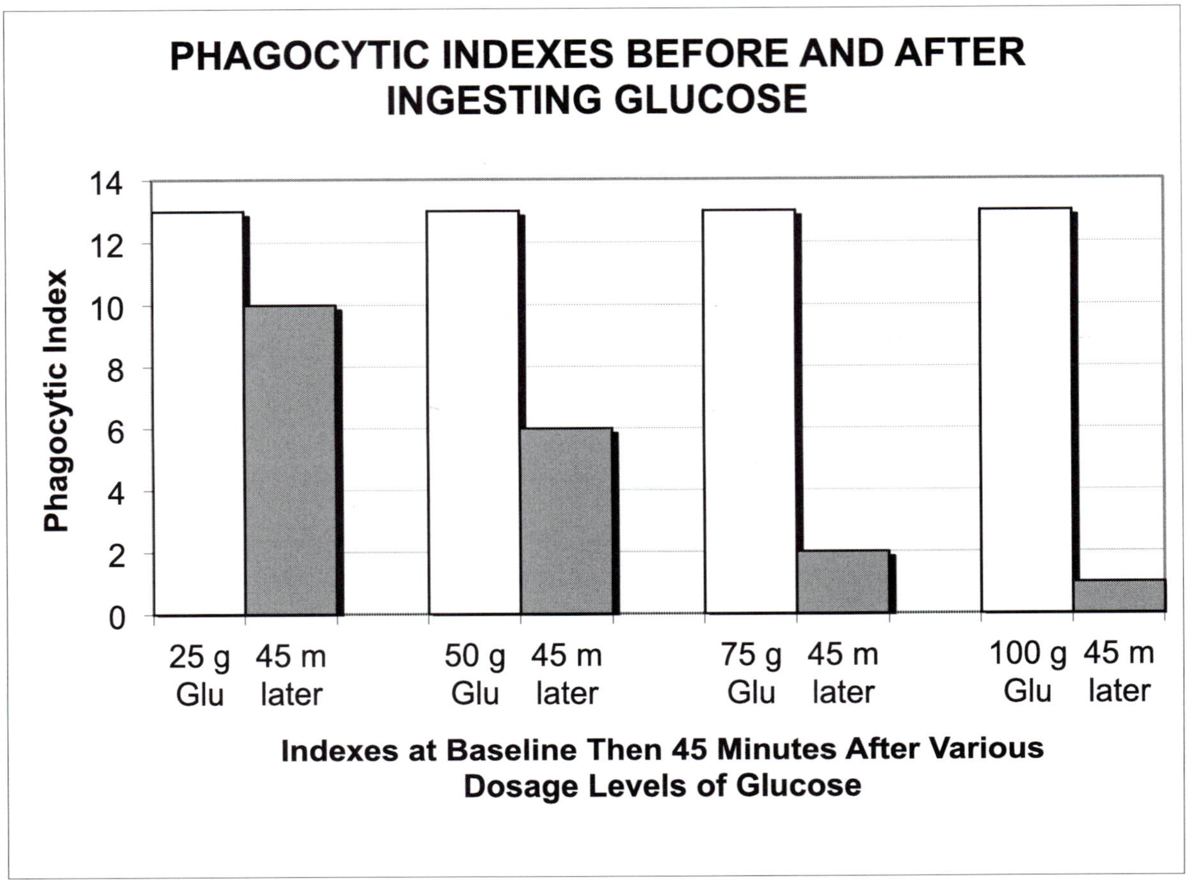

Discussion: **[It appears from Table II that a pseudodiabetic person could ingest approx. 15-20 gm of glucose with no appreciable reduction of phagocytic activity.]** As less glucose was consumed, the BSL did not rise as high as with greater doses. Phase microscopic observation revealed leukocytes at normal sugar levels were very active with pseudopods extending in all directions in search of foreign objects. Cells from higher than normal BSL conditions, however, were altered in form with increased numbers of fat vacuoles present resulting in slower, less efficient action toward foreign objects.
Summary:
· **Data suggest that in Db patients higher BSLs correspond with lowered phagocytic indexes.**
· **In non-diabetic subjects it was also shown that 45 min's after oral glucose consumption the phagocytic index was proportionally decreased.**

Article #50

Calcium and phosphorus release from intact human enamel under anaerobic conditions

Steinman RR. J South Calif Dent Assn 32(10):384-387, 1964

Proteolysis of intact human enamel has been shown to occur under anaerobic conditions which markedly increased its surface porosity [ref]. Similar proteolysis has been shown to occur with wool keratin under reducing conditions [ref]. **It is generally accepted that the first loss of enamel is from the prism sheath and interprismatic material, which are made up of both minerals and protein. The following experiment was to show what effect, if any, an anaerobic atmosphere may have upon the mineral component of enamel.**

General preparation of specimens: Freshly extracted teeth were immediately frozen, then the molars were divided into 4 equal parts with others divided into 2 equal parts. Dentin, cementum, and the cut enamel surfaces were sealed off with a layer of wax and specimens placed in test tubes with 0.5 ml water. Odd numbered samples were kept anaerobic under CO_2 and the same sample sections were re-used using even numbers to eliminate specimen selection bias.

STUDY 1: Phosphorus determinations: Specimens were incubated 48 hrs at room temperature then 0.5 ml ethanol added to each tube and agitated several minutes. Phosphorus contents were determined by the method of Russell and Allen. The tests were repeated in series B in which even numbers were anaerobic (Table II). To determine whether of organic or inorganic origin, series B was repeated with even numbers run anaerobically, then the solutions obtained were first evaporated then extracted with acetone to remove any organic phosphorus present. Values for aerobic, anaerobic, and acetone extraction of anaerobic samples are shown in Table III.

Results:

Table I – Phosphorus determinations **aerobically** vs. **anaerobically**

Average aerobic reading	.059	0.90 μg
Average anaerobic reading	.216	3.28 μg

Table II – Repeat **P** determinations with specimens in opposite environments

Average aerobic reading	.079	0.13 μg
Average anaerobic reading	.400	7.76 μg

Table III – Repeat **P** determinations plus acetone extraction of anaerobic samples

Average aerobic reading	.365	5.20 μg
Average anaerobic reading	1.43	20.56 μg

Table V – **Calcium** determinations aerobically vs. anaerobically

Average aerobic reading	100%	
Average anaerobic reading		40%

Note the consistent increase in calcium in the anaerobically treated specimens.

STUDY 2: Measuring possible fluoride interference effects: To determine F effects upon anaerobic P and Ca release, previous samples were immersed in sodium silicofluoride for 20 min's, rinsed, and incubated anaerobically for 48 hrs at room temp. Calcium was measured by its whitish precipitation from acetic acid and ammonium oxalate. Phosphorus determinations were conducted as described previously.

Results:

Table IV – **Fluoride inhibition** effects on **aerobic Ca release** and **P release.**

Average **P** release, with fluoride	.201	3.6 μg
Average **P** release, without fluoride	.369	6.72 μg
Average **Ca** release, with fluoride	100%	...
Average **Ca** release, without fluoride	77%	...

Note: Paper chromatography of some samples failed to show any fluoride effect on anaerobic protein release from enamel.

Discussion: **The present report shows that under anaerobic conditions P and Ca are released in significantly greater amounts than under aerobic conditions. Preliminary evidence suggests that this mineral loss is from the interprismatic area between the rods. These findings coupled with a previous report of anaerobic amino acid release would support the proteolysis chelation theory of dental caries. Chelation could also be occurring. The pH was 7.8-8.1 suggesting that an acid is not involved. It seems reasonable that enamel plus water would produce pH slightly on the alkaline side of neutral. It is significant that enamel sections treated aerobically with sodium silicofluoride decreased P and Ca release from enamel. Also observed was that mineral loss was less than that found under aerobic conditions. The first step by microorganisms is removal of interprismatic material to a significant depth to produce surface porosity. This apparently can be accomplished without acids or enzymes in anaerobic environments such as in pits and fissures or beneath plaque**.

Conclusions:

- **Intact human enamel in an anaerobic environment in water alone can release significant P and Ca.**
- **P released under anaerobic conditions appears to come from the inorganic portion of the enamel.**
- **Fluoride-treated enamel sections released less mineral than specimens under anaerobic conditions.**

Article #51

The possible role of carbon dioxide in initiating dental caries

Steinman RR. J South Calif Dent Assn 33(1):28-31, 1965

One theory of initial carious attack on enamel is lactic acid activity. Another is that an enzyme is involved. There seems general agreement that the initial in-depth attack is against the inter-rod material. Only molecules the size of water, silver nitrate, or methanol can diffuse readily into intact enamel. Lactic acid is larger and may have more difficulty, capable of some erosion rather than outright caries. Enzymes are larger yet and most likely are unable to enter dense, intact enamel. By contrast, CO_2 when dissolved in water forms carbonic acid in which calcium carbonate is soluble. If this molecule can dissolve enamel, specifically between the rods, a probable mechanism for initiating caries may be suggested. Plaque material is composed of some anaerobic bacteria and exists at least partly under anaerobic conditions produced probably by generation of CO_2 from carbohydrate metabolism. This requires a more rapid metabolism such as that following penetration of sugar into the plaque.

Previously it was shown that CO_2 induced release of minerals from intact enamel. This study was to determine if only anaerobic conditions are necessary or if a specifically CO_2 atmosphere aids mineral release.

STUDY 1: Freshly extracted, frozen teeth were sectioned into 4 equal size parts and their uninvolved surfaces coated with wax. These pieces were kept anaerobic by displacement of air with either H_2 or CO_2. 2 groups of specimens from the same teeth were incubated for 48 hrs in 0.5 ml water. Each 1-ml of water diluent per sample was analyzed for P.

Group 1– was in a H_2 atmosphere

Group 2– was incubated aerobically

Results:

Group 1– 1.0 μg P

Group 2– 1.1 μg P
Groups 1 and 2– same Ca release for both
It would appear that CO_2 is necessary in the anaerobic environment to remove mineral from intact enamel.
STUDY 2: To determine P release in the CO_2 atmosphere relative to time, 10 anaerobic tooth specimens were used per P determination after 6, 12, 24, 48, and 72 hrs.
Results: **Table I - showed the following linear relationship**

Hours	6	12	24	48	72
μg P released	2.7	2.8	3.7	5.0	6.3

STUDY 3: To determine P release under various CO_2 concentration or varying O_2 tension, using 10 different specimens per test as previously but for 48 hrs.
Results: **Table II - showed P release relative to O_2 %**

O_2 %	100	60	21	10	5	2	0
μg P released	0.8	1.3	0.8	2.2	4.2	4.2	3.8

STUDY 4: To determine enamel surface dissolution and dye penetration under anaerobic conditions, specimens were kept in CO_2 from 2 days to 2 weeks then placed in 1% methylene blue for ≤ 2 hrs. Sections were analyzed microscopically.
Results: Fig. 3 shows enamel surface darkly stained by methylene blue stopping abruptly at the wax-protected zone. Fig. 4 shows deeper streaks of penetration into interprismatic areas. Penetration appeared similar in both cut and uncut surfaces.
Discussion: **Anaerobic conditions involving CO_2 simulate oral physiological conditions beneath plaque and in the depths of grooves. However, incubating specimens in H_2 may not closely resemble biological conditions. Minerals under anaerobic conditions appear to be lost from deeper enamel portions and interprismatic spaces, causing porosity great enough to allow ingress of larger molecules that normally could not enter intact enamel. Caries may thus be initiated by this ingress of destructive material.**

Anaerobic P release from intact enamel is time-dependent up to nearly 72 hrs. It appears inversely related to O_2 content between 21% and 5% or directly to CO_2 content. **Maximum P release occurred at 5% CO_2, suggesting enamel dissolution by bacteria thrives in less than a totally anaerobic environment.**

H_2 can penetrate enamel well enough but cannot release minerals. CO_2 can both readily diffuse into dense, intact enamel and produce a release of minerals. This part of caries initiation may be consistent with the carbonic acid theory.
Conclusions:
· **Human enamel P release under anaerobic conditions appears time-related.**
· **P release is inversely related to O_2 tension, or directly related to CO_2 concentration.**
· **Histological observations suggest mineral loss in a CO_2 atmosphere is from the interprismatic spaces.**

Article #52

The chemical control of the release of calcium, phosphorus and amino acids from human dental enamel

Steinman RR. J South Calif Dent Assn 33(5):230-234, 1965

Dental caries involves both mineral and organic structure loss from the tooth. F ↓ mineral loss and ↓ dental caries. Glimcher suggests the affinity of organic to inorganic tooth components may involve unstable electrostatic to stable covalent bonds. Might these bonds have an effect on resistance?

Plaque contains bacterial enzymes, toxins, lactic and other acids, and CO_2. Whatever binds the mineral and organic components of enamel needs to be effective against both lactic acid and CO_2 as well as water.

Mineral release appears to be influenced more by certain ions than by the pH of the solution. e.g. 1% ferrous salt solution will dramatically reduce P release at a given pH compared to release in a CO_2 atmosphere. The protein may be bound so as to prevent release under anaerobic conditions. Also Ca may be bound independently of the P. Apparently at least 3 components of enamel must be simultaneously bound to resist attack. **It was the purpose of this paper to reveal the binding method used by Ca, P and protein to resist adverse CO_2, O_2 and pH conditions.**

STUDY 1: Enamel particles removed from human teeth with a diamond bur were thoroughly mixed, weighed in 125-mg amounts, and placed in consecutively numbered test tubes. Series 1 was incubated in a CO_2 atmosphere 72 hrs with 0.5 ml water. Series 2 was identical but without CO_2. After 72 hrs, 0.5 ml ethanol was added to each tube and centrifuged 10 min's at 2400 rpm for chromatographic analysis.

Results: Fig 1 **shows darker bands for anaerobic specimens, indicating more amino acid release.**

STUDY 2: To another similar series, chemicals were added in 2 to 5 mg amounts and incubated 72 hrs in a CO_2 atmosphere. 0.5 ml ethanol was added to each of the tubes which were then centrifuged and the supernatant analyzed chromatographically.

Results: Table I indicates results as follows:

The one chemical which decreased amino acid release was 1,3-difluoro-2,4-dinitrobenzene.

Those having no effect were silver pentafluoropropionate, sulfanilyl fluoride, 1-chloro-2,4-dinitrobenzene, tetra(p-fluorophenyl), ferrous chloride, ferric chloride, zirconium tetrafluoride, and disodium ethylene tetra-acetate.

Increasing the release of amino acids were sodium silicofluoride, carbonic anhydrase, tetrafluoroantimonous acid, and ferric ammonium sulfate.

Since the 1,3-difluoro-4,6-dinitrobenzene practically eliminated the release and was easier to handle and compatible with other reagents, it was chosen for further work relative to binding enamel minerals.

STUDY 3: The presence of Ca was determined as previously outlined.

Results: Table II shows P and Ca release from enamel under CO_2 atmosphere, colorimetrically analyzed at 500 mμ:

Chemical	**μg**	**Ca release**	**Optical density**
Control	19.3	...	0.77
NaF	38.1	reduced	0.01*
FeF_2	4.7	reduced	0.03*
$FeCl_2$	3.8	increased	2.00

***From this it appears the F ion reduced Ca release and the Fe ion reduced P release. Further work revealed that a combination of 1,3-difluoro-4,6-dinitrobenzene and ferrous fluoride markedly reduced amino acids, Ca and P released from enamel.** Could this be effective enough to block enamel surface destruction and resist methylene blue penetration?

STUDY 4: Freshly extracted teeth were divided into 2 parts and all except a narrow window of enamel covered with wax. Experiment 1 – exposed one piece to saturated 1,3-difluoro-4,6-dinitrobenzene and ferrous fluoride and the other in water as a control. After 2 weeks both were placed in methylene blue for 2 hrs and analyzed.

Results: The usual deep penetration of dye was observed in the control but none in the experimental sample

STUDY 5: Another sample in CO_2 for 6 days was placed in pH 3.3 lactic acid for 20 hrs and tested with methylene blue penetration.

Results: No penetration was noted in the experimental sample, but there was penetration in the control. Fig 3 shows the dramatic results.

Discussion: **Resistance to dental caries might relate to chemical stability of enamel chemical bonds. Preliminary work showed that if only one of the components, Ca, P, or protein were stabilized, enamel would still become porous in CO_2 and water. This indicated necessity of binding all major components of enamel simultaneously. Another study showed that the protein of silk may be made resistant to hydrolysis by treating with 1,3-difluoro-4,6-dinitrobenzene. This was found true for enamel protein except when pre-treated with a fluoride such as NaF. Fluoride ion seems to stabilize the calcium. The ferrous ion seems to stabilize the P. All three components were effectively bound by using saturated 1,3-difluoro-4,6-dinitrobenzene and ferrous fluoride.**

Practical aspects may deny clinical use of these reagents. The same ions which the reagents might bind are also found abundantly in the plaque itself and diminish chances of reagent ions reaching the enamel in an active state. The reagents are quite insoluble and would need to be dissolved to react with enamel. They are also highly toxic which discourages continued use by the patient. And the reaction occurs slowly. Still the best method of caries resistance is to control the patient's diet.

Conclusions:

- **An in vitro means of binding enamel Ca, P and amino acids appears possible.**
- **These mineral-binding reagents prevented enamel porosity which normally would have occurred in lactic acid or in a CO_2 and water environment.**

Article #53

The possible chemical reactions between human enamel and carbon dioxide

Steinman RR. J South Calif Dent Assn 33(9)434-436, Sep 1965

Calcium in the enamel is present partly as $CaCO_3$ and $CaPO_4$. Protein components are soluble 0.17%, peptides 0.15%, and insoluble 0.18% dry wt. The insoluble portion could be keratinous in nature (collagen).

A bacterial end-product, CO_2, is reported to accompany release of enamel amino acids, Ca and P compared with release by control samples under aerobic circumstances.

Insoluble carbonates such as $CaCO_3$ may be brought into solution by treating their aqueous suspensions with an excess of CO_2 [ref]. The release of $Ca_3(PO_4)_2$, in a similar manner, may be as $CaHPO_4$. In this way, mineral release in a carbon dioxide environment may be explained in terms of ↑ solubility. One might suspect that release of protein material under anaerobic conditions would be from the water soluble fractions which are phosphoproteins [ref] and peptides. **The purpose of this study was to determine the character of the protein affected by amino acid release.**

STUDY 1: Fresh orthodontically extracted bicuspids were immediately frozen for preservation, then divided into 2 or 4 parts. All surfaces except the intact enamel were covered with wax and specimens placed in individual test tubes with 0.5 ml 0.25 N NaOH for 24 hrs.

Results: This release of P from phosphoproteins was recorded in Table I as 2.4 μg from NaOH samples and 0.4 μg from water controls.

STUDY 2: Phosvitin, a phosphoprotein from egg yolk, contains 9.7% P. 20 mg/ml aliquots were placed in test tubes, half of which were incubated in a CO_2 atmosphere and the other half aerobically.

Results: Paper chromatograms revealed no increased release of amino acids from either group. It appears phosphoproteins are not significantly affected by a CO_2 atmosphere.

STUDY 3: Enamel pieces prepared as above were incubated aerobically 24 hrs then removed from solution. Odd numbered test tubes were frozen to prevent changes and even numbered tubes incubated 48 hrs. anaerobically in a CO_2 atmosphere

Results: **Chromatograms with ninhydrin reagent revealed no change in amino acid release under these anaerobic conditions.**

STUDY 4: All enamel pieces were incubated 48 hrs in a CO_2 atmosphere, half frozen until later and some of the remaining incubated an additional 24 hrs aerobically at 37° C while others were incubated 24 hrs aerobically at 2° C.

Results: Chromatograms with ninhydrin reagent revealed disappearance of amino acids in the 37° C aerobic group but still present in the 2° C aerobic group.

Discussion: It appears from this that the phosphoprotein of enamel is unstable in a NaOH solution and that a CO_2 atmosphere does not adversely affect its stability. However, the administration of NaOH to experimental animals did cause an increase in dental caries. Phosphoproteins may play a role in caries resistance but how cannot be answered at this time. Since no increase in amino acids was noticed in anaerobically incubated specimens and had no demonstrable effect upon phosphoproteins or phosvitin, **it appears logical that the organic portion affected is the peptide fraction. The peptide fraction is probably the most labile and could be the organic fraction whose loss could possibly open the enamel surface for penetration of even larger deleterious molecules. CO_2, because of its nature and small size may play a very important role in enamel surface destruction.**

Conclusions:

- **CO_2 probably causes breakdown of the peptide protein fraction of the enamel in the form of amino acids.**
- It probably has little direct effect upon the phosphoprotein fraction of the enamel.

Article #54

Some chemical characteristics of the loosely bound amino acids of human enamel

Steinman RR. J South Calif Dent Assn 33(10):462-467, Oct 1965

Protein molecules are very complex and contain many reactive groups. Subtle changes in the molecule cause denaturation, breaking only the weaker chemical bonds, and are reversible. The labile nature of some human protein enamel has been suggested in connection with amino acid (AA) release under anaerobic conditions and AA disappearance upon further aerobic incubation. **It was the purpose of this study to determine some of the chemical and physical conditions that might affect AA reactions and characterize the reactions involved.**

STUDY: Fresh human orthodontically extracted bicuspids and caries-free 3rd molars were immediately frozen until use. Specimens were divided into 2 or 4 parts and wax placed over all surfaces except intact enamel. These were placed in test tubes with the enamel surface at the bottom.

Results: It was apparent that under aerobic conditions the release of amino acids occurred at 2° C or in 50% ethanol or 10^{-2} M KCN. It was apparent that the disappearance of AAs during anaerobic incubation following anaerobic incubation did not occur at 2° C or with 10^{-2} M KCN. It appears that proline encourages disappearance of AAs during aerobic incubation following anaerobic release of the AAs. After proline will no longer encourage disappearance of AAs, it is apparent that phosvitin does encourage disappearance of AAs during aerobic incubation. It appears that the AA pattern is similar from both enamel and dentin and that removal of 1/3 of the enamel did not alter the release of AA from the enamel. No release of AA from phosvitin under anaerobic conditions was observed. It appears that ethylene oxide does not prevent the release of amino acids during anaerobic incubation but prevents disappearance of AAs during subsequent aerobic incubation.

Discussion: **Release of AAs under anaerobic conditions and their disappearance following an aerobic incubation is different from denaturation in that it is slow whereas denaturation is rapid. The freeing of AAs or their subsequent disappearance is not usually taken as an indication of denaturation and renaturation. However, since the reactions are occurring extracellularly, the most logical explanation is that it involves a process of denaturation and renaturation.** Another possibility is that a balanced state may normally exist between the protein and surrounding AAs such that by various means this balance is tipped in favor of freeing AAs under adverse conditions. The disappearance of the AAs is probably not the result of microbial action because the unsterilized saliva showed no diminution of AAs upon incubation. **Enamel might have an exchange of AAs with either the saliva or underlying dentin. The similarity of the amino acid pattern of the enamel and dentin and the small amount of amino acids released if no underlying dentin is present would favor the suggestion that the amino acid exchange is with the underlying dentin. This needs more study to be certain.**

Conclusions:

- **It is suggested that release of AAs such as under these milder study conditions can be a reflection of denaturation and that their disappearance is the result of renaturation.**
- **The AA pattern of saliva is significantly enough different from that of enamel and dentin that it is not suspected that AAs found following anaerobic incubation were of any salivary origin.**

Article #55

A possible physiological mechanism of resistance to dental caries

Steinman RR. J South Calif Dent Assn 33(11):514-516, Nov 1965

Recent work [refs] has shown the destructive potential of CO_2, an end product of much metabolism, upon intact enamel. It attacks both the protein and mineral components of enamel. Also reported [ref] is the change from positive to a more negative potential under anaerobic conditions of microbial growth, such as found in pits and fissures. The odontoblastic layer of the dentin maintains a negative potential [ref].

Metabolism influences potential differences between the enamel and pulp. When the tooth is cooled, both the metabolism slows and the potential falls. Conversely, when the tooth is warmed back up the potential again rises. **It was the purpose of this experiment to determine if an artificially maintained electrical potential would in any way prevent enamel surface destruction by CO_2.**

STUDY1: Fresh caries-free orthodontically extracted lower bicuspids were immediately frozen until use. One half the root was removed, pulp tissue removed, and the crown and remaining root forced into a 3" piece of polyethylene tubing so the crown was flush with the end. The flush end was placed at the bottom of a test tube, with 0.5 ml water. Another 0.5 ml was filled at the upward-facing pulp end of the tubing. One copper wire each was inserted into the water at each end of the tooth and connected to a 1.5 V dry cell. One was set up with the negative terminal connected to the pulp wire and another with the positive terminal connected to the pulp wire. This complete assembly of teeth was placed into a sealed jar made anaerobic by replacing the air with CO_2. After 8 days the solutions at the bottom of the test tubes were chromatographically analyzed for amino acids.

Results: Fig. 2 is a **chromatogram showing the presence of AAs from having the positive electrode at the pulp and the lack of amino acids when the negative terminal went to the pulp.**

STUDY 2: The above teeth were subjected to methylene blue dye for one hour.

Results: Fig 3 shows **obvious staining of the specimen with the positive pulp terminal indicating development of enamel surface porosity, while the one with the negative pulp terminal showed no penetration indicating its enamel surface had remained intact.**

Discussion: **Anaerobic growth in pits, fissures, and beneath plaque would suggest a low electrical potential due to significant amounts of CO_2 generated from bacterial metabolism. Cellular metabolism greatly influences environmental redox potentials by reducing O_2 tension and shifting to a more negative potential. Histochemically it has been shown that odontoblasts whose processes extend to the enamel exhibit increased concentrations of acetylcholine esterase and succinic dehydrogenase indicating their higher metabolic activity. This may explain why the pulp potential is negative relative to the enamel surface. Chilling or warming the tooth affects the metabolic rate and degree of difference in electrical potential. One way the metabolism could aid in keeping the enamel surface intact is by maintaining the optimal electrical potential. This study supports the work of Eggers-Lura and Yardeni that an oxidation reduction potential may be involved in dental caries susceptibility or resistance. It shows one way metabolism may play a role in maintaining surface enamel intact against destructive forces that might be present in the plaque.**

Conclusions:

· **Correct electrical potential may help preserve surface enamel against destruction by agents such as CO_2 and water.**

· **The pulp of the normally metabolizing tooth is negative to the enamel surface and may help preserve enamel integrity.**

Article #56

The possible character of the protein-mineral bond on dental enamel and how it may be stabilized

Steinman RR. J South Calif Dent Assn 34(4):67-72, Feb 1966

Although older teeth release less amino acids than do younger ones, total nitrogen content varies only slightly with age or from one individual to another [ref]. Recent reports from this laboratory [refs] demonstrated free or loosely bound AAs under anaerobic conditions, also under aerobic conditions at 2 C or in 50% ethanol. Later it was shown that even though enamel had 48 hours anaerobic exposure, it no longer demonstrated free AAs if followed by 24 hrs of aerobic incubation.

Steven reported the presence of loosely bound amino acids associated with collagen and gelatin and can be released with a mixture of ammonium hydroxide and acetone at pH 11. **Leimgruber suggested the type of bonding between enamel mineral and protein may be the key to resistance. Meckel showed that the presence of an organic film can reduce the amount of demineralization and suggested the organic cuticle may play a role in enamel resistance. Binding characteristics of ion exchange resins would suggest that a very weak bond probably exists between the protein cuticle and the mineral of the enamel. In what way might nature stabilize these bonds in caries-immune teeth? How might the bond between the enamel mineral and protein be stabilized?** It was the purpose of this study to attempt to find a partial answer.

STUDY 1: 0.5 ml of 1mg/100 ml water mixture of AAs listed by Steven was placed in each test tube. To this were added $Ca_3(PO_4)_2$, $CaCO_3$, keratin, etc. and incubated 24 hrs. followed by ninhydrin chromatographic analysis.

Results: When 0.5 ml of AA mixture was incubated **aerobically 24 hrs at 37° C** with 5 mg **$Ca_3(PO4)_2$, no disappearance of AAs occurred**. When the 0.5 ml mixture was incubated with 0.3 mg **keratin, no disappearance** of AAs was observed. But if the 0.5 ml AA moisture was incubated with 5 mg of **$Ca_3(PO_4)_2$ plus 0.3 mg of keratin for 24 hrs at 37° C, the AAs would disappear.**

Table I - Conditions of AA disappearance in the presence of keratin and $Ca_3(PO_4)_2$

No.	Condition	Result
1	50% ethanol (aerobic)	No disappearance
2	2° C (aerobic))	No disappearance
3	37° C (aerobic)	**Disappearance**
4	CO_2	No disappearance
5	37° C (aerobic)	**Disappearance**
6	H_2	No disappearance

Table II - Salts besides $Ca_3(PO4)_2$ were tried with negative results as shown below

No.	Condition	Result
7	$CaCl_2$	No disappearance
8	$CH_2(COO)_2Ca$	No disappearance
9	$CaCO_3$	No disappearance
10	Control AAs only	No disappearance
11	K_2HPO_4	No disappearance
12	Na_2HPO_4	No disappearance
13	KH_2PO_4	No disappearance

[One might wonder what anaerobic results would have shown, since that may more closely represent the clinical condition.]

Mucin, elastin, hyaluronic acid, and chondroitin sulfate were also found associated with disappearance of AAs besides keratin. Possibly the dipolar nature of free

AAs allowed bonding between protein (keratin) and the $Ca_3(PO_4)_2$. Additional anaerobic incubation did not release these AAs, indicating they were more securely bound to the $Ca_3(PO_4)_2$. The following study was conducted to ascertain if such AAs or their modification could help stabilize enamel against unfavorable clinical conditions.
STUDY 2: Freshly extracted teeth (for orthodontic reasons) were immediately frozen until used. Teeth were divided into at least 2 parts and all surfaces coated with wax except for intact enamel. These samples were incubated with various AA combinations with F salts under various conditions were challenged with pH $\leq$ 3.2 lactic acid $\geq$ 30 min's, then tested for amount of P released, Ca released, and enamel surface damage (under a dissecting microscope).
STUDY 3: All previous tooth pieces were placed in either saliva or hog gastric mucin for 10 min's, then dried gently with tissue. (Saliva assured the presence of loosely bound protein on the enamel surface). These specimens were placed in test tubes and incubated aerobically with FeF_2 24 hrs at 50° C with various AAs.
Results: The following AAs were found most protective against acid dissolution: Alanine, threonine, glutamate, valine, and lysine. In the presence of AAs among several other F salts tried, sodium fluorosilicate seemed superior. The best AA modifications at 37° C in air with sodium fluorosilicate (Na_2SiF_6) were valine methyl ester HCl, lysine methyl ester dihydrochloride, and glutamate HCl. STUDY 4: The experiment involved the following basic formula:
Enamel + DL valine methyl ester HCl + 37° C in air + Na_2SiF_6 for 2 hr.

The tie-up of enamel was tested by placing the tooth samples in 0.5 ml pH 1.8 lactic acid for 30 min's, then determining the P and Ca as previously described.
Results: The average P released from treated tooth samples was 17 μg compared with 41 μg for untreated controls. Fig. 2 shows marked turbidity in the test tube from white calcium oxalate precipitate for the untreated specimen compared with clear solution for the treated one. Fig 3 shows significant macroscopically observable etching of an untreated tooth specimen, and marked methylene blue penetration on another untreated sample compared to its treated counterpart.
Discussion: **Fluoride has been used for years topically and systemically to reduce dental caries, generally assumed beneficial because of the associated decrease in enamel solubility against pH 4.5 lactic acid. The F probably has no stabilizing effect upon the protein of the enamel, however. A previous paper [ref] showed that protein and mineral can be stabilized with a combination of ferrous fluoride and 1,3-difluoro-4,6-dinitrobenzene better than with a F solution alone. Drawbacks are that the treatment requires days and the materials are toxic. This technique, however, did show stabilization of protein in addition to the mineral, and greatly increased the resistance of the enamel surface to acid attack.**

This present study suggests a method of stabilizing enamel's protein as well as its mineral components and requires no more than an hour. Bipolar AAs in certain combinations are believed necessary for the reaction and circumvent the need for a 50° C temperature and O_2 atmosphere. Because extraneous molecules might interfere, clinical rubber dam isolation would be necessary. At least one hour of treatment time is necessary for practical stabilization to occur.

Currently it can be assumed that enamel proteins and minerals are bound together by AAs. Since stabilization does not occur if the teeth are polished, a layer

of protein is essential upon the enamel surface. Also, since stabilization does not occur at 2°C, which was found consistent with disappearance of amino acids in this study, it seems further plausible.

Conclusions:

- **Apparently modifications of AAs aid enamel stabilization by possibly binding its protein and mineral components.**
- **Teeth treated with certain AA modifications appear to possess resistance to acid dissolution not found in teeth treated by the usually prescribed fluoride techniques.**

Article #57

The inherent chemical instability of dental care

Steinman RR. J South Calif Dent Assn 34(5):247-249, May 1966

A certain amount of chemical instability inherent to biological systems seems important to allow the appropriate reversibility necessary for life-supporting exchange of material with the environment. Tissues are thus able to grow, repair physical damage, maintain functional integrity, and eliminate waste material away from their vital centers.

Dental enamel is recognized as the hardest tissue in the body and usually thought of as quite chemically stable. At the molecular level, however, hydroxyapatite is in an ionic state of dynamic exchange with protein, which implies some degree of inherent instability. It is reported that factors such as a CO_2 atmosphere at room temperature or 50% ethanol solution at 2° C can encourage release of AAs from intact enamel surfaces [ref]. Also, the reduction of solubility following standard F treatments suggests enamel reactivity can be modified and partially controlled.

Steinman [ref] reported the importance of chemically tying up the mineral and protein elements of enamel to achieve stability against noxious bacterial products. Despite certain limitations of toxicity and length of time to administer, a possible technique for achieving enamel stability was presented.

A more recent report [ref] described another technique for stabilizing enamel against rather strong lactic acid solutions. This consisted of pre-treatment of enamel with mucin or saliva followed by a combination of Na_2SiF_6 plus a modified AA such as lysine methyl ester dihydrochloride for 1 hr at 37°C.

Reports by Weiss and Bibby [refs] have shown that application of a surface protein to bovine enamel reduced its susceptibility to attack, and that the protein layer was compatible with fluoride treatments in such a way that both together increased resistance greater than either alone.

Steinman [ref] had observed that acid resistance was greater if mucin or salivary protein preceded the fluoride-lysine methyl ester dihydrochloride treatment rather than administered simultaneously, which pointed out the possibility that certain agents may have different effects if used before, simultaneous with, or after each other. This experiment was designed to determine these factors upon the stabilization process.

STUDY: Freshly extracted teeth were preserved by freezing until used, then divided into ≥2 pieces which were coated with wax to expose only intact enamel surfaces. Pieces from the same teeth served as controls. **The basic enamel stabilization procedure consisted of a 10-minute exposure to salivary (mucin) protein followed by 1 hr aerobic exposure to 6 mg Na_2SiF_6 plus 2 mg lysine methyl ester HCl.**

Results: Variations on this theme were carried out with results as follows (**Table II**):

Time	Beneficial	Ineffective	Detrimental
10 min's during protein pre-treatment	None	Histamine, cholesterol palmitate, glutathione (red), ATP, Co acetate, FeF_2	Urea
1-hr stabilization procedure	None	Same as above	Urea, choline, $CaSO_4$, starch, $MgCl_2$, Zn acetate
20 min's after stabilization	None	Same as above	Acetyl chloride, methyl chloride

Methyl iodide partly reversed tooth resistance and acetyl chloride more totally reversed it (Fig. 1). The average release of PO_4 from the stabilized piece of enamel was 12.6 μg compared to 43.3 μg released from acetyl-chloride-treated pieces.

Discussion: **Previous studies showed that a lack of O_2 or the presence of H_2 or argon will encourage the release of amino acids from intact human enamel, suggesting the partial chemically unstable nature of enamel. The organic fraction of enamel is obviously important in resistance to acid attack. Could it be that dental caries susceptibility is merely an expression of the chemical instability of enamel? It would appear that the quality and type of bonding which is present in the enamel determines the amount of mineral release more than the pH of the attacking acid. Consquently, if the reactivity of the enamel could be curbed, dental caries would be thereby controlled.**

Conclusions:

· Stabilization of enamel appears best achieved under strictly controlled conditions.

· Beyond the basic enamel stabilizing mixture previously presented, no added chemical tried was found to further enhance its effectiveness.

· The type of mineral-protein bonding may be the determining factor in the amount of mineral release from intact enamel.

Article #58

The movement of acriflavine hydrochloride through molars of rats in health and disease

Steinman RR. J Dent Res 46:162, Abstr #493, 1967

The present study was made to determine the route of acriflavine HCl (A-MCI) from an intraperitoneal injection through molars of 21-45 day old rats fed either a cariogenic diet and infected with Strep FA1 or Purina chow from date of weaning until sacrificed. The dosage of A-MCI was 50 mg/kg body wt. The time varied from 5 min's to 1 wk. Jaws were frozen immediately following sacrifice of animals and sectioned while frozen, then mounted in glycerine and viewed through a microscope under UV light on color film. **The A-MCI reached the odontoblastic layer in 5 min's, following the odontoblastic tubules to the DEJ in 10 min's, diffused into surrounding dentin and enamel during the first hr, and largely disappeared from the tooth over the next 7 days.** After 2 days on a cariogenic diet, in the dentin beneath the depth of the occlusal grooves, reduced A-MCI penetration was observed. These animals were sacrificed 1 hr post-injection. **Of the glycolytic microbial products tested, CO_2 inhibited the movement of A-MCI into the tooth but lactic acid had no effect upon the ingress of A-MCI. Mechanical pulp exposures with a ½ round bur**

resulted in marked reduction of A-MCI into the dentin adjacent to the infected area while the normal movement of A-MCI occurred from the adjacent pulp tissue into the dentin.

Article #59

The movement of acriflavine hydrochloride through molars of rats on a cariogenic and noncariogenic diet

Steinman RR. J South Calif Dent Assn 35(4):151-157, 1967

Various techniques have been tried to demonstrate fluid movement through hard structures of teeth. [See ref's for Fish, Bodecker, Lefkowitz, Volker and Sognnaes, Armstrong and Barnum, Sognnaes, Shaw, Bogoroch]. Bodecker further suggested that the fluid may play a role in resistance to dental caries. Acriflavine HCl and other fluorescing dyes have been used to study fluid movement through other body organs. Acriflavine HCl from an intraperitoneal injection in rats was detected in odontoblastic tubules at the DEJ in < 10 min's, and through the enamel in < 1 hour with gradual disappearance over the following 7-10 days. **The purpose of this study was to determine if (1) there is an alteration of distribution of acriflavine prior to actual cavitation, (2) fluorescing dye is influenced by metabolism, and (3) microbial products external to the tooth affect normal acriflavine movement through the tooth.**

STUDY 1: To determine if distribution of acriflavine dye may be altered in areas of the tooth which may later show cavitation, more than 200 21-day-old rats were divided randomly into two groups.

Group 1– On a high-sucrose cariogenic diet were experimentally infected by swabbing their mouth with streptococci FA1 bacteria.

Group 2– Controls were placed on a Purina laboratory chow noncariogenic diet.

50 mg/kg body wt. was injected intraperitoneally. After 1 hr the jaws were mounted in ice and sectioned for microscopic examination. Specimens were taken at time intervals from immediately following pulp exposure to 3 weeks after.

STUDY 2: To determine if metabolism were involved in dye distribution and what effect CO_2 and lactic acid would have.

Group 1– Rats were anesthetized and cavities made in their molars with a ¼ round bur exposing the pulp. Acriflavine was injected i.p. an hour prior to jaw freezing and sectioning.

Group 2– The upper posterior teeth were isolated with a metal jig to allow upper incisors and molars to be exposed to wet cotton saturated with a constant stream of CO_2, or 10^{-3} M KCN, or pH 2.3 lactic acid for 2-3 hours. Acriflavine was injected i.p. an hour prior to jaw freezing and sectioning.

Results: Acriflavine dye reached the odontoblastic layer within 5 min's and to the DEJ within 10 min's. Dye gradually spread into the dentin and enamel within an hour and gradually disappeared over the next 7-10 days. **Within 2 days an almost complete absence of fluorescence was seen in dentin beneath the depth of occlusal grooves from rats on the cariogenic diet (Fig 2A). Within 3-4 wks a breakdown of enamel occurred above this area of stasis.** A yellow-orange color from food or microbial products gradually moved through the enamel and into the dentin above this area. **Fig 3 showed teeth from a cariogenic diet with fluorescence moving into the dentin beside areas where cariogenic food filled the occlusal enamel groove. There was a marked**

reduction of fluorescence in dentin between the depth of the groove and the nearest portion of the pulp chamber. Fig 4 showed teeth from a noncariogenic diet with normal fluorescence in areas where cariogenic food filled the occlusal enamel groove and in dentin between the depth of the groove and the nearest portion of the pulp chamber.

Normal movement of acriflavine in the dentinal tubules was inhibited by KCN and CO_2 in the 2-3 hr specimens. Fig. 5A shows lack of dye movement into the cusp of the upper molar treated with KCN, which was similar to the inhibition of dye penetration produced by CO_2. Applying pH 2.3 lactic acid had no effect upon acriflavine movement into odontoblastic tubules. The pulps exposed with a ¼ round bur gradually necrosed and practically no acriflavine was observed in the dentinal tubules next to this area. Fig. 6 is of a tooth from a noncariogenic diet for 16 days which had a pulp exposure 2 days previously. There was a notable lack of dye in tubules next to the necrotic pulp tissue.

Discussion: Since normal tooth material fluoresces anyway, how does it differ from acriflavine dye? Acriflavine fluorescence can be distinguished by intensity, location, and color compared with sections free of acriflavine. Intensity is related to the amount of acriflavine present. Soft tissues such as pulp and odontoblastic tubules show practically no fluorescence. Acriflavine is a brighter green than dentin, and some microphotographs even show dentin to be black in certain areas in cariogenic diet subjects.

The speed of distribution and pathway of dye up the odontoblastic tubules suggests active fluid movement rather than passive diffusion through the tooth. Areas of no dye penetration in dentin beneath occlusal grooves suggests a cessation of normal fluid transport preceding actual cavitation by several weeks. This alteration may be brought about by some microbial product, probably an end product of carbohydrate metabolism. Lactic acid did not alter distribution of acriflavine, but CO_2, which is an end product of CHO metabolism, did inhibit acriflavine transport. CO_2 may also play a role in demineralization [ref]. These findings indicate that dental caries may exhibit alteration of fluid transport within the affected tissue.

What is the role of this fluid transport? Was Bodecker correct in suggesting that it plays an important role in resistance? Results of this study would seem to corroborate that suggestion.

Conclusions:

- **CO_2, a microbial product, is capable of inhibiting fluid transport in the tooth.**
- **KCN inhibition of fluid transport would suggest energy is essential to dental fluid movement.**

Article #60

The pharmacologic control of dental caries in the rat

Steinman RR. J Dent Res 47:196, Abstr #634, 1968

Previous studies with rats on a cariogenic diet injected with acriflavine HCL (50 mg/kg ip) showed that the fluorescent dye failed to move from the pulp through the odontoblastic tubules to the enamel beneath some occlusal grooves. Last observation showed dental caries to be present above these areas of fluid inhibition. Further work demonstrated in animals on a cariogenic diet that the administration of Urecholine produced a stimulation of fluid movement through that dentin directly opposite carious enamel. **To determine what effect urecholine might have upon the incidence of**

dental caries, 21 male Sprague-Dawley rats had their major salivary glands removed at 22 days of age and placed on a cariogenic diet. 12 of the rats were given urecholine (0.1 mg/kg ip) every other day for 8 weeks. The teeth were examined under a dissecting microscope and the caries scored by the method of Shaw. **Average caries score of the experimental group = 31.8, the control = 58.7** (p value = 0.0003).

Bradykinin (0.2 mg/kg ip) was found to cause the fluid to move from enamel surface practically to the pulp. Bradykinin administered once a week to 11 male Sprague-Dawley rats 3-15 wks of age produced an average caries score of 17 while 9 control animals on the same diet had a score of 1 (p = 0.00003). **From these studies it would appear that the incidence of dental caries in the rat may be profoundly influenced by the administration of certain pharmacologic agents. It is suggested that these drugs might act by influencing fluid movement through the dentin.**

Article #61

Pharmacologic control of dentinal fluid movement and dental caries in rats

Steinman RR. J Dent Res 47(5):720-724, 1968

Steinman previously reported [ref] that systemically-introduced dye could penetrate to the DEJ of rats'teeth within 10 min's. In rats on a cariogenic diet, fluid movement beneath occlusal grooves was severely depressed prior to cavitation. Fluid movement required an intact pulp and appeared to require metabolic energy. The purpose of this study of 225 21-day-old Sprague-Dawley rats **was to determine if dentinal fluid movement could be altered by pharmacologic agents and if an alteration in fluid movement would affect incidence of dental caries in rats.**

STUDY 1: This was a **short-term** experiment to determine effects of a specific chemical agent on fluid movement from 1 to 3 hrs. All rat jaws were immediately frozen, later sectioned and viewed under UV light.

Group 1 – **50** were given a noncariogenic diet

Group 2 – **100** were placed on a cariogenic diet for 3 wks.

Series 1 – Drugs were applied to maxillary teeth for 3 hrs, as follows:

Atropine sulfate

Methacholine bromide

Bethanechol chloride

Series 2 – Acriflavine was injected intraperitoneally, the bethanechol was given 10 min's later.

Rats were killed after 1 hr. Control rats received only acriflavine and the dye distribution was compared with molars of the experimental rats.

STUDY 2: This was a **long-term** experiment to determine effects of the drug on dental caries incidence.

Group 1

Series 1 – **21** male rats with submaxillary, sublingual, and parotid salivary glands removed, were placed on a cariogenic diet.

12 were given bethanechol intraperitoneally every other day for 8 wks, then their teeth scored for caries lesions by the method of Shaw

9 served as Controls.

Series 2 – **15** rats were placed on a noncariogenic diet for 10 wks.

8 were given i.p. injection of bradykinin 1 hr before microscopic examination

7 controls were given only acriflavine at the same time.

Group 2 – **16** rats were placed on a noncariogenic diet for 10 wks..

Series 1 - 8 rats were given an i.p. injection of bradykinin with acriflavine 1 hr before they were killed.

Series 2 - 8 Controls were given only acriflavine dye.

Group 3 – **20** rats on noncariogenic diet

Series 1 – 11 were given i.p. bradykinin once weekly for 15 wks then killed for analysis.

Series 2 - 9 were the Controls

Results: In short-term experiments with rats on the cariogenic diet, upper teeth exposed to **parasympathetic stimulants showed evidence of fluid stimulation** (regions of inhibition and yellow-orange fluorescing material were no longer present in the dentin or enamel). Similar results were observed in rats given the parasympathetic stimulant intraperitoneally. **Atropine was found to reduce the amount of acriflavine dye into the tooth.**

In short-term experiments with rats missing all their major salivary glands, experimental rats showed a Mean Caries Score of 31.8 compared to controls with 58.7 (Table 1)[?]. No 1st or 2nd molars of control rats were free from caries, but 23 1st and 2nd molars of experimental rats were free from caries.

Intraperitoneally-injected bradykinin was found to encourage reverse fluid movement from the external surface of the tooth toward the pulp in rats on the noncariogenic diet. Bradykinin given regularly to rats on a noncariogenic diet for 15 wks was found to produce a Mean Caries Score of 17. 0 in experimental rats and only 1.0 in Controls.

Discussion: **In a recent in vivo study of human teeth, Bergman and Linden demonstrated a centrifugal flow of fluid from the interior to the enamel surface. From the present investigation and a previous report [ref], the following points can be made: (1) Fluorescent dye originating from i.p. injections does not diffuse into the dentin en masse but moves up individual odontoblastic processes to the DEJ. (2) Vital pulp is essential for the dye movement, which can be inhibited by application of KCN to the teeth. (3) A parasympathetic stimulant encouraged dye movement from pulp to DEJ and a parasympathetic depressant inhibited fluid movement, suggesting that movement of fluorescent dye from pulp to DEJ is a demonstration of active transport. Altered permeability cannot be excluded as an explanation. Under circumstances with salivary gland removal, the incidence of dental caries could not be attributed to salivary gland stimulation and more logically could be attributed to an effect on the pulp of the tooth.**

Bradykinin is a polypeptide that greatly increases capillary permeability which permits peptide and even some protein release from the vascular system. Its action causing movement of fluid from outside to deep within the tooth might be the result of a change in osmotic relationship between the pulp and dentin.

Failure of fluid movement preceding cavitation may be influenced by some microbial product. CO_2 appears to inhibit normal fluid movement, bethanechol and other parasympathetic agents stimulated it, but lactic acid has not been observed to alter fluid movement. Regular stimulation was associated with a significant decrease of dental caries in rats on a cariogenic diet.

Change in fluid movement into the tooth by administering bradykinin was found to produce caries in rats on a noncariogenic diet. It would appear that the health of the teeth depends in large measure on the normal fluid movement within the tooth.

Conclusions:

- **Dentinal fluid movement can be altered by certain pharmacologic agents.**
- **Parasympathetic stimulants appear to encourage the movement of fluid from inside the tooth out toward the enamel.**
- **This stimulation was found to reduce the incidence of dental caries.**
- **Bradykinin, a sympathetic drug, encouraged movement of fluid from outside the tooth toward the pulp and produced caries in rats on a noncariogenic diet.**

Article # 62

Evidence suggesting the existence of a hypothalamic-parotid gland endocrine axis

Leonora J, Steinman RR. Endocrinology 83:807-815, 1968

Published data over the past 80 years suggests that salivary glands may possess, in part, an endocrine function or that their morphological and physiological state is dependent upon endocrine hormones. **In 1934, Ogata [ref] reported that bovine salivary glands exhibited a hormone-like activity and proposed a salivary gland endocrine theory. Similar studies were published by Takizawa and Hukusima [refs]. The hormone-like substance called parotin was isolated from bovine parotid glands and finally prepared in a "homogeneous crystalline form" in 1949. It was suggested that it decreased serum Ca levels, enhanced calcification of teeth and bone, and increased uptake of labeled inorganic phosphorus (^{32}P) in incisors and femur bones of rats. Subsequent Japanese work suggested bovine parotid gland parotin exists in α and β forms [refs]. In the present study, evidence suggests that the parotid gland does function in part as an endocrine gland and that it is under the direct control of the hypothalamus. The parotid hormone (PH) may stimulate the movement of fluid through odontoblastic tubules in the dentin of rat molars.**

STUDY: Rabbit hypothalami were homogenized with HCl, mixed with acetone, centrifuged for 15 min's, and the supernatant freeze-dried. Samples were adjusted to a pH of 7.0. Bioassay was conducted with reference to a known concentration of hypothalamic powder.

Other tissue extracts were obtained from rabbit heart, brain, liver, thyroid, and pituitary glands. Parotid glands were partially homogenized and pH adjusted to 8.5. After more thorough homogenization, the parotid tissue was centrifuged, the supernatant twice precipitated with acetone and recovered by filtration, and stored under dessication.

21-day-old male Sprague-Dawley rats and 25-day-old hypophysectomized rats were placed on a high sugar cariogenic diet. After anesthetization, acriflavine fluorescent dye was administered intraperitoneally. 10 min's later various tissue extracts were introduced via the jugular vein, each administered over a 35-min period. 5 min's following that, the teeth were prepared and analyzed.

Results:

Two areas within a tooth were selected to determine whether acriflavine was transported by fluid movement from the pulp toward the enamel. Fluorescent dye arrived in the pulp of a tooth from intraperitoneal injections then moved up the individual odontoblastic tubules to the DEJ. Under UV microscopy, tubules fluoresced a brilliant green color when dye was present. In black and white photomicrographs this appeared as thin gray-white lines not seen in non-fluorescing areas. The effect of crude hypothalamic extract (HE) on fluid movement in the dentinal odontoblastic tubules and on salivation in intact and sialoadenectomized male rats is shown in **Table 1**.

Rat preparation	I.V. material injected	Dose (mg protein)	Fluid movement No. animals	Salivation No. animals
Intact	Saline		0 / 3	0 / 3
	ST*		0 / 3	0 / 3
	HE** in ST	6.4	14 / 14	14 / 14
	HE in saline	3.2	1 / 4	1 / 4
	HE in saline	0.8	4 / 4	1 / 4
	HE in saline	0.4	9 / 9	1 / 9
	HE in saline	0.2	2 / 4	0 / 4
Ligated salivary gland ducts	HE in ST	6.4	5 / 5	0 / 5
Sialoadenectomized	HE in ST	6.4	0 / 6	0 / 6

*0.075 M sodium sulfite + 0.03 M sodium tetrathionate, **Hypothalamic Extract

Distribution of acriflavine in odontoblastic tubules occurred similarly whether HE was dissolved in saline or ST. Because of this, subsequent bioassays were done using saline as the vehicle. Since maximal stimulation, as visualized by fluorescent odontoblastic tubules, was found using only 0.4 mg protein, this amount of protein was used for subsequent bioassays. **Ligation of salivary gland ducts revealed that fluid movement in odontoblastic tubules was not dependent on salivation. Sialoadenectomization eliminated observable fluid movement indicating that the hypothalamic factor responsible for fluid movement did not exert its effect directly on the odontoblastic cells but through action on one or all the salivary glands.** The effect of crude HE on each salivary gland on fluid movement in male rat odontoblastic tubules is shown in Table 2.

Table 2 - effect of crude HE on each salivary gland on fluid movement in male rat odontoblastic tubules

Salivary gland present	HE Dose* (mg protein)	Fluid movement No. Animals	Salivation No. animals
Parotid	0.2	2 / 2	...
	6.4	8 / 8	8 / 8
Submaxillary	6.4	0 / 5	5 / 5
Sublingual	6.4	0 / 5	5 / 5

*HE dissolved in 0.075 M sodium sulfite + 0.03 M sodium tetrathionate

Fluid movement occurred when the parotid gland was present (shown in fig. 5,6) but not when either the submaxillary or sublingual gland alone was present (fig. 7). This suggests dependency upon a hypothalamic-parotid gland axis and that it is the parotid gland which releases a factor, possibly a hormone, causing fluid movement.

Table 3 - The effect of various tissue extracts and Pitressin on fluid movement

Tissue extract	Dose (mg protein)	Fluid movement No. Animals
Pituitary	1	0 / 3
Thyroid	4	0 / 3
Brain	3	0 / 4
Heart	4	0 / 3
Liver	10	0 / 4
Pitressin	0.05 IU	0 / 7

Neither the above tissue extracts nor Pitressin at these levels was seen to cause fluid movement. **In a group of parotidectomized rats, very good fluid stimulation was obtained with an extract of acetone-dried parotid glands, found still effective when the dose was reduced to 13 mg of protein.**

Table 4 - Effects of crude HE on fluid movement in hypophysectomized male rats

Preparation	Dose (mg protein)	Fluid movement No. animals
Saline		0 / 2
HE* in saline	1.6	0 / 4
	7.2	5 / 5

*Administered 5 days after hypophysectomy

Results in Table 4 indicate the hypothalamic factor exerted its effect directly on the parotid gland and bypassed the pituitary gland. (The marked elevation in HE dose required may be due to the disrupted hormonal balance in the hypophysectomized animal.)

Discussion: **Tables 1 and 2 show that HE contains a factor which exerts direct action on the parotid gland to synthesize and/or to secrete a hormone carried by systemic circulation to the teeth where the parotid hormone apparently stimulates dentinal fluid movement. Evidence that this is not from mere passive diffusion is that it follows specific channels to the DEJ and is inhibited by KCN on the teeth. It is unlikely that KCN would inhibit passive diffusion.** Parotid hormone may either stimulate active fluid transport or alter odontoblastic cell membrane permeability to allow its movement. At present, the function or composition of this fluid is unknown. **Since fluid movement is observed in rats in which all the salivary ducts are completely ligated, apparently the parotid hormone diffuses from the capillaries to the odontoblasts at the DEJ. The reduced sensitivity (1/18th) of the parotid gland to the HE under these conditions suggests that proper sensitivity relies on the intact hypothalamic-parotid axis system for optimum performance.**

This probably is the first evidence suggesting that a hypothalamic factor bypasses the pituitary to activate another endocrine gland to synthesize and/or release another hormone which has an effect elsewhere in the body.

Probably the hormone is a peptide similar to other releasing factors isolated from hypothalamic tissue. Present information suggests that the hypothalamic factor is not sialogen.

The name "parotin releasing factor" (PRF) is suggested for the hypothalamic factor which stimulates the parotid. Parotin was isolated in "pure form" by Ito [ref] and reported with a molecular weight of 132,000. Fractionation based on ammonium sulfate and pH is now recognized not to be sufficiently critical for isolating pure hormone preparations and it is felt the molecular weight may more accurately be less than this reported value.

We administered PRF to rats having all but their submaxillary glands removed and found no fluid movement. This suggests (1) the submaxillary gland does not contain the same hormone as the parotid gland, and (2) the parotid gland activity reported in this paper is not the same as the parotin described by the Japanese investigators.

Current research in our laboratory includes (1) isolation of PRF and the parotid hormone causing fluid movement and 2) a search for a quantitative bioassay procedure to evaluate these biologically active principles.

Article (abstract) #63

Suppression of dental caries by chemical activation of the hypothalamic-parotid endocrine axis

Steinmann RR, Leonora J. J Dent Res 48:S207, Abstr #666, 1969

Preliminary evidence suggests that the direction of fluid movement through the dentin plays a major role in resistance to dental caries. Fluid movement is controlled by the hypothalamic-parotid gland axis. **Components of the ornithine cycle, particularly urea, stimulate the hypothalamic-parotid axis to activate fluid movement through the odontoblastic processes of dentin. This study was to determine whether a continuous chemical activation of the hypothalamic-parotid axis with subcutaneous administration of exogenous urea or citrulline would decrease the incidence of dental caries in rats maintained on a high-sucrose cariogenic diet for 13 weeks.**

STUDY: 76 21-day-old male Sprague-Dawley rats were divided into groups.
Group 1– 20 received saline subcutaneously 3x/day
Group 2– 17 received urea 20 mg/100 gm body wt. subcutaneously 2x/day
Group 3– 13 received urea 80 mg/100 gm body wt. subcutaneously 3x/day
Group 4– 12 received urea 240 mg/100 gm body wt. subcutaneously 3x/day
Group 5– 14 received citrulline 60 mg/100 gm body wt. subcutaneously 2x/day

Results: The average numbers of cavities after 13 weeks were:
Group 1– 15.6 $\pm$ 1.7
Group 2– 9.9 $\pm$ 1.3
Group 3– 4.5 $\pm$ 1.3
Group 4– 1.8 $\pm$ 0.3
Group 5– 11.2 $\pm$ 1.5

Conclusions: **Group 4 with urea 240 mg/100 gm body wt. subcutaneously 3x/day showed the lowest caries rate but showed evidence of stress indicated by enlarged adrenals, spleen and kidneys, and lower body weight than the controls in Group 1. Group 3 with urea 80 mg/100 gm body wt. subcutaneously 3x/day showed low caries rate with little or no evidence of stress.**

Article #64

Effect of diet on dentinal fluid movement in germfree and nongermfree rats

Sanchez A, Steinman RR, Leonora J. Am J Clin Nutr 23:686-690, 1970

Data indicate that bacteria in the presence of a high sugar diet multiply more rapidly and produce a greater amount of acid which attacks the tooth surface. **It is commonly accepted that bacteria are primarily responsible for the initiation of dental caries. If this were totally true, bacteria should grow more rapidly, produce even greater amounts of acid, and cause more decay on diets supplemented with nutrients such as vitamins, minerals, or amino acids. On the contrary, dietary supplementation with lysine, phosphate, or one of a number of vitamins decreases the incidence of dental caries.** Evidence is accumulating that physiological processes occur in the tooth, however it is unclear whether these processes are at all related to microbial action. Fluid transport appears to be present in the hard tissues of teeth, somewhat parallel to that seen in other body tissues and has been demonstrated to move outward (centrifugally) from the pulp through the enamel [refs]. Recently this has been shown to be controlled both neurally and hormonally [refs].

Parasympathetic stimulation [ref] of fluid transport appears to reduce the incidence of dental caries in rats on a high-sucrose diet. Activation of the hypothalamus-parotid gland endocrine axis [ref], which also stimulates dentinal fluid movement, reduced caries incidence as much as 99% [ref]. The fluid movement process can be reversed with sympathetic stimulators such as bradykinin. This reversed the direction of fluid from the outside inward (centripetally), resulting in a highly significant caries increase in experimental animals [ref].

Stasis appears to occur in the dentin beneath occlusal grooves of teeth as early as 2 or 3 days after animals are fed a high-sucrose diet [ref]. (Studies have shown that stasis of dentinal fluid precedes actual cavitation by several weeks.) No stasis was observed in corresponding areas of teeth in animals on a noncariogenic diet. The purpose of this study with germ-free and conventional laboratory rats **was to determine whether stasis of dentinal fluid is the result of dietary factors (systemic) or if it is from bacterial (local) action on the teeth.**

STUDY: 54 laboratory rats were divided into 2 groups, germfree and regular. Germfree rats were housed in sterile stainless steel units. 4 animals per week from each diet group were injected intraperitoneally with acriflavin fluorescent dye and sacrificed for jaw samples which were quickly frozen, sectioned, and viewed microscopically under UV light. Stasis would be indicated by the absence of fluorescence in the odontoblastic tubules. A value of 1.00 = all areas under the occlusal grooves showed fluid movement (fluorescence). 0 = no areas under the occlusal grooves had fluid movement fluorescence. These resulting fluid movement ratios were analyzed using the T test.

Group 1– 22 germfree (axenic) male Sprague-Dawley rats were fed an autoclaved cariogenic diet with all essential vitamins and minerals (experimental).

Group 2– 32 male Sprague-Dawley rats with the usual oral microflora were fed autoclaved Purina Chow (controls)

Results:

Animals and diet	No./group	Fluid movement ratio	Mean no. fluor. areas/animal
Germfree rats			
Purina chow	11	0.47 ± 0.05	0
Cariogenic diet	11	0.26 ±0.09	0
Conventional rats			
Purina chow	15	0.57 ±0.03	0.07 ± 0.07
Cariogenic diet	16	0.38 ±0.03	1.34 ±0.30

There was a highly significant reduction in dentinal fluid movement in the teeth of rats on the high-sucrose diet compared to those on a noncariogenic diet in both germfree and nongermfree groups.

No significant difference in dentinal fluid movement was noted between the germfree animals and those with the usual oral microflora on the same diet.

Discussion: **A yellow fluorescence was frequently found in the dentin beneath some of the occlusal grooves in animals on a high sucrose diet. This occurred approximately 2 weeks after animals were placed on the cariogenic diet and subsequent to fluid stasis in the dentinal processes, but was very seldom seen in**

animals on the control diet. Dental caries often is found in this area several weeks later. Data suggest that in animals with the usual microflora the processes of cavitation from the outer surface occur subsequent to a loss of fluid movement within the tooth. Briner and Rosen [ref] found that animals on a high-sucrose diet had hypomineralized areas beneath occlusal grooves which never became mineralized. Those on a noncariogenic diet, however, did remineralize. Failure of complete mineralization probably corresponds to the areas of dentinal fluid stasis noted in this study.

Conclusions:

· **Stasis of fluid movement found in the dentin of teeth in animals on a high-sucrose, cariogenic diet was not the result of microbial action but in some way related to the diet**

· **Data show that fluid movement is controlled by the hypothalamus-parotid gland endocrine axis.**

· **Certain elements of the diet possibly exert fluid movement effects through the hypothalamus.**

Article (abstract) #65

Relation between early changes in dentin and later dental caries

Steinman RR, Leonora J. J Dent Res 50:247, Abstr #780, Mar 1971

The purpose of this study **was to determine if a relationship exists between these changes and the later incidence of caries in rats on the same diets.**

STUDY: 21-day-old Sprague-Dawley rats were divided into 2 groups, a high-sucrose diet and a control group. Group 1– 60 were fed Purina lab chow; Group 2 – 56 were fed a 67% sucrose diet.

At 28 days, 23 Purina fed and 17 sucrose-diet-fed rats were given an i.p. injection of acriflavine. Shortly afterwards their jaws were frozen, sectioned, and examined under UV light for fluorescent areas in the odontoblastic processes of the teeth, or for any other abnormal changes in fluorescence. These sections were then placed in ninhydrin reagent for 18 hours and viewed under a light microscope. At 66 days, 1 group on each diet was sacrificed and their jaws treated as above. At 111 days, the remaining animals were sacrificed and their caries determined by the method of Shaw.

Results: Data for each group expressed as areas of reactivity are as follows:

	Purina chow	vs. Sucrose diet
At 28 days of age		
Presence of acriflavine	6.78	2.17
Altered fluorescence	0.26	5.82
Ninhydrin reactive areas	0.82	9.71
At 66 days of age		
Altered fluorescence	0.87	10.14
Ninhydrin reactive areas	0.29	8.79
At 111 days of age		
Caries present	0.13	10.4

Conclusion: **The changes statistically were diet-related, p = 0.001**

Article #66

Relationship of fluid transport through the dentin to the incidence of dental caries

Steinman RR, Leonora J. J Dent Res 50(6) Part 2:1536-1543, 1971

Susceptibility or resistance to dental caries is usually thought of in terms of structure, which is determined for the most part during calcification. A plausible theory also is that susceptibility to dental caries may be related to an altered metabolism in the tooth. **Tooth metabolism depends on the Embden-Meyerhof pathway in avascular dentin [ref] for supporting a rapid fluid transport system essential for nutrient uptake and waste removal. The health of the tooth may rely on the rate of fluid transport such that a reduction in the flow rate through the dentin may produce deleterious effects such as lactic acid accumulation in the tooth structure.**

The purpose of these experiments is to determine (1) if fluid transport rate is related to the incidence of dental caries, (2) if the transport rate can be altered by systemic means, and (3) what effect this might have on dental caries.

Male 21-day-old Sprague-Dawley rats were fed either a high-sucrose cariogenic diet or Purina laboratory chow

STUDY 1: **The rate of dentinal fluid movement (FM) was determined** on the 28th day of life both in the cariogenic diet group and their controls, also in the anesthetized and unanesthetized states. The rate at which intraperitoneally introduced dye moved into and out from the odontoblastic processes was the criterion.

Group 1– Cariogenic diet group
Group 2– Control noncariogenic group
Group 3– Anesthetized group
Group 4– Control unanesthetized group on lab chow diet

Unanesthetized rats (Group 4) on the laboratory chow were killed at 15, 30, 45, and 60 min's and rats on the cariogenic diet (Group 1) were killed at 45, 60, 70, 90, 135, and 180 min's. Each jaw was rapidly frozen, and coded. Sections were viewed microscopically under UV light, paying particular attention to whether acriflavin dye was present in the dentin areas beneath each occlusal groove. A ratio of the number of fluorescing occlusal grooves divided by the number of fluorescing-plus-nonfluorescing grooves = FMR (fluid movement ratio). [This may be the first published example of quantifying FMR using a fluorescence technique.]

STUDY 2: **The systemic effects of urea and citrulline on FM were studied** in rats on the cariogenic diet. On the 28th day of age, these compounds were infused through the subclavian vein or internal carotid artery gradually over a period of 35 min's, then after 10 min's the jaws were processed as previously.

Group 1– Urea group on cariogenic diet
Group 2– Citrulline group on cariogenic diet

The total dose of each compound was administered gradually over a 35 min period, then after 10 min's the jaws were processed as described in Study 1 above.

STUDY 3: Various multiple doses of urea and citrulline were administered subcutaneously or intraperitoneally for 91 days to rats fed on the high-sucrose cariogenic diet ad libitum during the experimental period

Group 1– 20 rats received saline 0.5 ml/100 gm body wt. 0.9% subcutaneously as controls
Group 2– 17 rats received urea 20 mg/100 gm body wt. intraperitoneally twice a day
Group 3– 14 rats received urea 80 mg/100 gm body wt subcutaneously three times a day.
Group 4– 14 rats received urea 240 mg/100 gm body wt subcutaneously three times a day

Phase 1– studied the incidence of dental caries at 111 days of age in 25 rats compared with the incidence in 23 rats maintained on lab chow.

Phase 2– studied the relationship between dentinal FM to incidence of dental caries.

Rats were weighed twice a week for the first 8 wks, then once per week thereafter. At the end of the experiment the jaws were removed, coded, and scored for caries by the method of Shaw. The adrenal glands, testes, ventral prostate, thymus, thyroid, submaxillary glands, spleen, kidneys, and pituitary gland were dissected and weighed on a torsion balance.

STUDY 4: This experiment was **to study the mechanism whereby daily systemic administration of urea results in a reduced incidence of dental caries**. 40 21-day-old male rats were placed on a cariogenic diet for 6 wks.

Group 1– 20 rats were injected with urea 240 mg/100 gm body wt. subcutaneously 3x/day

Group 2– 20 rats received saline in the same volume and frequency as controls

Injections were continued for 3 wks while rats were on the cariogenic diet. The blood and saliva samples were taken at 45, 140, and 180 minutes after an injection of urea or saline. Blood samples were collected, centrifuged, and the plasma saved. Immediately afterwards, pilocarpine was administered subcutaneously to induce salivation. The urea content of each plasma and saliva sample was determined by the method of Chaney and Marbach [ref].

Two hours after the last injection of urea or saline, on the last day of the experiment, blood obtained via heart punctures from each group of rats was pooled and centrifuged. The supernatant plasma was bioassayed for FM-promoting activity as in Study 2 above.

Results:

Fluorescent dye appeared to move in and disappear from the odontoblastic processes at a faster rate in the unanesthetized rats fed laboratory chow than in the unanesthetized rats fed the cariogenic diet.

FIG. 1 - Bar graphs for unanesthetized rats in Fig. 1 show the FMR rising to 0.55 in 30 min's then dropping off after 50 min's for controls compared with a slower rise to only 0.4 and dropping off after 90 min's for the cariogenic-diet group. In anesthetized (pentobarbital) rats the control group FMR rose to 0.45 in 45 min's dropping back after 60 min's compared to a much slower rise to 0.6 then gradually fading out after 180 min's for the cariogenic-diet group. **Pentobarbital sodium anesthesia dramatically enhanced the suppressive effect of the cariogenic diet on the rate of FM.**

TABLE 1 - Comparison of the effectiveness of urea and citrulline to stimulate fluid movement by intra-arterial or intravenous infusion

Compound	Dose (mM)	Fluid Movement: Common carotid artery	Fluid Movement: Subclavian vein	Significance
Noninfused	...	0.11 ±0.02 (14)	...	...
Saline (control)	155.0	0.14 ±0.02 (21)	0.14 ±0.02 (18)	NS
Urea	6.25	0.25 ±0.05 (12)	...	<0.03
	12.5	0.42 ±0.03 (12)	...	<0.001
	25.0	0.66 ±0.04 (11)	...	<0.001
	25.0	...	0.22 ±0.04 (5)	<0.05
	50.0	...	0.48 ±0.07 (5)	<0.001
	100.0	...	0.76 ±0.03 (10)	<0.001
Citrulline	6.25	0.31 ±0.04 (7)	...	<0.001
	12.5	0.46 ±0.04 (9)	...	<0.001
	25.0	0.66 ±0.04 (9)	...	<0.001
	12.5	...	0.21 ±0.02 (13)	0.02
	5.0	...	0.49 ±0.03 (16)	<0.001
	0.0	...	0.76 ±0.02 (8)	<0.001

These data indicate the capacity for urea and citrulline to stimulate FM

A proportional increase of fluid movement was noted with increasing doses of either urea or citrulline. Infusion through the internal carotid artery is 2-4x more effective than through intravenous infusion.

TABLE 2 - Effect of subcutaneous injection of urea and citrulline on incidence of dental caries in male rats

Chemical	Dose Mg/100g body weight	Injec-tions per day	Caries score	Per cent Reduc-tion	Statis-tical Signify-cance	No. rats
Saline	...	3	33.3 ±4.2	...	...	20
Urea	20	2	22.5 ±2.0	33	0.02	17
	80	3	9.0 ±2.3	73	0.002	13
	240	3	3.5 ±0.7	90	0.001	12
Citrulline	60	2	23.9 ±4.9	29	0.16	14

A significant reduction in dental caries was obtained with the higher doses of urea. The decrease in caries incidence obtained with citrulline was equivalent to that obtained with the lowest dose of urea.

The relationship of the FMR to dental caries incidence is shown in Fig. 2 below.

FIG. 2 - Fluid movement ratio (FMR) for rats at 28 days of age

```
     0     0.1    0.2    0.3    0.4    0.5    0.6    0.7    0.8    0.9    1.0
P    ------------------------------------------>
C    -------------->
```

Number of caries for rats at 111 days of age

```
     0      1      2      3      4      5      6      7      8      9      10
P    ->
C    ---------------------------------------------------------------------------->
```

P = Purina lab chow diet; C = Cariogenic diet

A high FM ratio is associated with a low incidence of decay, and vice versa, i.e. a marked inverse ratio. p = <0.001

TABLE 3 - Effect of chronic administration of urea and citrulline on various organs and glands in male rats

Chemical agent	Dose mg/ 100g	Inject's per day	Body Wt. (gm*)	Adrenal Glands (gm*)	Testes (gm*)	Prostate (gm*)	Thymus (gm*)	Thyroid (gm*)	Submax Gland (gm*)	Spleen (gm*)	Kidney (gm*)	Pituitary (gm*)
Saline control	...	3	409	10.0	781	109	193	3.7	164	166	716	2.4
Urea	20	2	412	10.4	839	130	203	...	...	...	705	...
	80	3	373	11.9	844	115	148	3.5	180	247	797	2.7
	240	3	322	21.1	960	105	134	3.7	174	692	914	3.3
Citrulline	60	2	416	12.4	809	130	148	4.0	177	170	803	2.6

*Organ and gland weights are expressed as mg/100 gm of body weight

Note: Urea values at the 20 mg/100 gm dose level were not significantly different from the saline Control. Citrulline values were not statistically significant from the Control except for the thymus wt. loss and kidney wt. gain. Range values around the mean in the original publication were not included above due to insufficient space.

Table 4 - Comparison of urea concentration in the plasma and saliva at various times in rats receiving either saline or urea by injection 3x/day

Materials injected subcutaneously	Bleeding time Post-injection	Urea concentration (mg%) Plasma	Saliva
Saline Control	45 min	18.5 (20)	12.1 (20)
	120	15	...
Urea	45	29.6 (14)	25.3 (14)
	120.0	20.0	...
	180	17.3 (20)	11.7 (20)

Range values around the mean in the original publication were not included above due to insufficient space.

TABLE 5 - Plasma level of FM-promoting principle after subcutaneous injection of saline or urea

Materials Injected intravenously	Dose (ml) plasma + saline	Fluid movement	Level of significance
Saline control	0 + 2	0.14 ±0.02 (18)	...
Plasma control*	2 + 0	0.16 ±0.02 (16)	NS
Plasma experimental**	0.5 + 1.5	0.23 ±0.03 (10)	0.01
	1.0 + 1.00	0.29 ±0.03 (10)	0.002
	2.0 + 0.00	0.30 ±0.03 (10)	0.002

*Obtained by heart puncture from saline-injected rats
**Obtained by heart puncture from urea-injected rats

Discussion:

FM suppression. Data show that the FM rate through odontoblastic processes is significantly affected by the diet (Fig. 1). A cariogenic diet significantly suppressed FM compared with the control, and pentobarbital sodium anesthesia potentiated the suppressive effect of the high sugar diet.

FM suppression is discernible as early as 2 days following a cariogenic diet.

FM activation. However in short 45-min experiments, the suppressive effect can be overcome by systemic administration of urea or citrulline through intravenous or intra-arterial infusion (Table 1). With these chemical agents, it is possible to manipulate FM to a level equal to or greater than observed in Purina chow fed rats. Since the intra-arterial infusion was significantly more effective in re-establishing

FM than the intravenous infusion, these compounds exercise their effect on FM by activating a mechanism in the central nervous system.

When urea and citrulline were continually administered for 13-16 weeks, there was significant reduction in the dental caries rate. Urea was significantly more effective than citrulline because urea is a terminal metabolic product whereas citrulline can yet be diverted into other metabolic pathways.

The correlation between suppressed FM and increased dental decay suggests that the FMR is important for dental caries resistance. McClure reported that a diet containing only 1-2% urea significantly reduced caries. The beneficial systemic effect of urea is emphasized by examination of the blood and saliva urea levels in rats receiving the highest doses of urea 45 min to 3 hrs following injection (Table 4).

Systemic mechanism. The idea that urea must exercise its effect through a systemic mechanism rather than through a surface reaction is confirmed by the following observations. Others have shown that a reduction in food consumption is often associated with a decrease in dental caries. However, rats under stress may have a reduction in food consumption but have an increase in dental decay. In this experiment, the rats receiving the highest dose of urea were under stress, indicated by increased adrenal and pituitary weights as well as reduced thymus and body weights (Table 3). More evidence for the systemic effect of urea is apparent from the FM response of 28-day-old rats to plasma obtained from urea- and saline-injected rats is compared (Table 5). The intravenous infusion of 2 ml of control plasma from the saline-injected rats had no significant effect on the suppressed FMR whereas only 0.5 ml of plasma from urea-injected rats caused a significant rise in the FMR.

Evidence of hormonal involvement. The inevitable conclusion from these data is that a hormonal factor, not urea, is the responsible factor. Other yet unpublished evidence shows that urea and other compounds of the ornithine cycle and carbamyl aspartate of the pyrimidine cycle exercise their effect on FM through the hypothalamus. Under the influence of urea, the hypothalamus secretes the hypothalamic parotid hormone-releasing factor (PRF) which stimulates the parotid gland. The parotid gland secretes a parotid hormone that stimulates FM by acting on the odontoblasts. Surgical interruption of this endocrine axis, such as parotidectomy, renders these compounds ineffective in stimulating FM. Effectiveness is dependent on an intact endocrine axis. Evidence for the existence of the hypothalamic-parotid gland endocrine axis has been published previously.

Protective function of FM. Bone is a relatively vascularized structure whereas dentin is avascular and dependent on a rapid fluid transport system for nutrient uptake and waste removal. Teeth are exposed to the atmosphere and the aerobic environment may be of importance in influencing metabolic pathways [refs]. In deep occlusal grooves and beneath plaque there is a more anaerobic environment which could adversely affect metabolic pathways. Teeth in experimental animals on a high-sucrose diet showed hypomineralized areas in the enamel and dentin adjacent to the stagnant food and might be explained as a consequence of reduced fluid transport along with a shift to a more anaerobic metabolism and the accumulation of lactic acid in the dentin. These changes prepare the tooth for

successful attacks from unfavorable external factors. External conditions may produce dental caries partly by first influencing the metabolism within the tooth.
Conclusions:
· **The rate of fluid transport was suppressed significantly by rats on a high sucrose diet compared to controls on Purina lab chow.**
· **Dentinal fluid transport may be stimulated by the systemic administration of urea or citrulline.**
· **Systemic administration of urea to rats on a high-sucrose diet significantly reduced the dental caries rate.**
· **Reduction of dental caries rate may be the result of stimulation of the dentin fluid transport (DFT) system produced by the hypothalamic-parotid endocrine axis.**
[This is a key article because it not only brought in critical new evidence but tied it in with previous findings, lining up facts to support the concept of an active hypothalamic-parotid hormonal axis]

Article #67

Studies of the parotid hormone in the pig

Steinman RR. Personal notes, ca 1971

Rat studies have shown that the parotid hormone stimulates DFT in the dentin of molars. The high sucrose cariogenic diet suppresses DFT and is associated with dental caries. Suppression can be reversed with certain compounds such as carbamyl phosphate, which stimulated DFT with a decrease in dental caries rate. This is thought to occur by release of a parotid hormone into blood circulation. Our studies suggest that parotid hormone plays an essential role in maintaining function of DFT in rat teeth, therefore is an important determinant in dental health maintenance. Might this also be true in the pig?

Research literature shows the following animals have been observed by various investigators to have dental caries: human, monkey, rat, hamster, mouse, Mongolian gerbil, hibernating arctic ground squirrel, horses, dogs, bears, elephants, and rabbits. Plaque of most species of zoo animals contains streptococci and actinomyces. One suggestion is that the problem may occur because these animals are domesticated, however sheep or cattle were not reported to have caries and the reason offered is that they are grass eaters. Also absent from this list is any report of caries in swine.

The pig was introduced into dental research in 1962 (Weaver ME, Sorenson FM, Jump EB. The miniature pig as an experimental animal in dental research. Arch Oral Biol 7:17-24, 1962). The article stated the advantages of the pig for research. Its embryological development is comparable to man. Its physiology is similar to humans. It possesses both deciduous and permanent teeth. The hormones found in the pig have their counterparts in man. Flora from pig saliva and tooth scrapings also appear similar to man's. The following references include research involving swine:

Dentinal fluid studies of swine teeth. Acta Odont Scand 23:411-421, 1965
Induction of pulp polyps in swine teeth. J Dent Res 45:414, 1966
Trabecular pattern in the jawbone of swine. Angle Orthodont 38:205-210, 1968
Eruption pattern of permanent teeth in the mini pig. Arch Oral Biol 14:323-331, 1969
Calcification pattern of the teeth of the pig. Arch Oral Biol 16:639-648, 1971
Eruption of the deciduous teeth of mini pigs. Arch Oral Biol 14:323-331

Eruption of permanent teeth in the mini pig. Anat Rec 154:81-86
No studies of caries were found under the heading "swine." ["porcine?"]

The most susceptible areas of the tooth are the developmental grooves—the pits and fissures. The occlusal surfaces of the permanent molars contain pits and fissures 1-3 mm deep. Why, with all the dental surface irregularities and oral flora similar to man's is there no caries reported? What is the basis for resistance to caries in the pig? Does the parotid hormone play an important role?

Studies of dental caries with animals has been confined to those animals which have dental caries. It might be very profitable to study the teeth of an animal that has teeth highly resistant to dental caries, not accounted for by their anatomy.

ERUPTION SCHEDULE FOR SWINE (MINI PIGS)

	0	10	20	30	40	50	60	70	80	90 weeks
Deciduous										
1st molar				X						
2nd molar		X-------	--------	--------	--------	--------	→			
3rd molar	X-------	--------	--------	--------	--------	--------	→			
4th molar	X-------	--------	--------	--------	--------	--------	→			

	0	10	20	30	40	50	60	70	80	90 weeks
Permanent										
1st molar			X							
2nd molar						X				
3rd molar										(116 wks) → X

The mandibular 4th deciduous molar has deep grooves which would be very good for caries research. 18 deciduous mandibular molars were examined and found to have no caries. Also 22 permanent mandibular molars were examined without caries.

Article (abstract) #68

Lactic acid concentration in various tooth structures in rats maintained on either a cariogenic or noncariogenic diet

Steinman RR, Leonora J, Shiroma E, Dwyer T. J Dent Res 54(2):419, Abstr, 1975

In our laboratory a tenfold difference in incidence of dental caries is usually observed between animals maintained on a high sucrose diet and those fed Purina lab chow. Impacted food residues from occlusal grooves of weanling white rats maintained either on noncariogenic Purina chow or on a cariogenic high-sucrose diet contained comparable concentrations of lactic acid [ref]. Microbial acid production in an incubated mixture of ground Purina chow and saliva was significantly higher than that when a high-sucrose diet and saliva mixture was incubated. This lack of correlation between acidogenic potential and cariogenicity of the diet suggests that metabolic factors within the tooth determine the onset and course of the carious process. The Embden-Meyerhof metabolic pathway has been reported to exist in dentin [ref]. The end product of this pathway is lactic acid. Since the amounts on the external surfaces of the tooth are not different between regular and cariogenic diets, any difference in dentin or pulp would likely be a reflection of metabolic differences within the tissue. **The purpose of this study was to examine the correlation between the lactic acid content of various tooth structures and dietary intake, whether Purina lab chow or a high-sucrose diet.**

STUDY: 250 male 21-day-old Sprague-Dawley rats were divided into groups. 150 rats were maintained on a 62% sucrose diet for 7-12 days and 100 controls were fed Purina chow. Jaws were immediately frozen and sectioned for analysis. Using a dissecting microscope, the pulp, the dentin from the cusp tips, and the dentin from beneath the occlusal grooves were mechanically removed from the enamel and immediately freeze-dried. Samples were weighed and lactic acid microdeterminations made using a modification of Barker's and Summerson's method [ref].

Results:

Concentration of lactic acid in various structures of rat molars

	Lactic acid (µg/mg)				
Sample	High sucrose diet		Purina lab chow		p values
Dentin/cusp tip	1.15	(20)	1.57	(18)	0.003
Dentin/beneath occlusal grooves	1.47	(18)	1.68	(15)	0.03
Pulp	2.59	(18)	2.09	(23)	0.001

Numbers in parenthesis indicate the number of determinations

There was significantly more lactic acid in the cusp-tip dentin of control rats than from those on the high-sucrose diet. However, the differences were less noticeable in the dentin beneath occlusal grooves. There was significantly more lactic acid in the pulp of rats fed the high-sucrose diet than pulps in control rats.

Conclusions:

· **Since differences in the amount of lactic acid on the external surface of the tooth were essentially similar, the observed differences in the dentin and in the pulp are probably a reflection of a difference in metabolism within the dental tissues.**

· **Resistance or susceptibility to dental caries may well be a reflection of the metabolic (physiologic) state of the teeth.**

Article #69

Effect of infusing selected chemical compounds on dentinal fluid movement in the rat

Steinman RR, Leonora J. J Dent Res 54(3):567-569, 1975

Previous studies have shown that active fluid movement (FM) occurs in the odontoblastic processes of rat dentin [refs]. FM is suppressed in rats on a cariogenic diet [refs]. Reversal of this suppression has been reported to occur from an infusion of citrulline or subcutaneous administration of urea. **Since the relationship of these compounds to the urea-ornithine cycle suggests the possibility that related compounds might be similarly effective, the purpose of this study was to explore the effects of other congeners on dentinal FM.**

STUDY: 240 male 21-day-old Sprague-Dawley rats were separated into 7 experimental groups and 1 control group. All rats were maintained on a cariogenic diet containing 62% sucrose. Carbamyl phosphate, carbamyl-DL-aspartic acid, guanidine, KCN, and urea were tested for their stimulatory action on dentinal FM. Rats were injected intraperitoneally with acriflavine dye to trace fluid movement. The various chemical agents were introduced through the left internal carotid artery. The total dose of each compound was administered gradually during a 35-min period. After 10 min's the jaws were immediately debrided and frozen for sectioning. The presence of acriflavine was observed microscopically under UV illumination. The fluid movement rate (FMR) was calculated by the formula: Fluorescing occlusal grooves / fluorescing + nonfluorescing grooves = FMR.

Results:

It was found that carbamyl phosphate, carbamyl-DL-aspartic acid, guanidine, KCN, and urea all stimulate dentinal FM.

Most effective - Carbamyl phosphate and carbamyl-DL-aspartic acid
Less effective – KCN
Least effective – Guanidine, L-asparagine, and reagent grade urea

Discussion:

We believe the stimulatory effect of urea was due to its contamination with NaCN since it is approximately 30 times more potent than reagent grade urea. This finding does not negate the previous concept of a systemic mechanism of defense.

The infusion of all these compounds apparently stimulates the hypothalamus to secrete the parotid hormone releasing factor (PRF) which in turn induces the secretion of the parotid hormone. Parotid hormone is responsible for the activation of the FM mechanism in the odontoblasts. This is supported by preliminary findings that indicate carbamyl-DL-aspartic acid is effective in stimulating FM only when the hypothalamic-parotid endocrine axis is intact. If the axis is interrupted either by making a lesion in the hypothalamus or by bilateral extirpation of the parotid glands, carbamyl-DL-aspartic acid is ineffective in stimulating FM. This suggests that dentinal FM is under hormonal control.

Conclusions:

- **Equimolar concentrations of carbamyl phosphate and carbamyl-DL-aspartic acid were equally effective in inducing FM.**
- **Other ornithine cycle congeners KCN, guanidine, L-asparagine, and reagent grade urea also induced FM at higher concentration.**
- ***A previously reported action of urea was most likely attributable to contamination with NaCN.***
- **The cariostatic role of these active compounds should be tested.**

Article #70

Effect of selected dietary additives on the incidence of dental caries in the rat

Steinman RR, Leonora J. J Dent Res 54(3):570-577, 1975

In the previous study it was found that chemical compounds having the carbamyl group stimulated dentinal FM. The purpose of this investigation was to test these chemicals alone and in combination with other dietary additives for their possible cariostatic activity.

STUDY: 1,840 male 21-day-old Sprague-Dawley rats were separated into 2 experimental sections of 793 and 1107. Experimental rats were fed a cariogenic diet containing 62% sucrose supplemented with one or more dietary additives. The principal additives were compounds related to the carbamyl group. These included carbamyl phosphate, carbamyl-DL-aspartic acid, L-asparagine, sodium cyanate, and guanidine. Bone meal and desiccated eggshell meal were included as additives in concentrations ranging from 1-4%. Zinc and chromium are trace elements involved in the metabolism of sugar, and molybdenum is known for its caries suppressive effect. These were added to the diet as zinc sulfate, molybdic acid, and potassium chromate in concentrations ranging from 250-1000 ppm, 10-40 ppm, and 4-16 ppm, respectively. These concentrations have been shown to be both efficacious and yet innocuous in rats and humans. At the end of 13 weeks the rats in the first experiment were fasted overnight, bled via heart puncture into heparinized syringes, autopsied, and the jaws removed. Teeth were coded, mixed, and scored at random, done blind in relation to treatment. Rats in the 2nd experiment were not fasted before being bled. Ca:PO4 ratios were obtained from an independent laboratory and summarized in Table 5.

Results:

TABLE 1

Effectiveness of various selected dietary supplements in suppressing dental caries

Group No.	Agent/Compound	Dose (mM)	Caries Scores	(No. samples)
1	**Control-Cariogenic diet**		**9.2**	(175)
2	**Control-Purina diet**		**0.9**	(42)
3	Carbamyl Phosphate	0.78	12.2	(22)
4	"	1.56	9.6	(43)
5	"	6.25	3.3	(65)
6	"	12.50	1.8	(51)
7	Carbamyl-DL-Aspartic Acid	1.56	7.4	(22)
8	"	6.25	7.9	(42)
9	"	25.00	3.2	(22)
10	L-Asparagine	6.25	7.8	(22)
11	"	25.00	5.2	(20)
12	Guanidine HCl	6.25	9.5	(22)
13	Sodium Cyanate	6.25	8.7	(22)
14	"	25.00	4.1	(44)
15	"	50.00	2.3	(42)
16	1% Bone Meal		16.0	(22)
17	2% Bone Meal		13.2	(22)
18	4% Bone Meal		12.9	(22)
19	1% Eggshell Meal		5.0	(21)
20	2% Eggshell Meal		4.0	(20)
21	4% Eggshell Meal		4.0	(20)
22	¼ concentration -Trace Elements		4.5	(22)
23	½ concentration -Trace Elements		3.1	(21)
24	Full concentration -Trace Elements		1.9	(63)

TABLE 2

Caries suppression resulting from chemical compounds + bone meal or eggshell and trace elements

Group No.	Agent/Compound	Dose (mM)	Caries Scores	(No. samples)
	Carbamyl Phosphate	0.78		
25	+1% Bone Meal		9.2	(22)
26	+2% Bone Meal		5.8	(21)
27	+1% Eggshell Meal		1.0	(22)
28	+2% Eggshell Meal		1.4	(21)
	Carbamyl Phosphate	1.56		
29	+1% Bone Meal		3.5	(20)
30	+2% Bone Meal		2.0	(21)
31	+1% Eggshell Meal		1.0	(20)
32	+2% Eggshell Meal		1.0	(22)
	Carbamyl Phosphate	6.25		
33	+1% Bone Meal		3.0	(21)
34	+2% Bone Meal		3.9	(42)
35	+1% Eggshell Meal		1.0	(41)
36	+2% Eggshell Meal		1.6	(42)
37	+4% Eggshell Meal		0.5	(22)
	Carbamyl Phosphate			

38	+ Full concentration -Trace Elements		2.2	(43)
	Carbamyl-DL-Aspartic Acid	6.25		
39	+1% Eggshell Meal		5.1	(21)
40	+2% Eggshell Meal		2.8	(22)
41	+4% Eggshell Meal		3.1	(20)
	Carbamyl-DL-Aspartic Acid	6.25		
42	+ Full concentration -Trace Elements		2.8	(44)

TABLE 3

Caries suppression resulting from chemical compounds + bone meal or eggshell and trace elements

Group No.	Agent/Compound	Dose (mM)	Caries Scores	(No. samples)
	Carbamyl Phosphate	0.78		
43	+2% Bone Meal + ¼ Trace Elements		6.9	(21)
44	+2% Bone Meal + ½ Trace Elements		4.9	(21)
45	+2% Eggshell Meal + ¼ Trace Elements		0.8	(21)
46	+2% Eggshell Meal + ½ Trace Elements		2.3	(21)
	Carbamyl Phosphate	1.56		
47	+2% Bone Meal + ¼ Trace Elements		5.8	(22)
48	+2% Bone Meal + ½ Trace Elements		1.7	(22)
49	+2% Eggshell Meal + ¼ Trace Elements		0.0	(22)
50	+2% Eggshell Meal + ½ Trace Elements		7.7	(22)
	L-Asparagine	6.25		
51	+2% Bone Meal + ¼ Trace Elements		10.6	(20)
52	+2% Bone Meal + ½ Trace Elements		6.1	(22)
53	+2% Eggshell Meal + ¼ Trace Elements		1.1	(22)
54	+2% Eggshell Meal + ½ Trace Elements		0.9	(22)
	Guanidine HCl	6.25		
55	+2% Bone Meal + ¼ Trace Elements		4.2	(22)
56	+2% Bone Meal + ½ Trace Elements		8.7	(22)
57	+2% Eggshell Meal + ¼ Trace Elements		1.1	(22)
58	+2% Eggshell Meal + ½ Trace Elements		0.5	(22)

TABLE 4

Effectiveness of either bone meal or eggshell meal plus trace elements in suppressing dental caries

Group No.	Agent/Compound	Caries Scores	(No. samples)
59	+2% Bone Meal + ¼ Trace Elements	5.1	(22)
60	+2% Bone Meal + ½ Trace Elements	13.2	(22)
61	+2% Bone Meal + Full Trace Elements	4.8	(20)
62	+2% Bone Meal + ¼ Trace Elements	2.1	(22)
63	+2% Bone Meal + ½ Trace Elements	2.4	(19)
64	+2% Bone Meal + Full Trace Elements	1.5	(22)

Note: All above statistical p values for Tables 1-5 were « 0.05. See original paper for specific values.

TABLE 5

Caries attack rates and $Ca:PO_4$ ratios for various dietary regimens

Diet	$Ca:PO_4$ ratios (mol)	Caries Attack Rates
High Sugar	0.89:1	9.2 ±1.0
Purina Chow	1.19:1	0.9 ±0.3
1% Eggshell Meal	1.70:1	5.0 ±2.1
2% Eggshell Meal	2.26:1	4.0 ±1.7
1% Bone Meal	1.12:1	16.0 ±3.5
2% Bone Meal	1.31:1	13.2 ±4.8

Note: The above Ca:PO4 ratios were calculated on a molar basis

When added alone to the cariogenic diet, carbamyl phosphate was effective at high dose levels in reducing the incidence of dental caries (Table 1 Groups 3-6,). The addition of eggshell meal acted synergistically with carbamyl phosphate to

suppress dental caries (Table 2 Groups 27, 28, 31, 35, 36, 37). Thus 0.78 mM carbamyl phosphate combined with eggshell meal was more effective than 12.5 mM carbamyl phosphate alone (Table 1 Group 6, and Table 2 Groups 27, 28). The efficacy of carbamyl phosphate with eggshell meal was further increased by supplementation with trace elements (Table 3 Groups 45, 49). The addition of trace elements at ¼ concentration completely suppressed dental decay (Group 49, Table 3). Increasing trace elements to ½ concentration went beyond optimum and was less effective (Table 3 Groups 46, 50)

Neither L-asparagine nor guanidine were cariostatic as the sole dietary supplement (Table 1 Groups 10-12). When combined with eggshell meal and trace elements, however, both compounds showed marked cariostatic activity (Table 3 Groups 53, 54, 57, 58).

As the sole additive to a cariogenic diet, bone meal apparently increased the incidence of dental caries (Table 1 Groups 16-18). [However, compared to Control Group 1, it apparently reduced incidence ~50%] Trace elements at increasing dose levels progressively reduced the caries rate (Table 1 Groups 22-24). Adding bone meal to trace elements substantially elevated their cariostatic effect (Table 4 Groups 62-64).

Discussion:

Carbamyl phosphate. Carbamyl phosphate proved to be the most effective compound when used as the only supplement to the diet. Carbamyl-DL-aspartic acid was not as effective. Since sodium cyanate can act as a carbamylating agent in vitro [ref], its cariostatic effect may be similarly mediated in vivo. Its effect was only ¼ that of carbamyl phosphate.

If carbamyl phosphate were applied to the prevention and control of caries in humans, the dose would extrapolate to about 150 mg daily. At this level it would not seem to have adverse effects.

Eggshell meal. The cariostatic efficacy of eggshell meal was surprising since the dietary addition of calcium carbonate alone does not reduce dental caries [refs]. Apparently eggshell contains a substance which weakly stimulates fluid movement. The potentiating effect of eggshell meal on the action of carbamyl phosphate and to a lesser extent on carbamyl-DL-aspartic acid makes it possible to reduce the effective anticariogenic dose levels of these compounds.

Trace elements (TE): Optimum dose levels exist among carbamyl phosphate, eggshell meal, and trace elements. Whereas TE at ¼ concentration enhanced their combined effectiveness to reduce caries, TE elevated to ½ concentration provoked a rise in caries score. TE added to a cariogenic diet not already having these elements produced a definite cariostatic effect. Chromium may affect glucose homeostasis such that deficiency produces impaired glucose tolerance [refs]. Zinc may be involved with the normal production and action of insulin [ref] and Zn deficiency would impair blood glucose homeostasis. Preliminary data from our laboratory suggest that insulin stimulates fluid movement by inducing a sharp rise in the blood titer of parotid hormone activity. The role of molybdenum in dental caries is not clear although there are indications that it may potentiate the effect of fluoride [ref].

Bone meal: Substitution of bone meal for eggshell meal substantially reduced the effectiveness of carbamyl phosphate, L-asparagine, and guanidine when combined with TE.

Conclusions:

· Striking reductions in caries incidence were observed in rats receiving carbamyl phosphate in their diet.
· This effect was enhanced in combination with eggshell meal and/or trace elements.
· Combinations of eggshell meal and trace elements alone and with L-asparagine or guanidine also induced marked reduction in caries incidence.
· Cariostatic efficacy of carbamyl phosphate, carbamyl-DL-aspartic acid, L-asparagine, guanidine, and sodium cyanate is particularly significant in view of the activity in stimulating fluid movement within the odontoblastic processes via the recently discovered hypothalamic-parotid gland endocrine axis.
· These results mark a possible new approach to caries prevention dietarily through systemic alterations enhancing the tooth's own defensive capabilities.
[A comprehensive, challenging research project with potentially important results]

Article #71

Acidogenic potential of cariogenic and noncariogenic diets in the rat

Steinman RR, Leonora J. J Dent Res 54(3):578-580, 1975

The previous study showed that the cariogenic potential of a high sucrose diet could be nullified by suitable dietary supplements. Carbamyl phosphate, eggshell meal, and selected trace elements reduced the caries rate to normal noncariogenic-diet control levels. This effect was attributed to enhanced resistance within the tooth itself. **Since there was potential for dietary elements to affect the acidogenic potential of the external oral environment, this investigation was to compare residual lactic acid in the occlusal grooves of rats on cariogenic vs. noncariogenic diets, also to determine acidogenic potential of various food and rat saliva mixtures.**

STUDY 1: Lactic acid determination of occlusal groove food residues.
333 male 21-day-old Sprague-Dawley rats were divided into groups.
Group 1– 150 rats were fed a 62% sucrose diet.
Group 2- 100 control rats were fed a regular Purina chow diet. After 7-12 days the jaws were removed, immediately frozen, and sectioned for examination. The combined occlusal-groove food residues from each group were mechanically collected under a dissecting microscope and lyophilized. Samples were weighed, then 11 lactic acid determinations per group were made and the data analyzed using Student's T test.
STUDY 2: pH of various food-saliva mixtures.
Group 1– 55 rats were placed on a 62%-sucrose diet
Group 2– 28 control rats were fed regular Purina chow.

Salivary flow was induced using subcutaneous pilocarpine, and collected samples of sucrose-fed rats were divided into 7 aliquots of 5 ml. 4 aliquots were each mixed with 100 gm of the 62%-sucrose diet. 3 aliquots were mixed with 100 mg of the 62% sucrose diet mixed with 1.56 mM carbamyl phosphate, 2% eggshell meal, zinc, molybdenum, and chromium. Saliva from the control Purina chow fed rats was portioned into 4 aliquots of 5 ml and each mixed with 100 mg of ground Purina lab chow. All saliva samples were then incubated at 37 C for 24 hours under continuous agitation. pH measurements of each sample were made at 1, 4, 7 , 18, and 24 hrs.

Results:

The concentration of lactic acid in food collected from dental occlusal grooves of rats on a high-sucrose diet was not significantly different from controls

on a Purina chow diet. The terminal titratable acidity observed in saliva incubated with the high-sugar diet, however, was significantly less than that from either the Purina diet controls or the supplemented sucrose diets (Table 2).

Discussion:

Although sucrose is recognized as an effective cariogenic agent, Thachet et al suggest it is not wholly related to its acidogenic potential because Purina chow fed rats are sometimes seen to sustain greater acid production than high-sucrose fed rats. Apparently microbial acid production reflects the nutritive quality of the metabolizable substrate. Noncariogenic foods with saliva, for example, are potentially destructive in irradiated [ref], desalivated [ref] rats as well as those treated with bradykinin [ref] or hydrogen peroxide [ref]. Although acid in the external environment is necessary for the pathogenesis of dental caries, evidence shows that the internal metabolic state is decisive in determining whether the tooth actually succumbs to the carious process.

Conclusions:

· Impacted food residues from occlusal grooves of white rats on either noncariogenic Purina chow or cariogenic high-sucrose diets contained comparable amounts of lactic acid.

· Microbial acid production from ground Purina chow mixed with saliva was statistically the same as acid production from a high-sucrose diet mixed with saliva.

· Less acid was produced by an unsupplemented high-sucrose diet mixed with saliva.

· This lack of correlation between acidogenic potential and cariogenicity of the diet suggests that factors within the tooth determine its resistance to the onset and course of the carious process.

Article #72

Physiological basis for resistance to dental caries—a new look

Steinman RR. Texas Dent J 93:(12)6-8, 1975

Dr. Steinman and his wife each have had numerous dental restorations but their children ages 22, 26, and 28 had only one pit restoration among them. The regimen was (1) no between-meals snacks, (2) sucrose consumption reduced to only 12-15 lbs/person/year, and (3) all cereals and breads were whole grain. Essentially the diet was devoid of refined foods. [Despite possible benefits of community water fluoridation during development of the children's teeth, these radiographs illustrate significant contrast between the children's and parent's caries rates.]

It is suggested that resistance to dental caries depends upon normal physiologic processes operating in the tooth from pulp to enamel surface. Inherent metabolic and fluid transport processes normally prevent the ingress of external noxious material and, when altered, allow lowered resistance to dental caries.

Dental caries continues to present a major human health problem. **Jenkins [ref] stated, "The comparative or complete failure of all methods of caries prevention on a community scale implies that their basis is wrong or that they have failed to consider all important factors." One neglected factor is the possibility that resistance to dental caries is largely systemic and mediated through the tooth. It is the purpose of this paper to examine systemically this host-parasite relationship.**

The External Environment: Acid is produced in the oral environment from presence of food, saliva, and bacteria. **Saliva with carbohydrates and other foods produces**

significant amounts of acid. Observations in our laboratory showed rat saliva with either Purina lab chow or a high-sugar cariogenic diet was not related to incidence of dental caries. In fact, incubation studies showed greater acid production most often in the least cariogenic diet. It appears that acid in the oral environment is destructive regardless of diet. Acid may explain *how* the tooth decays but does not explain *why* it decays.

The Caries Process: The first evidence of demineralization is seen at the surface of the enamel and may also be evident in the dentin [ref]. Inflammatory cells have been observed in the pulp adjacent to the changes in enamel [ref]. These changes are also observed in the molars of rats placed on a cariogenic diet [ref] suggesting that the carious process occurs in depth. **Evidence indicates that even early superficial caries is associated with direct pulpal responses.**

The Tooth: Enamel: The nature of the caries process suggests that the major problem facing the tooth is to prevent penetration of deleterious external material. We would suggest that this is accomplished by certain physiological processes in the enamel, dentin, and pulp which produce movement of fluid from inside the tooth outward to the enamel surface [ref]. *In vivo* absence of inward marginal leakage around restorations compared with *in vitro* leakage in the same person or animal would support this concept [ref]. Rats placed on a cariogenic diet for one week showed copious penetration of methylene blue dye into their dental enamel surfaces whereas controls on a noncariogenic Purina chow diet did not [ref]. Thus, the first line of dental defense appears to be physiological, involving movement of fluid through the enamel from inside to the outer surfaces.

Dentin: Dentin has been shown to contain all the necessary glycolytic enzymes in significant amounts for the rapid metabolism important to a transport mechanism [ref]. Investigators since 1927 (Fish) have demonstrated movement of fluid through dentin. We have concluded from our studies that the fluid transport rate is under control of the hypothalamic-parotid gland endocrine axis. The fluid transport rate is suppressed by a high-sucrose diet, leading to dental caries. **When this rate is again stimulated, the caries rate was seen to be reduced. Administration of bradykinin suppressed the fluid transport resulting in a caries rate equivalent to that seen in high-sugar-fed rats** [ref]. Thus, the rate and direction of fluid transport in the dentin significantly affects the health of the tooth.

Pulp: **The hydrostatic pressure in the pulp of teeth is higher than found in most other tissues of the body [ref]. Hydrostatic pressure in the pulp immediately fell to zero when blood vessels to the teeth were ligated, and significant caries resulted in laboratory rats [ref]. It is our opinion that the relatively high hydrostatic pulp pressure assists the hormonally-regulated transport system for normal egress of fluid through the odontoblast and its processes.**

Diet: Experimental animals that would not normally experience dental caries on a regular Purina chow diet can be induced to have appreciable dental caries similar to animals eating a high-sucrose cariogenic diet if given irradiation [ref], hydrogen peroxide [ref], or bradykinin [ref]. Conversely, caries can be reduced 95-100% [ref] in animals on a high-sucrose diet if their dentinal fluid transport is stimulated. The external environment is consistently destructive in terms of acid, but apparently whether dental caries occurs is largely dependent upon normal physiologic host resistance. When physiological disharmony occurs, dental caries may result if noxious material is able to penetrate the enamel. **Carlos observed, "We tend to assume that if all the conditions outside the tooth are favorable for caries initiation, then the solubilizing agents will more or less naturally enter the tooth and the dissolution products will more or less naturally get out. I suspect that these assumptions are not tenable…." We agree that ultimately the success of external attacks on the tooth is likely determined from within the tooth.**

Article #73

Physiologic resistance to dental caries

Steinman RR, Leonora J. J Missouri Dent Assn. 57(3):14-21, 1977

For the last 100 years the popular approach to dental caries has been limited to the external surface of the tooth. Nothing of importance is considered to occur within the tooth once it erupts. Two reasons for this article are that incidence of dental caries is as prevalent today as 100 years ago and a critical search of the literature shows important physiologic and metabolic activity is occurring within teeth.

One may select from one of two approaches to dental caries studies, (1) accept each theory based on internal consistency with its supporting data, or (2) assemble all pertinent available data like puzzle pieces and judge what would be the most valid theory considering the total picture. The first approach can lead to cyclic reasoning because the theory is correct based on the data which is correct based on the theory, etc. The second approach takes all factors into account and would seem more capable of reaching a correct, reasonable conclusion.

A conclusion from available data is that 3 conditions must be present for dental caries, (1) the proper microbe, (2) available microbe nutrients, and (3) caries-susceptible teeth. This would imply an equilibrium such that if resistance is weak, caries will occur, but if strong enough the tooth will not decay.

Assuming dental caries is the result of interaction between the tooth and its external environment, 3 experimental approaches are possible. (1) Leave the internal resistance constant but manipulate the tooth's external conditions, such as when using fluoride [ref], chlorohexidine [ref], or antibiotics [ref]. (2) Leave the external environment constant but manipulate the internal resistance of the tooth, such as by systemically introducing bradykinin [ref], hydrogen peroxide [ref], or blocking the dental vascular supply [ref]. (3) Manipulate both the resistance of the teeth and their external environment such as by controlling dietary factors (which affect both dental metabolism and external microbial growth) or by removing major salivary glands (which alters the tooth's internal physiology and its external environment).

The External Environment: When the 3 conditions are present for caries to occur, acid is produced in significant amounts. When various cariogenic and noncariogenic foods were experimentally mixed with rat saliva and incubated, no significant pH differences were noted. When these diets were fed to rats, there was no relationship observed between the acid produced and the incidence of dental caries. **It appears that the external environment is destructive regardless of diet.**

The Carious Process: Caries occurs with inflammatory responses observed in the pulp simultaneously with external enamel demineralization.

The Tooth: Ingress of external deleterious material involves internal physiologic processes in enamel, dentin and the pulp. Methylene blue dye was not observed to

penetrate the outer intact enamel of experimental rats fed regular Purina lab chow but did penetrate in copious amounts when changed to a high-sugar diet for one week. These conditions paralleled the incidence of caries and supports the theory that the first line of defense for the tooth is a physiologic outward micro-flow of fluid through the enamel.
Dentin: Histochemical localization of ground sections of dentin confirms the presence of amounts of glycolytic enzymes significant enough to support rapid metabolism [refs]. Lactic acid build-up in molar dentin of regular Purina-fed rats was significantly greater than found in high-sucrose-fed rat molars, adding confirmation for the presence of dentinal glycolytic metabolic pathways. **The appearance of chondroitin 4-(^{35}S) sulphate in young rat molars one hour following intraperitoneal administration of sodium (^{35}S) sulphate [ref] provides chemical evidence for a rapid dentinal metabolism.** Movement of fluid through the dentin and enamel has been reported by Fish [ref] and others since the 1920s. **Plasma proteins have also been identified in human dentin [ref].** We have concluded from our studies that control of the rate of fluid transport through dentin is via the hypothalamic-parotid gland endocrine axis [ref]. **The role of cyclic AMP as the second messenger in the action of several hormones suggests the importance hormones might play in everyday function of teeth when it is considered that 2-3x more cyclic AMP was found in monkey pulp tissue than in surrounding gingival tissues [ref]. When the fluid transport mechanism was stimulated there was significant reduction in caries [ref], but when bradykinin was administered to produce a reversal of fluid transport in rats fed a regular Purina chow diet, there was an incidence of caries equal to that seen in high-sucrose diet fed rats. Thus, the rate and direction of fluid transport through the dentin appears to have significantly affected health of the tooth.**
Pulp: **The arrangement of the capillary bed adjacent to the odontoblasts apparently permits rapid exchange between capillaries and odontoblasts, but this relationship is absent in deeper portions of the pulp. It appears that the pulp is designed for a rapid transfer from capillaries to odontoblasts, further enhanced by occasional pores found in the endothelial cells [ref].** Normal hydrostatic pressure in the pulp exceeds that of other body tissues. When this pressure was experimentally eliminated by ligating pulpal blood vessels, there was a significant caries increase in rat teeth [ref]. Fluid probably cannot move through dentin and enamel without normal hydrostatic pressure from the pulp. It is our opinion that physiologic pulpal hydrostatic pressure assists the hormonally regulated fluid transfer mechanism via the odontoblasts and their processes.

There is a more rapid rate of metabolism in the dentin [ref] and pulp [ref] in the coronal portion of the tooth than the root portion [ref]. The periphery of the pulp is significantly more active than the central portion [refs]. Activity seems greater in the portion of the pulp adjacent to the enamel cap, and less activity is found in the floor of the pulp chamber.

The transport system through tooth structure serves two purposes, (1) it supplies nutrients for the metabolic processes occurring in teeth, and (2) it plays an important role in the defense of the teeth. A fundamental requirement for metabolism and defense is a proper nutrient supply to all these tissues.
Effect of diet: Animals fed regular Purina laboratory chow do not have appreciable dental caries. However, if they are irradiated [ref], given hydrogen peroxide [ref], or

administered bradykinin [ref], their caries incidence was found similar to that of animals on a high-sucrose cariogenic diet. The high caries rate observed in rats maintained on a high-sucrose diet was shown to be reversed 95-100% by stimulating the fluid transport system [refs]. In both cases, the microbes had available nutrients, which suggests the external environment is destructive regardless of the diet, and further indicates that physiologic activity within the tooth is what largely determines the incidence of caries.

Nutrition: **There are 2 essentials in any metabolic process, (1) a supply of nutrients and (2) regulation of the rate of metabolism. An optimum rate of metabolism is essential to maintain cellular structure and function. This requires a continuous exchange of nutrients and waste products and the pace varies according to tissue needs. The first essential demands necessary are the dietary nutrients, their proper absorption, and appropriate transfer to the sites of utilization. It is well to note that altering the supply of carbohydrate [ref], fat [ref], protein [ref], and vitamins A [ref], B [ref], trace elements [ref], and minerals [ref] has been found to influence the incidence of post-eruptive dental caries.**

In general, the regulation of the rate of metabolism in various tissues, including the teeth, is under hormonal control. Thyroxin [ref], insulin [ref], and testosterone [ref], have been found to alter the incidence of dental caries. Bradykinin, a tissue hormone, can also adversely affect teeth. Besides hormones, stress [ref], heredity [ref], and physical status [ref], have been shown to influence incidence of caries.

In health, intricate control mechanisms operate in harmony. In disease, disharmony is to be found. When disharmony occurs in teeth, dental caries can occur. The defense of the tooth depends upon a functional balance of these systems for optimum health. [See line drawing in full original article, "What it takes to maintain a tooth in health," Fig. 1]

Article #74

The control of dental caries by manipulating dentinal fluid movement

Steinman RR. J Missouri Dent Assn. 57(5):14-20, 1977

Why is dentinal fluid movement important? Let us first take a brief look at the dental environment-- with microbes and food incubated at close to 37° C. **Any carbohydrate incubated in the same way will produce essentially the same amount of acid yet if these mixtures are fed to animals they do not produce the same amounts of dental caries. For example, in our laboratory a high sucrose cariogenic diet when incubated in rat saliva was found to produce significantly less acid than a regular Purina laboratory chow diet. However, the high sucrose diet produced 10 times the decay.** Why is fluid transport in the dentin essential? **Consider first of all that enzymes of the Embden-Meyerhof metabolic pathway are present in the dentin in amounts capable of metabolic rates found in the heart or liver on a protein weight basis**. Transport would be essential to maintain metabolism in dentin.

Mineral Exchange in the Dentin

Isotope tracer studies show that no calcified tissue areas of teeth are inaccessible to mineral nutrients. The mineral exchange rate is less in dentin than in bone, and in enamel slower than in dentin. Factors altering the mineral content of teeth are luxation [ref], long-standing rickets [ref], and diet [refs]. The major difference between bone and dentin is that bone has capillaries while dentin is totally avascular. This makes fluid transport more critical in dentin to bring nutrients into the tooth structure for metabolism and to maintain the structure.

Dentinal Fluid Transport

Investigators from the days of Fish [ref] in the early twenties have shown the vital connection between the dentin and the pulp. The chemical composition of the dentinal fluid has also been reported [refs]. What we have found is that the rate of dentinal fluid transport is under the control of hormones and that it plays an important role in maintaining the health of the teeth.

Endocrine Control of Fluid Transport Through the Dentin

As reported in the literature, our work has shown that active fluid movement occurs in the odontoblastic processes of the rat molar (7 refs). **The hypothalamic-parotid gland endocrine axis controls the rate of dentinal fluid transport in the teeth** [ref]. The rate of fluid transport in rats on a high sucrose cariogenic diet is about 1/2 the rate observed in rats on Purina lab chow [ref]. If the rate of fluid transport were increased, a reduction in dental caries occurred [refs]. **Carbamyl phosphate, a key compound in the formation of urea and in pyrimidine synthesis in the body, was found to be a potent stimulator** of the hypothalamic-parotid gland endocrine axis, which in turn increases the rate of fluid transport in the dentin. Other related compounds have been reported as well. Data presented here will be limited to the effects of carbamyl phosphate, bone meal, eggshell, and trace elements upon the incidence of dental caries when added to a high-sucrose (60-62%) diet.

Group 1 – Control rats on the cariogenic diet without any additives. Caries score = 9.2

Group 2 – Controls on Purina lab chow. Caries score 0.9 ±0.3. Our goal is to reduce the amount of decay to that found in this Purina-fed group and still have the animals eating at least 60% sucrose in their diet.

Groups 3, 4, 5, 6 - Carbamyl phosphate at various levels in the diet. As amounts increased there was a corresponding decrease in dental caries (and concomitant decrease in body wt.)

Groups 16, 17, 18 – Bone meal alone was found surprisingly ineffective in reducing dental caries, and in fact produced a significant increase in dental caries at the 1% dose level.

Groups 19, 20, 21 – Eggshell meal tended to reduce dental caries but not statistically significant.

Groups 22, 23, 24. The Trace Elements

The 1/4 concentrations for each were Zn 250 ppm, Mo 10 ppm, Cr 4 ppm. The 1/2 concentrations were double these amounts. As amounts increased there was a corresponding decrease in dental caries, and the growth rate was significantly reduced.

Results:

TABLE 1 – Effectiveness of various selected dietary supplements in suppressing dental caries

Group No.	Agent/Compound	Dose (mM)	Caries Scores	(No. samples)
1	**Control-Cariogenic diet**		**9.2**	(175)
2	**Control-Purina diet**		**0.9**	(42)
3	Carbamyl Phosphate	0.78	12.2	(22)
4	"	1.56	9.6	(43)
5	"	6.25	3.3	(65)
6	"	12.50	1.8	(51)
16	1% Bone Meal		16.0	(22)
17	2% Bone Meal		13.2	(22)

18	4% Bone Meal	12.9	(22)
19	1% Eggshell Meal	5.0	(21)
20	2% Eggshell Meal	4.0	(20)
21	4% Eggshell Meal	4.0	(20)
22	¼ concentration -Trace Elements	4.5	(22)
23	½ concentration -Trace Elements	3.1	(21)
24	Full concentration -Trace Elements	1.9	(63)

TABLE 2 – Caries suppression resulting from chemical compounds + bone meal or eggshell and trace elements

Group No.	Agent/Compound	Dose (mM)	Caries Scores	(No. samples)
	Carbamyl Phosphate	0.78		
25	+1% Bone Meal		9.2	(22)
26	+2% Bone Meal		5.8	(21)
27	+1% Eggshell Meal		1.0	(22)
28	+2% Eggshell Meal		1.4	(21)
	Carbamyl Phosphate	1.56		
29	+1% Bone Meal		3.5	(20)
30	+2% Bone Meal		2.0	(21)
31	+1% Eggshell Meal		1.0	(20)
32	+2% Eggshell Meal		1.0	(22)
	Carbamyl Phosphate	6.25		
33	+1% Bone Meal		3.0	(21)
34	+2% Bone Meal		3.9	(42)
35	+1% Eggshell Meal		1.0	(41)
36	+2% Eggshell Meal		1.6	(42)
37	+4% Eggshell Meal		0.5	(22)

TABLE 3 – Caries suppression resulting from chemical compounds + bone meal or eggshell and trace elements

Group No.	Agent/Compound	Dose (mM)	Caries Scores	(No. samples)
	Carbamyl Phosphate	0.78		
43	+2% Bone Meal + ¼ Trace Elements		6.9	(21)
44	+2% Bone Meal + ½ Trace Elements		4.9	(21)
45	+2% Eggshell Meal + ¼ Trace Elements		0.8	(21)
46	+2% Eggshell Meal + ½ Trace Elements		2.3	(21)
	Carbamyl Phosphate	1.56		
47	+2% Bone Meal + ¼ Trace Elements		5.8	(22)
48	+2% Bone Meal + ½ Trace Elements		1.7	(22)
49	+2% Eggshell Meal + ¼ Trace Elements		0.0	(22)
50	+2% Eggshell Meal + ½ Trace Elements		7.7	(22)

TABLE 4

Effectiveness of either bone meal or eggshell meal + trace elements in suppressing dental caries

Group No.	Agent/Compound	Caries Scores	(No. samples)
59	+2% Bone Meal + ¼ Trace Elements	5.1	(22)
60	+2% Bone Meal + ½ Trace Elements	13.2	(22)
61	+2% Bone Meal + Full Trace Elements	4.8	(20)
62	+2% Bone Meal + ¼ Trace Elements	2.1	(22)
63	+2% Bone Meal + ½ Trace Elements	2.4	(19)
64	+2% Bone Meal + Full Trace Elements	1.5	(22)

Note 1: All above statistical p values for Tables 1-5 were « 0.05. See original papers for specific values.
Note 2: All the above subjects in Tables 1-5 were fed a cariogenic diet.

Groups 25-28 (Table 2) had carbamyl phosphate added at the 0.78 mM level which was ineffective. No significant reduction was observed with bone meal but with eggshell a highly significant reduction was obtained. Group 27 was equivalent to Purina controls. Increasing carbamyl phosphate to 1.56 mM reduced dental caries with both bone meal and eggshell meal. Eggshell was found superior with both groups 31 and 32, equivalent to the caries rate in Purina-fed controls. A further increase in carbamyl phosphate to 6.25 mM showed no further reduction in dental caries, but eggshell was again shown superior. Groups 35 and 37 were equivalent to Purina-fed controls. In this experimental series, no significant growth reduction was observed. When trace elements were added to eggshell and carbamyl phosphate, a further reduction in dental caries was observed. Note groups 45 and 49. No dental caries was found in group 49. The bone meal groups did not experience the low caries rate of eggshell fed groups. Growth rates were reduced with trace elements alone but became normal when eggshell and carbamyl phosphate were added. Groups 59-61 (Table 4) had bone meal and trace elements added to the high sucrose diet. There was no reduction in dental caries, neither was there an improvement in growth compared to adding trace elements alone. Groups 62-64 (Table 4) had trace elements added to the eggshell. This combination produced excellent growth and significant dental caries reduction, again showing the superiority of eggshell additive.

Discussion:

The observed reduction in dental caries incidence can not be explained as the result of diluting the sugar content of the diet since eggshell and bone meal were used in equal amounts with widely differing dental caries rates.

Is the observed reduction in dental caries due to an alteration of environmental acidity? We measured acid production of 3 food mixtures and rat saliva. **A mixture of Purina lab chow, eggshell meal, carbamyl phosphate, trace elements (the combination which produced perfect teeth) and the high sucrose control diet were incubated with rat saliva. We found that the Purina chow incubated with rat saliva and the mixture which produced perfect teeth incubated with rat saliva produced more acid in 24 hrs incubation than did the high sucrose control diet incubated with rat saliva. The difference in dental caries rates by these two diets appears to have no relation to the amount of acidity produced. From the microbe's point of view, the better the diet the more acid it can make.**

In another experiment, the amounts of lactic acid in the occlusal grooves of Purina-fed controls and high-sucrose fed rats were measured. No significant difference was found in concentration of lactic acid in the grooves of molars from these two widely differing diets. Lactic acid is associated with caries in the grooves of teeth. Again, the difference in dental caries is NOT related to the amount of acid.

Although it is obvious that the amount of acid gives no indication of the amount of dental caries to be expected, this in no way negates the destructive nature of the external environment but suggests that the external environment remains potentially destructive regardless of the diet.

We observed that the rate of fluid transport is about ½ in the teeth of high sucrose fed animals compared to the teeth of Purina fed animals [ref]. We further observed that there is significantly more lactic acid in the dentin of Purina fed animals than in the dentin of animals fed the high sucrose diet. O'Day and Bavetta reported a lower content of collagen in the teeth of animals fed a high sucrose diet compared to the collagen in the teeth of Purina fed animals. Studies by Francis and Briner [ref], and Briner and Rosen [ref], reported differences in mineral content in teeth of animals on a high sucrose diet and on Purina lab chow. It is our opinion

that these internal differences are directly or indirectly responsible for the observed differences in the incidence of dental caries.

We used two approaches to the problem of dental caries. (1) While still remaining on the high sucrose diet which suppressed the rate of fluid transport in dentin, certain dietary additives were found to stimulate the rate of fluid transport to levels found in Purina-fed control animals. (2) Minerals and trace elements were added to improve the nutritive content of the diet. Neither approach solved the problem alone but resulted in highly effective reduction of dental caries when combined.

Conclusions

· **Two problems in the high sucrose diet were corrected, (1) the reduced rate of dentinal fluid transport associated with the high sucrose diet was stimulated, and (2) the nutritive value of the diet was improved by the addition of minerals and trace elements.**

· **Normal dentinal fluid transport is important but it must also carry the right material. Dental caries susceptibility appears to result from poor nutrition both during tooth formation and after eruption.**

Article #75

The clinical significance of the physiologic approach to the control of dental caries

Steinman RR. J Missouri Dent Assn. 57(7):15-18, 1977

Dental caries is an infectious disease. This presupposes a favorable environment for the infecting agent. In areas of limited food supply in the oral cavity and under conditions of starvation the bacteria do not have adequate nutrition for growth, and therefore less dental caries is observed. Dental caries is observed under conditions of adequate food for the bacteria in association with susceptibility of the host. Susceptibility is a reflection of the poor biologic state of the host as affected by nutrition, heredity, hormonal balance, stress, etc.

In the two preceding articles the importance of the physiologic processes occurring in the teeth were presented. It is important to remember that there is a rapid rate of metabolism occurring in the teeth and that nature is not known to waste energy. In other tissues normal metabolism is usually associated with health, and abnormal metabolism associated with disease. The purpose of this article is to show the clinical significance of these observations.

Food, saliva, and bacteria accumulating as plaque on the tooth surface produce significant amounts of acid. No program of prevention would be complete without a plaque control program. However, it is equally important that due consideration be given to the internal factors of resistance.

Purina Laboratory chow is composed of a wide variety of unrefined foods and very rich in essential nutrients. The growth rate and the condition of the teeth of animals fed this diet suggest that it contains an excellent combination of nutrients.

To study the role of some specific nutrients in relation to decay, a diet made up largely of refined foods is necessary. We have formulated such a diet [ref] which gives good growth and good teeth comparable to those found in Purina fed animals. Besides refined foods, it contains minerals, vitamins, and trace elements. Also added are phosphorus, iodine, fluoride, pyridoxine, zinc, molybdenum, and chromium. There is adequate protein, some fat, and more than 60% sucrose. Carbamyl phosphate was included to overcome the suppressive effect of this high a sucrose concentration on fluid movement in the teeth. Eggshell meal was also incorporated. Judging from the condition of the teeth and the growth of the animals, this is an excellent diet.

By removing specific nutrients from this diet and observing the effect upon the incidence of dental caries, the relationship between specific nutrients and dental caries can be observed. As specific nutrients were removed from this diet, an increase in dental caries was observed. When 2 or 3 additives were removed, the decay rate was further increased.

TABLE I – The importance of complete nutrition in the prevention of dental caries

Diet	Caries Score
Purina Laboratory Chow	0.9
High sucrose diet + Zn, Mbd, Cr + Carbamyl phosphate + Eggshell meal	0.0
High sucrose diet - Zn, Mbd, Cr + Carbamyl phosphate + Eggshell meal	1.0
High sucrose diet + Zn, Mbd, Cr - Carbamyl phosphate + Eggshell meal	2.1
High sucrose diet - Zn, Mbd, Cr - Carbamyl phosphate + Eggshell meal	4.0
High sucrose diet - Zn, Mbd, Cr + Carbamyl phosphate -Eggshell meal	3.3
High sucrose diet + Zn, Mbd, Cr -Carbamyl phosphate - Eggshell meal	4.5
High sucrose diet - Zn, Mbd, Cr - Carbamyl phosphate -Eggshell meal	9.2

The combination of ingredients giving perfect teeth in this study has been repeated a number of times and has shown consistently to produce teeth equal to the teeth of Purina fed rats.

Many specific nutrients when deficient can increase dental caries incidence including fluoride, pyridoxine, vitamin A, phosphorus, protein, and fat. Replacing sucrose in the diet with starch also was found to decrease the incidence of caries. It is apparent that a prominent part of resistance to dental caries is to eat a wide variety of unrefined foods naturally rich in vitamins, minerals, and trace elements.

Incidence of dental caries is further influenced by the hormonal balance of the host. Thyroxin, insulin, testosterone, corticosteroids, and the tissue hormone, bradykinin, have all been shown to influence the health of the teeth.

In general, the poorer the dietary value of vitamins, minerals, and trace elements and the more frequently this poor feeding is consumed, the more decay may be observed. Or the more nutrients that are removed from food the more dental caries may be encouraged. Other factors are hormonal balance, demand of the body for nutrients during periods of stress or rapid growth, and heredity.

Prevalent characteristics of caries-prone patients are:

1. Eating foods with low nutritive value. Sugary between-meal snacks are too often almost totally deprived of vitamins, minerals, and trace elements.

2. Diluting the nutritive value of food by addition of sucrose in large amounts or draining cooking water from vegetables.

3. Consuming white flour which contains less pantothenic acid, pyridoxine, zinc, molybdenum, chromium, fluoride and phosphate than natural whole wheat.

4. Possibly suffering from an endocrine imbalance.

Conclusions:

·Total nutrient value is the key to good nutrition and the prevention of dental caries.

·The poorer the diet, the more frequently it is usually consumed; the more nutritious the diet, the less decay is likely.

·Many nutrients affect the health of teeth and no one nutrient is responsible for the health of the teeth.

·Two patients with dental caries may not be suffering from the same problem.

·The best source of necessary nutrients is to be found in a variety of fruits, vegetables, grains, legumes, nuts, eggs, milk.

·Refined foods do not have the vitamins, minerals, and trace elements so necessary for good dental health.

·Resistance to dental caries depends upon all known and unknown nutrients found naturally in foods.

·For abundant health and beautiful teeth, select your food wisely.

Article #76

Is caries susceptibility an internal problem of the tooth?

Steinman RR. Quintessence Int 10:95-99, 1978

Does the tooth as a whole play a part in susceptibility or is it a surface phenomenon involving only the plaque-enamel interface?

A key to dental caries resistance is the oral environment as seen from the marked increase in dental caries upon removal of the salivary glands surgically, or their atrophy by disease or irradiation. It is possible that the salivary glands play a role in maintaining the health of the teeth in ways other than by the production of saliva. All the enzymes of the Embden-Meyerhof metabolic pathway are found in the dentin in an amount that gives it the capability of a rapid rate of metabolism [refs]. The end product of this metabolic pathway is lactic acid.

In 28-day-old Purina-fed rats significantly more lactic acid was found in the dentin of their molars than was found in the dentin of molars of animals fed the high sucrose cariogenic diet. The probable source of this acid was from the metabolizing dentin. This disparity may be a reflection of different rates of metabolism in dentin depending upon the diet of the animal.

Metabolic activity is eliminated in endodontically treated teeth. This leaves only the external oral environment to be involved in any caries process. Four studies were found in the dental literature relating the incidence of dental caries to endodontic treatment. Two clinical reports reported that less caries occurred in endodontically treated human teeth compared to intact teeth in the same mouth [refs]. A third stated "endodontically treated teeth of irradiated patients remain functional for many years and show no increased vulnerability to decay"[ref].

Brown and Lefkowitz endodontically treated upper right and lower left rat first molars. On a cariogenic diet during the experimental period, the intact first molars showed twice the incidence of dental caries.

STUDY 1: To investigate the role of the pulp in caries resistance the upper right first molars and the lower left first molars of male 24 to 25-day-old rats were treated endodontically. These animals had their major salivary glands surgically removed and were placed on a high sucrose cariogenic diet for 8 wks. The caries score was determined by the method of Shaw.

Results: The endodontically treated teeth had a score of 1.2 ±0.5 while the intact first molars had a score of 5.0 ±1.2. An equal amount of caries was observed in the second molars whether adjacent to intact first molars or adjacent to the endodontically treated first molars.

Discussion: **To avoid possibility that the animals may avoid chewing with the treated teeth, a lower one from one side and an upper one from the other side of the mouth were treated. The salivary glands were removed to eliminate any local or systemic effect they might have on resistance. Since there was no difference in the incidence of dental caries in the second molars, regardless of their location relative to the intact or treated first molars, it appears that the environment in all quadrants was equally destructive. The difference in decay between treated and untreated molars was probably due to differences other than those found in the oral cavity.**

If the removal of the salivary glands had produced an equal increase in caries in both the intact first molars and the endodontically treated teeth, then the increase would largely be due to the absence of saliva in the oral cavity. However, four times more decay was found in the intact first molars compared to the treated first molars. The mode of action of the salivary glands must be due to more than just the production of saliva.

A factor found in the parotid salivary gland which may play a significant role is the parotid hormone of the hypothalamic-parotid gland endocrine axis [ref]. This hormone infused into rats on a high sucrose diet stimulated the rate of fluid transport through the dentin from the pulp outward (unpublished), resulting in as much as a 95-100% reduction in dental caries [refs]. Urecholine, a parasympathetic stimulant, was also found to reduce the incidence of dental caries in desalivated rats on a high sucrose cariogenic diet [ref].

Erosion vs. caries – Both erosion and caries are considered to be the result of action of acid upon the tooth. Erosion occurs at the surface of the tooth whereas caries is characterized by deep subsurface demineralization prior to cavitation. **Erosion may be limited to the surface because of normally operating fluid transport in the dentin. Under normal conditions the destructive material is prevented from penetrating deeply into the tooth. Dental caries is associated with a depressed rate of fluid transport, which allows the destructive material to penetrate deeply into the tooth. [Otherwise it would be more shallow and still remineralizable].**

Dental caries occurs in the occlusal grooves. Cavitation was not observed until several weeks after rats had been fed Purina chow or high sucrose cariogenic diets for 1 wk. Methylene blue dye was placed in their mouths for 6-7 hours and penetration characteristics into the teeth observed under a microscope. **Dye penetration through enamel and deeply into dentin was noted in animals on the cariogenic diet whereas**

no penetration was observed into dentin on those fed regular Purina chow. Two widely contrasting responses to the same external environment were observed, one with penetration and later dental caries, and the other with no penetration and excellent teeth.

What if the relation between the teeth and the external environment were altered by administration of various compounds in Purina fed animals so penetration into the dentin and pulp would occur?

STUDY 2: 10-wk-old rats with mature caries-free teeth showed food material in the occlusal grooves fluorescing yellow, orange, and red under UV light. One hour after an intraperitoneal injection of **bradykinin**, undecalcified sections of these teeth showed large amounts of orange fluorescing into the dentinal tubules and some even to the pulp. This rapid movement in mature intact teeth suggests that this fluorescing material was actually drawn into the tooth under these conditions. Bradykinin, a polypeptide, is a potent, vasodilating tissue hormone. When it was administered once a wk to 21-day-old Purina fed rats for 15 wks, incidence of dental caries equivalent to rats on high sucrose cariogenic diets resulted [ref]. It is assumed that associated with administration of bradykinin the pulp-dentin portion of the tooth was functioning abnormally. The resulting decay would support this suggestion, as the presence of disease is usually found to be related to abnormal function or metabolism.

STUDY 3: When Purina fed rats were given **hydrogen peroxide** by stomach tube from 21 to 26 days of age, methylene blue dye from bags placed in their cheek pouches penetrated through the tips of the cusps rather than through the enamel beneath the food found in the occlusal grooves [ref]. Shapiro et al found that hydrogen peroxide administered to rats by stomach tube for 8 wks on a Purina diet developed dental caries on their cusp tips [ref]. Action of the hydrogen peroxide is probably systemic since they are unable to vomit [ref]. **The point in common from both the administration of bradykinin and of hydrogen peroxide is that decay occurred at the site of penetration, whether beneath the food or at the cusp tip.**

What about administering compounds to decrease incidence of dental caries? When selected compounds were administered intravenously, the rate of fluid transport increased [ref]. When these compounds were added to the high-sucrose cariogenic diet, or administered by injection, a statistically significant reduction in dental caries was observed [refs]. This stimulation in fluid transport is thought to be brought about by the activation of the hypothalamic-parotid gland endocrine axis [ref]. Acid potential studies of these diets showed that ability of the bacteria in the saliva-food incubation mixture to produce acid was in no way impaired [ref]. In other words, the microbes were able to metabolize normally and produce lactic acid as usual with these diets, yet produced little or no dental caries.

<u>Conclusions</u>:

· **Since this system can be manipulated to control whether caries occurs regardless of diet, we conclude that the rate and direction of this transport system in the tooth is a major determining factor in susceptibility and resistance.**

· **It is apparent that the role of salivary glands includes biologically active material other than saliva.**

· **This active material is transported through the blood stream from the salivary glands to the pulp of the teeth.**

Article #77

<u>Susceptibility to dental caries</u>

Steinman RR, Leonora J, Tièche JM. Austral Dent J 24:222-224, 1979

What causes the tooth to be susceptible to caries? In our opinion dental caries occurs because the pulp is malfunctioning, thereby permitting destructive material which is ever present externally to move into the tooth and destroy it. **If the pulp is functioning normally, the destructive material remains outside the tooth and consequently is harmless. We believe that the pulp is the control center of the tooth. Our approach recognizes the importance of the external environment but states that the internal environment determines what effect the external environment will have on the tooth.**

Other approaches seem incomplete:

Caries-activity tests were designed to predict caries susceptibility. They give valuable information about the bacterial population in the oral cavity but tell nothing about the response of the tooth to this environment. Studies of acid produced by various food-saliva mixtures were designed to classify foods according to their caries potential. The assumed relationship between the acid produced by the food-saliva mixture and caries was not verified. Although sugar is involved, the amount of sugar in a diet has not been found to indicate the amount of caries to be associated with that diet [refs]. In all these studies the response of the tooth was not considered. It was thought to be an inert object in a destructive environment.

<u>The enamel</u> serves as a barrier to the destructive oral environment. Fluoride reduces incidence of dental caries by decreasing enamel solubility. However, solubility can be reduced by certain ions as much or more than can be achieved with a 0.1% solution of NaF and yet have no effect on caries incidence [ref]. For example, lead reduces enamel solubility but has been found to be associated with an increased incidence of caries [ref]. A recent study of 148 individuals with a DMF varying from 0-28 showed a tendency for the caries-resistant participants to have the highest apparent solubility in acid. Although the idea of enamel solubility in acid as a measure of caries susceptibility is attractive, not all evidence supports it. **Enamel may be more than just a mechanical barrier**. A recent study concluded that "porosity of tooth enamel in no way signifies caries-prone enamel" [ref]. Enamel receives physiological support from the dentin and the pulp. If this support is disturbed, by whatever means, the tooth becomes susceptible to caries. This relationship can be disturbed in animals on a noncariogenic diet with the intraperitoneal administration of bradykinin [ref]. The resulting incidence of caries is similar to that found in animals fed a high sucrose diet. Similar results were found following the administration of hydrogen peroxide by stomach tube to young rats [refs].

<u>The pulp</u>. If a disturbed pulp is the basis of caries susceptibility, endodontic treatment should completely eliminate any abnormal activity within the tooth. Caries occurring subsequent to endodontic treatment would be the result of only the external environment acting upon the tooth. Very few studies [refs] have been conducted to determine if there is a difference between endodontically treated teeth and intact teeth in the same mouth of individuals with caries or with animals subsisting on a cariogenic diet. These studies agree that **fewer lesions occur in endodontically treated teeth compared with those found in intact teeth. We have found that endodontic treatment is also highly**

effective in reducing the incidence of caries in desalivated animals compared with intact teeth in the same mouth regardless of diet [ref].

Saliva and caries susceptibility. **No other manipulation in man or animals increases incidence of caries as does the destruction of the salivary glands, whether by surgical removal, irradiation, or by disease. The salivary glands serve an endocrine [refs] as well as an exocrine function.** What is the effect of saliva on the external environment of the tooth? Saliva was found to reduce the incidence of caries in endodontically treated teeth compared to controls, but the difference was minimal [ref]. Caries reduction from saliva alone in this study was found similar to that found when saliva from immune individuals was added to the drinking water of desalivated animals [ref]. These differences were not statistically different.

The parotid hormone. **The high metabolic capability of dentin [ref] suggests the importance of dentinal fluid transport**. This transport can be affected by hormonal, nutritional, and chemical factors. **In view of the important regulatory functions exhibited by hormones on numerous physiologic processes, hormonal control of dentinal fluid transport appears as a logical extension.** Published evidence [ref] suggests the existence of a hypothalamic-parotid endocrine axis whose function, in part, is the regulation of the dentinal fluid transport mechanism. **Parotid hormone has been isolated in essentially pure form and found to be an effective stimulator of dentinal fluid transport [ref]. Ingestion of a high sucrose cariogenic diet by rats for 1 wk suppressed dentinal fluid transport, presumably by exercising a suppressive effect on the function of the hypothalamic-parotid endocrine axis [refs]. This effect can be overcome with an intravenous infusion of carbamyl phosphate. The effects of dietary high sucrose can also be reversed if rats are fed carbamyl phosphate and other dietary additives for 3 mos. A significant reduction in the caries incidence was achieved compared to controls on the unsupplemented diet [ref].**

Is the effect of foods systemic or local? The observed variation in the incidence of caries associated with alterations in human diets imposed by war time restrictions [refs], by the availability of local foods [ref], or imposed by institutional regimes [ref], or by variations in experimental diets fed to rats [refs] are usually interpreted as being the result of an alteration in the oral environment rather than due to a systemic effect. It may be equally valid to suggest that the effect could be systemic since the local and systemic environments were not separated. In our experiment with dietary supplements [ref] the cariogenicity of the high sucrose diet was markedly reduced by trace elements, carbamyl phosphate, and eggshell meal. **The question is whether this reduction in caries was systemic or local in action. Foods come in contact with the teeth in the oral cavity as well as nourish the host. The effect can be separated by endodontic treatment. We found no difference in the incidence of dental caries in the endodontically treated teeth of animals fed the unsupplemented diet. Nor was there a difference between the endodontically treated teeth of desalivated animals fed either the supplemented or unsupplemented diet [ref]. In this study, the reduction in the incidence of caries associated with supplementation appears to be due to a systemic response.**

Conclusions:

· **Information presented concerning the enamel, the pulp, the effect of endodontic treatment on the incidence of caries, the saliva, the parotid hormone, dentinal fluid**

transport, and supplementation of the diet, seems to imply that a malfunctioning pulp is the physical basis of caries susceptibility.

*This article was subsequently reprinted in 1980 as a direct copy with permission from the *Australian Dental Journal*, as **Susceptibility to dental caries, the pulp plays a major role,** Steinman RR, Leonora J, Tièche JM. Oral Health 70(7):43-44, 1980

Article #78

The biological approach to the health and disease of teeth

Steinman RR. Unpublished teaching syllabus, 1979

The observation from the Vipeholm study [ref] that sugars in solution are less cariogenic than sugars in solid form suggests that part of the problem is local. The amount of damage locally depends upon how long the sugary food remains in the oral cavity, or how long it sticks to the teeth, or how long it remains in pits and fissures. Sugars and carbohydrates are essential for the production of acid in relation to the teeth for caries activity. It is one of the essential nutrients for the bacteria as well as the host. If food were not present in the oral cavity, dental caries would be no problem, but who wants to be fed by a stomach tube even if this would eliminate dental caries?

Plaque, acid production, and caries: A major feature of the external environment essential to initiate the disease is the **plaque** in which the food and the bacteria combine to produce acid, which is thought to be essential for the carious processes. Various techniques have been tried in an effort to classify the cariogenicity of foods in relation to **acid production**. The amount of acid produced by incubating various foods in human saliva [refs] showed that in general the **nutritive value was more closely related to acid production than the carbohydrate content of the food.** Decalcification of enamel incubated in a food-saliva mixture [ref] **gave no direct relation between the amount of acid produced in the saliva and the amount of accompanying enamel decalcification**. Even the measurement of acid production in **plaque after eating snacks gave no clear-cut picture** as to the cariogenicity of various snacks [ref]. These various techniques give information as to the amount of acid produced under these conditions, but do not tell how much decay will be produced. However, it seems certain **that wherever food, saliva and bacteria accumulate, acid is produced in measurable amounts which may be destructive.**

Acid determinations in rat teeth vs. caries: To further clarify the relation between acid production and caries, rat saliva was collected and incubated with widely differing rat diets [ref]. Associated with the diets was a ten-fold difference in caries observed in animals fed these diets. **The saliva-food incubation produced significantly more acid in the diets associated with the lowest amount of caries.** A determination of the acid in the occlusal grooves of rats on two widely differing diets showed **no significant difference in acid but again ten times more decay in one group as found in the other group**.

It must be concluded, however, that wherever food, saliva and bacteria accumulate in the oral cavity, **acid is produced in destructive amounts regardless of the diet. The presence or the amount of acid on the external surface of the tooth does not tell us how much caries will be present. Since wide variations in caries are observed under varying conditions of acid concentration on the external surface of**

the tooth, perhaps one should consider susceptibility, what it is, and how it is manifested.

Sucrose vs. starch: A number of workers have found that when the sucrose in a cariogenic diet is replaced with starch, there is a reduction in dental caries (many refs). When the sucrose is replaced in increments, **the reduction in decay occurs when the concentration of sucrose falls below 20% to 0%.** The only difference in these diets is in the type of carbohydrate whether sucrose or starch. In agreement with these animal studies, **patients with fructose intolerance avoid sucrose and consume starch as their source of carbohydrate in their diet** [refs]. Their **incidence of caries was found to be very low**. Since there was found to be no difference in acid production in the incubation studies with starch compared with sucrose, for example, and yet there is a significant difference in caries when these two carbohydrates are compared. **Could it be that some of the problem is systemic?** Let's take a look. What effect does an excess of sugar have on the host? Two approaches to the problem have been taken. First, let us look at what effect an excess of sugar has upon the host in relation to dental caries. Second, let us look at what effect micronutrients added to a diet, which has an excess of sugar, has upon the incidence of dental caries.

Pre-eruptive exposure to excess sugar: An excess of sugar while the pre-eruptive teeth are calcifying may have an adverse effect upon these forming teeth. Various sugars were administered to preweanling rats. During this period of time the teeth are not in the oral cavity but inside the jaws in the process of calcification. Any major effect would most probably be systemic. The added sugars were administered by eye dropper, by injection, and by addition to a formula during the suckling period. All animals were placed on a high-sucrose cariogenic diet at weaning. Thirteen weeks later the animals were sacrificed and their teeth examined by the method of Shaw, et al. **The animals receiving the added sucrose, the Karo corn syrup, the dextromaltose, or the fructose, had about twice the amount of dental caries as the rats receiving only water or lactose** (many refs). Thus, **an excess of rapidly digested and absorbed sugar did have a detrimental effect upon the later caries experience of the teeth after they were in the oral cavity. Lactose which is hydrolyzed and absorbed more slowly than the other sugars did not cause the marked increase in dental caries as observed with the other sugars.**

Phosphate: A further study [ref] showed that the **animals had a 20-30% reduction in phosphate blood level following the administration of sugar. This was associated with a 10% decrease in the phosphate level of the teeth developed during the administration of the sugar. This suggests that a phosphate deficiency was imposed on the host by an excess of sugar administered during the calcification of the teeth (because carbohydrate must be phosphorylated to be metabolized).**

Post-eruptive exposure to excess sugar: Let us now look at the effect of an excess of sugar in the post-eruptive period of the teeth. **In a study of foods of the average American diet including desserts, it was found that this diet produced a caries score of 13.6. If the desserts were omitted from the diet, the caries score was 1.5** [ref]. **When an equal mixture of glucose and fructose was administered intraperitoneally in an amount equivalent to the amount of sucrose in the desserts, the caries score was 10.9 or equivalent to that found when the desserts were fed in the diet to the animals [ref]. The added sugar by injection most probably altered the incidence of**

dental caries by systemic means. In other words, the excess of sugar had a detrimental effect upon the host systemically [ref].

Trace elements: In the previous studies, the effect upon the incidence of dental caries of an excess of sugar administered systemically was observed. Let us next consider what effect the addition of **micronutrients** to a synthetic diet with an excess of sugar might have upon the host relative to the incidence of dental caries. In 1948, Sognnaes [ref] formulated a **synthetic diet which was assumed to have in it all the known essential nutrients. It contained, however, 66% sucrose.** This diet was **found to be cariogenic** with rats in comparison to the almost caries-free animals fed Purina laboratory chow. In an effort to determine the nature of the cariostatic agent in the natural diet, Purina chow was ashed and added in the amount of 4% reagent salt mixture of the synthetic diet [ref]. This resulted in a dramatic reduction in the incidence of dental caries. We have found that the enrichment of a similar high-sucrose cariogenic diet with Zn, Mo, Cr, eggshell meal and carbamyl phosphate produced a very dramatic reduction in dental caries compared with animals on the diet without the enrichment [ref]. When some of the enriching material was omitted from the diet, less reduction in the incidence of dental caries was observed. [i.e. ↓ micronutrients compounded caries incidence associated with ↑ sugar diet]

From these 2 separate approaches it appears that an excess of sugar creates a relative deficiency of micronutrients in the host. The body requires micronutrients to utilize the sugars. If an excess of sugar is present in the diet and if the associated micronutrients are not present in the food, then a relative deficiency develops which appears to be associated with an increased susceptibility to dental caries. **This was observed during the post-eruptive period. (The sugar being digested and absorbed much more rapidly than the starch creates a more acute relative deficiency of micronutrients as shown by the greater amount of dental caries** associated with the sugar in the diet compared to an equivalent amount of starch. In short, the diet with an excess of **added sucrose may create a demand for more micronutrients**.) [Sugar overwhelms micronutrient benefits]

Importance of dietary role: What is the practical significance of all of this experimental data? What advice should we give to our patients? Unfortunately, there is no consensus of opinion upon this important question. There are those who suggest that the dentist should ignore the nutritional problems of the patient, that not enough is really known about the relationship between dental disease and diet, and that we should wait for more definitive information. Let us drag our feet no longer.

Let me refer you to **"Dietary Goals for the United States, February 1977, prepared by the staff of the select committee on Nutrition and Human Needs, U.S. Senate." Very briefly, what do they recommend in 1977 which is of special interest to the dental profession that fits into what we have just presented? Listen to their recommendations:**

1. Reduce the consumption of sugar by 40%

2. Increase the carbohydrate content of the diet by increasing the consumption of foods containing starch, such as whole grains, vegetables and fruits. Fresh fruits and vegetables are emphasized.

3. Replace the refined cereal products of bread, etc. with the whole grain variety.

What will this do? It will reduce the amount of sucrose and increase the amount of starch in the diet, but of greater importance, it will increase the amount of micronutrients in the diet which are so essential for the health of the teeth and the body. Of course, there are other recommendations which would be of benefit to the patient, but are less directly related to oral health problems.

It is our duty as members of the health team to do our part in giving this information to the patient. It is then the responsibility of the patient to make their own decision as to whether they will accept or reject the advice given. In the final analysis, it is the patients' responsibility, not the professions, to maintain health. Unless the patients are willing to cooperate and live by healthful principles, the doctor can do no more than give the patient palliative relief. But how can they know unless you tell them?

WHAT ABOUT CEREALS AND DENTAL CARIES?

Since cereals are a major part of our diet, this question has some importance in our daily life. Like other components of the diet, cereals may affect the oral environment. They may also affect the internal environment of the body, or nutritional state of the host. Our first observations will be concerned with the possible effect of cereals in the oral environment.

In an effort to classify foods as to their cariogenicity, food-saliva mixtures have been incubated for various periods of time to determine the pH and the amount of acid present. **In general, the unrefined cereals produce more acid than their refined counterparts** [ref]. When teeth or powdered enamel are placed in similar mixtures over various periods of time, **the refined cereal mixtures produced significantly more decalcification** [refs]. From these studies it might be **suggested that the whole grain products are less cariogenic than their counterparts that are refined**.

In 2 studies, the replacing of white flour or refined cereals with the whole grain counterparts resulted in a significant decrease in caries [refs]. In an experiment using soft, cooked human foods there was no consistent difference between refined and whole grain products. Apparently other factors overshadowed any effect the grain segment of the diet might have made. However, there was found a relationship between the physical state of the animal and its teeth [ref]. In two other studies the difference in caries was so low it was considered not significant. These results were not too impressive [refs].

In several of these studies, 10-30% sucrose was added. This uniformly produced a highly significant increase in dental caries (many refs). Grain foods are high in starch and when replaced with sucrose a marked increase in caries was observed.

In diets deficient in lysine the addition of lysine significantly reduced dental caries [ref]. The addition of oat hulls and other hulls in the amount of 5-20% produced a significant decrease in dental caries. This was thought to be due to several compounds that possess strong bactericidal properties [refs]. **Phosphate supplementation was found to significantly reduce dental caries** [refs].

In feeding various packaged cereals as the sole source of nutrient [ref], no parallel was found between sugar content and caries. The experiments were for only 28 days and some groups lost weight during the experimental period. In one study using white bread, starch and gluten, the cariogenicity of these foods did not appear to be directly related to stickiness [ref].

Conclusions:

· Caries rates from animal studies in which cereals constituted the major portion of the diet suggest that whole grain cereals were less cariogenic than their refined counterparts.
· If refined cereal diets were supplemented with phosphates, the caries rate was dramatically reduced.
· If diets were supplemented with 10-30% sugar, dental caries occurred at about the same rate as that found in animals on the usual high sucrose cariogenic diets.
· Caries depends largely on what else is in the diet besides sucrose and cereals (cariogenicity of a high sucrose diet can be nullified by appropriate amounts of proper supplements).
· Caries-prone individuals may need to be more careful in their food choices and eating frequency than those with no caries problem.

Article #79

The effect of desalivation upon pulpal function and dental caries in rats

Steinman RR, Leonora J, Singh RJ. J Dent Res 59(2):176-185, 1980

The current consensus is that acid of bacterial origin is a primary factor in the induction of dental caries and that enamel is the primary determinant of susceptibility or resistance to caries. Decay is assumed to be a reflection of the amount of acid which penetrates into the enamel--the more acid the more decay. Rather than a mere surface phenomenon, recent studies have shown that the carious process occurs in depth. If true, the internal rather than the external environment may be the ultimate determinant of dental caries susceptibility.

A significant amount of dental literature (22 refs) emphasizes the existence of a dentinal fluid transport (DFT) system that begins in the pulp at the level of the odontoblasts and extends through the dentin via cytoplasmic extensions contained in narrow canaliculi [refs]. Bodecker [refs] coined the term "dental lymph" to distinguish this fluid from other body fluids. A subcutaneous injection of dye results in accumulation of dye into the tooth within 30 min's [refs]. Introducing dye in dry form directly into the pulp chamber resulted in its distribution over virtually the entire length of the odontoblastic processes. Further demonstrations of active fluid passage completely through the substance of the tooth were obtained with radionuclides ^{131}I, ^{32}P, ^{42}K, and ^{3}H. When administered intravenously these various tracer ions were transported from the pulpal blood supply, through dentin and enamel, out into the surrounding salivary environment [refs]. DFT in human teeth has been successfully demonstrated *in vivo.*

The dynamic nature of dentin is supported by the spectrum of enzymes it contains, such as acid phosphatase and alkaline phosphatase, hydrolytic and nonspecific esterases, and all the enzymes of the Embden-Meyerhof pathway [refs]. All these enzymes would indicate a high degree of cellular activity in dentinal tissue. Odontoblastic cells and their cytoplasmic processes are involved in secretory and exchange activities throughout all stages of dental development (10 refs). Many subcellular organelles within the odontoblasts involved in transport have been histologically identified as contributing to this activity. These, along with fenestrations reported in the terminal capillaries among the odontoblasts [refs] help explain the circulatory system's exchange mechanism with odontoblasts.

Furthermore, these structures are generally found exclusively in tissues involved with rapid fluid transfer [ref]. Dentin, being avascular, requires such a transport system within its structure to maintain functional integrity. In normal dental health, the direction of fluid pressure is primarily outward.

Hormonal, nutritional, and chemical factors can affect DFT. Since hormones influence regulation over other physiologic processes, hormonal control of DFT appears to be a logical extension. Published evidence [ref] suggests the existence of a hypothalamic-parotid endocrine axis (HPEA) whose function, in part, is regulation of the DFT mechanism. This parotid hormone has been isolated in essentially pure form and has been found effective in stimulating DFT with as little as 10 picograms [ref].

Ingestion of a high-sucrose diet by rats for 1 wk has been found to suppress DFT presumably by exercising a suppressive effect on the function of the HPEA [refs]. Despite the high-sucrose cariogenic diet, intravenous administration of carbamyl phosphate has been shown to overcome or reverse the high-sugar suppressive effect. Cariogenic diets supplemented with carbamyl phosphate and other dietary additives for 3 months showed significant reduction in decay compared to that observed in rats on the unsupplemented diet [ref]. DFT can also be suppressed in rats fed a noncariogenic diet by intraperitoneal injections of bradykinin or by stomach-tube administration of hydrogen peroxide, and in these cases was associated with a significant increase in dental caries rate.

It is not known whether submaxillary glands, like parotid glands, might possess endocrine activity affecting dental physiology. However, the endocrine potential of these glands has been established by isolation of a nerve-growth factor and a glucagon-like substance capable of mimicking the action of pancreatic glucagons [refs]. Destruction of the salivary glands by surgical removal, irradiation, or disease has been associated with increased incidence of decay. Desalivation eliminates not only saliva from the oral cavity but also any endocrine function.

The purpose of this study was to examine the possible relationship between pulpal function and dental caries under conditions of endodontic treatment or desalivation, and with or without a cariogenic diet, with or without cariostatic supplements.

STUDY:

215 male 21-day-old Sprague-Dawley rats were divided into 9 groups as follows:

Group 1– Intact controls with regard to salivary glands and 1st molars

Group 2– Total sialoadenectomy with intact 1st molars

Group 3– Intact with upper left and lower right 1st molars endodontically treated

Group 4– Total sialoadenectomy with endodontically treated upper left and lower right 1st molars. 96 were fed a high sucrose cariogenic diet supplemented with 250 ppm Zn, 10 ppm Mo, 4 ppm Cr, 50 ppm Mn, 2% desiccated eggshell meal and 1.56 mM carbamyl phosphate; 4 groups of 24 rats each

Group 5– Intact controls with regard to salivary glands and 1st molars

Group 6– Total sialoadenectomy with intact 1st molars

Group 7– Intact with upper left and lower right 1st molars endodontically treated

Group 8– Total sialoadenectomy with upper left and lower right 1st molars endodontically treated. 96 were fed a high sucrose cariogenic diet [ref]; 4 groups of 24 rats each

Group 9– 23 controls were fed regular Purina lab chow.

Diet consumption was quantified for each group. One each of the 4 serial groups was used successively weekly for 4 wks for each of the high sucrose diet groups. At 22 days of age the endodontic treatment and the removal of the major salivary glands were performed under Brevitol anesthesia. Endodontic treatment was aided by use of a sheet metal jig (fig. 1) which kept the mouth open and isolated upper incisors and molars from the rest of the oral cavity through specially placed slots. Entry was made with a 1/2 round bur to the pulp chambers and the pulps extirpated with a barbed broach. Cavit was injected with a syringe replacing all pulp tissue in the chambers and roots. Following endodontic treatment the major salivary glands were removed. Animals remained on their respective diets 14 wks and then were sacrificed, weighed, and their jaws removed, coded, and scored.

Results:

TABLE I Body weight, diet consumption & caries score as affected by operative procedure & diet

Group	Body wt, g	Diet/day, g	Operative Procedures: Surgery	Operative Procedures: Teeth	Caries score	Statistical significance
			UNSUPPLEMENTED DIET			
1	425	17.6	Intact	No endo	3.3	*
2	294	19.7	Desalivated	No endo	14.4	*
3	416	16.8	Intact	No endo	3.5	*
				Endo	0.5	*
4	322	18.3	Desalivated	No endo	15.7	*
				Endo	1.3	*
			SUPPLEMENTED DIET			
5	442	18.5	Intact	No endo	0.6	*
6	294	18.0	Desalivated	No endo	12.5	*
7	416	17.5	Intact	No endo	0.4	*
				Endo	0.4	*
8	313	18.0	Desalivated	No endo	13.7	*
				Endo	1.3	*
			PURINA LAB CHOW			
9	406	21.1	Intact	No endo	0.2	*

* All were $p < .001$

Desalivation caused a marked decrease in body weight not affected by endodontic treatment or high sucrose diet supplements. No correlation was apparent between incidence of caries and body weight even though marked differences in caries scores occurred.

Supplementation of the cariogenic diet of intact animals resulted in significant caries reduction (Groups 1 and 5).

Endodontic treatment of two 1st molars in intact rats fed the unsupplemented cariogenic diet significantly decreased the incidence of caries compared to that observed for intact 1st molars within the same mouth (Group 3 - Endo vs No endo).

Endodontic treatment of 1st molars in intact rats fed the supplemented cariogenic diet had little effect when compared to the incidence of decay in the remaining 1st molars within the same mouth (Group 7 - No endo vs. Endo).

Discussion:

The purpose of this study was to examine the association between pulpal function and the incidence of dental caries. **Comparison of Groups 1, 5, and 9 confirms our previous conclusion that a cariogenic diet supplemented with carbamyl phosphate,**

trace elements, and eggshell meal fed to intact rats, significantly decreased the incidence of decay, in fact approaching that noted in Purina-fed rats. The current study more clearly defines how supplementation of a cariogenic diet achieves cariostasis.

Sialoadenectomized rats fed the unsupplemented cariogenic diet experienced a 4-fold increase in decay compared to the intact rats (Groups 2 vs 1). Sialoadenectomy in rats fed the supplemented cariogenic diet produced a 20-fold increase in decay (Group 6 vs 5). It is clearly evident that sialoadenectomy nullifies the cariostatic effectiveness of supplementation to levels similar to desalivated rats on the unsupplemented cariogenic diet. Cariostatic efficacy seemed limited to intact rats. High caries scores from desalivated rats on the supplemented diet show that supplementation per se has no effect against the cariogenicity of the high sucrose diet. Rather, the cariostatic effect of the supplements must be through other, most likely systemic, means. These defense mechanisms may be associated with salivary functions such as saliva itself and/or hormonal secretion.

Results obtained from endodontic treatment on opposite-arch contralateral molars suggest that susceptibility of teeth rather than the oral environment is the primary determinant for cariogenesis. Rats fed the unsupplemented diet experienced a significant difference in caries incidence between intact and endodontically-treated teeth (Group 3) within the same mouth. Intact 1st molars were as susceptible to decay as the intact molars in Group 1 fed the same diet. However, the endodontically-treated teeth showed significantly less decay. ***Therefore, if the external environment is the primary determinant for cariogenesis, it is apparent that endodontically-treated teeth are significantly less susceptible to the environment than intact teeth.***

This striking difference in decay between intact and endodontically-treated 1st molars in the same mouth disappears when the diet is supplemented. ***The insignificant difference in decay between the intact and endodontically-treated molars is due to the cariostatic effectiveness of the supplemented diet on the intact molars. Regardless whether the diet is supplemented or not, it is clear that endodontia significantly decreases susceptibility of teeth to dental decay.***

When rats possessing both intact and endodontically-treated first molars were sialoadenectomized, it was found that intact molars experienced a significant increase in dental decay (Groups 4 and 8) regardless of diet. The effect of the sialoadenectomy on endodontically-treated teeth was minimal.

Although saliva is extremely important for many physiologic functions, it did not appear to have a significant role in controlling cariogenesis under the conditions of this experiment (Group 3 vs 4, and Group 7 vs 8).

The endodontically-treated teeth presented an interesting paradox compared to intact 1st molars in the same mouth. Data clearly suggest that the cariogenic response of intact molars can be manipulated by supplementing a cariogenic diet and by desalivation. The supplemented diet is only effective when pulpal and salivary gland functions are present. **Since the oral environment appears to be uniformly destructive and since the highest incidence of decay occurs in intact molars, it may be deduced that it is the pulp, to a most significant degree, that determines whether or not teeth will be susceptible to cariogenesis.**

Since the highest incidence of decay occurred in intact teeth of desalivated animals and the least in endodontically-treated teeth regardless of diet, it would appear that cariogenesis stemmed from a malfunctioning pulp as a result of desalivation.

The concept of pulpal involvement in cariostasis can also be deduced by the effects of the supplemented and unsupplemented diets on cariogenesis in intact rats. Since the incidence in intact teeth obtained with the unsupplemented diet (Group 1) lies between the low level obtained with the supplemented diet (Group 5) and the incidence in desalivated rats (Groups 2 and 6) regardless of diet, it suggests that pulpal function is significantly impaired, though not to the extent observed in sialoadenectomized rats. It can be argued that pulpal function is significantly more effective in rats fed the supplemented diet (Group 5) when compared to those fed the unsupplemented diet (Group 1).

Pulpal function can be manipulated even in Purina-fed rats. The weekly administration of bradykinin induced an incidence of decay in noncariogenic Purina-fed rats approximating that observed in rats fed a high-sucrose cariogenic diet. In these rats the direction of DFT (pulpal function) appeared to be severely impaired to the extent that fluorescent substances in the oral cavity penetrated deeply into the tooth structure, as observed by microscopic analysis.

It is our opinion that the key to caries resistance through the pulp is by keeping pulpal function at or near its optimal physiologic function. We suggest that two important systemic factors are (1) an optimal fluid transport mechanism which prevents the ingress of toxic substances, and (2) the parotid hormone which stimulates this mechanism to drive fluid outward through the dentin.

It is possible, though unlikely, to ascribe the dramatic reduction in caries associated with endodontic treatment to any effect Cavit might have had on the bacteria of the oral cavity.

A glucagon-like substance has been identified in homogenates of submaxillary glands from rats, mice, dogs, and humans. Secretion is similar to pancreatic glucagons because it is stimulated by arginine and low concentrations of glucose, and is inhibited by high concentrations of glucose. The submaxillary gland also serves as the source of nerve growth factor (NGF) and epidermal growth factor (EGF), both of which are recognized hormones and are not found uniquely in rodents.

The increased caries susceptibility associated with the unsupplemented diet and the desalivated animals was due to a malfunctioning pulp, possibly due to absence of hormonal factors normally associated with salivary glands that would encourage the pulp to operate normally.

Conclusions:

- **Supplementing a cariogenic diet with carbamyl phosphate, trace elements, and eggshell meal significantly decreased the incidence of decay.**
- **The cariostatic effectiveness is implemented only when the diet is fed to intact rats.**
- **The ↑ in dental caries associated with desalivation appears to be the result of a malfunctioning pulp due to elimination of endocrine factors secreted by salivary glands and to a lesser extent due to the absence of saliva in the oral cavity.**
- **Since endodontically-treated teeth are relatively resistant to the cariogenic process when compared to intact molars, evidence suggests that the pulp may have an**

essential role in determining susceptibility to decay in response to the composition of the diet and to desalivation.

Article #80

Isolation and partial characterization of a porcine parotid hormone that stimulates dentinal fluid transport

Tièche JM, Leonora J, Steinman RR. Endocrinology 106:1994-2005, 1980

Extensive data for many years have been published suggesting that salivary glands possess an endocrine function [refs] and/or their physiological states are dependent upon signals from other glands [refs]. Leonora and Steinman published evidence of a hypothalamic-parotid gland endocrine axis [ref] proposed at least partly to regulate a dentinal fluid transport (DFT) mechanism. Under the control of a hypothalamic parotid hormone-releasing factor, parotid glands secrete a parotid hormone (PH) that stimulates DFT through activation of odontoblastic cells. Histological studies of dental tissues show the existence of odontoblastic cell bodies at the pulp-dentin junction with cytoplasmic processes extending from the predentin area to the dentin-enamel junction through narrow canaliculi [refs]. Considerable evidence emphasizing the existence of DFT has been reported (21 refs). Using trypan blue or India ink administered subcutaneously, Fish in 1927 was able to demonstrate travel of dye to dentin in less than 30 min's. after injection [refs]. Similar findings were reported by Bodecker [refs] who used the term "dental lymph" to distinguish this fluid from other body fluids. Lefkowitz [ref] showed that only 13 min after introduction of dry dye into the dental pulp chamber it had been actively distributed virtually the entire length of the odontoblastic processes. He was further able to trace intravenously administered ^{131}I, ^{32}P, ^{42}K, and ^{3}H via fluid passage through dentin, enamel, and out into the surrounding salivary environment [refs]. DFT has been demonstrated *in vivo* in human teeth [refs]. Steinman [ref] developed a highly observable method of demonstrating DFT in rat teeth by fluorescence microscopy and found that DFT was inversely related to the cariogenicity of the diet. More recently, he showed that resistance to caries is reliant on an optimally functioning pulp and that primary factors for susceptibility of rat teeth to cariogenesis are dependent on its functional impairment [ref]. Susceptibility can be manipulated and/or affected by dietary changes only when pulpal and salivary gland structures are kept intact, regardless of the external oral environment. It appears that the role of salivary glands is not limited to saliva production but that they also play a fundamental hormonal role in DFT. Since experimental dietary and chemical measures promoting cariogenesis have an inverse effect on DFT [ref], we hypothesize that DFT, under the hormonal control of a parotid gland factor, may be responsible in part for the resistance of teeth to decay. The purpose of this study was to isolate, purify, and characterize a principle from porcine parotid glands which specifically controls DFT activity.

STUDY:

Fresh porcine parotid glands were obtained and ground in a meat grinder, covered with acetone, periodically stirred, and supernatant acetone decanted. The extraction process was repeated 4x leaving the insoluble residue, which was recovered by filtration and air dried. This yielded porcine parotid gland acetone-dried powder (PPGADP) which was extracted at pH 7.0 and 5.0 through several filtration and ultracentrifugation steps described in detail in this paper. The pH 5.0 extracts were pooled and neutralized with 1

N NaOH. After ultrafiltration the UM 05 concentrate of the PP-PM 30 filtrate was freeze-dried. Following ion exchange chromatography, the biologically active concentrate (CM52 active fraction) was freeze-dried. Aliquots from gel filtration were collected for bioassay and the most active fraction (G-50 active fraction) was freeze-dried. Further isolation occurred by analytical polyacrylamide disc gel electrophoresis (analytical PAGE) was accomplished to isolate contents of each each piece of gel for fluorescent determination of the proteins yielded. Each fraction was bioassayed for DFT-stimulating activity. The proteins were quantified using bovine serum albumin as the standard. Once the pure parotid hormone-A_β (PH-A_β) was quantified by amino acid analysis, it was selected as the standard for quantifying fractions in steps 4-6. From the purified fraction, the molecular weight (MW) was determined, amino acids analyzed and sequenced, and DFT-stimulating activity was bioassayed.

Results and discussion:

A parotid hormone (PH-A_β) was isolated and purified from porcine parotid glands. The biological effect of the hormone is the stimulation of a dentinal fluid transport (DFT) in molar teeth of rats. The method for purifying the PH-A_β includes extraction at pH7 and 5, ultrafiltration through Amicon membranes, ion exchange chromatography on carboxymethylcellulose, gel filtration on Sephadex G-50, and preparative electrophoresis in polyacrylamide gel. The PH-A_β is characterized as a glycoprotein having a molecular weight of 8100 and containing 2% hexose. The amino acid composition suggests a molecule rich in glycine (46%) and proline (27.7%). Alanine, glutamic acid, arginine, serine, aspartic acid, leucine, and lysine account for the remaining 26% of the residues. The isoelectric point is pH 7.50. **The partial N-terminal amino acid sequence was determined to be NH_2-Ala-Pro-Pro-Gly-Ala-Arg-Pro-Pro-Pro-Gly-Pro-Pro-Pro-Pro-Pro-Pro-(Glu)-(Pro-(Pro)-Arg-(Pro)-(Pro)-(Pro)-(Gly)-(Gly)-(Gly). A 5.5 x 10^7-fold increase in DFT activity has been achieved relative to the crude gland extract. As little as 9.7 pg PH-A_β are effective in stimulating DFT. The significance of the PH-A_β appears to be the maintenance of a functional DFT within teeth to allow the avascular dental tissues to meet their high metabolic requirements.**

Article #81

A radioimmunoassay procedure for quantitating parotid hormone

Tièche JM, Leonora J, Berk LS, Steinman RR. Biochem Biophys Res Comm 98:154-162, 1981

Abstract: **The methodology and characterization of a double antibody radioimmunoassay (RIA) for quantitating parotid hormone (PH) in biological fluids are reported. A specific antiserum against PH was raised in rabbits using PH conjugated to human serum albumin.** Its binding capacity and association constant were 22 µg/ml and $K_a = 1.01 \times 10^{-12}$ M^{-1}, respectively. **The sensitivity of the RIA was 1.5 pg PH when a sequential incubation schedule was used. This RIA makes possible the quantitation of PH in biological fluids and tissue extracts.**

Article #82

DFT, its cariostatic effect

Leonora J, Steinman, RR. Unpublished syllabus, ca 1981

The purpose of this lecture is to broaden your perspective on factors essential for maintaining optimal dental health. These factors include **dental fluid transport** (DFT) and **hormonal control of DFT**. Dental tissues share a characteristic unique to hard tissues in that vascular perfusion is limited. Vascularization stops at the pulp-dentin interface which leaves the rest of the tooth structure without a blood supply. Yet dentin maintains a high level of metabolic activity and remodeling capability, which involves an exchange process between the pulp blood supply and dentin. Because tissue perfusion is an important physiological process without which life-sustaining metabolic functions cannot exist, the questions which must be addressed are: How does dentinal perfusion occur and what is/are the mechanism(s) involved in sustaining optimal perfusion?

Dentinal Fluid Transport (DFT)

I. **Morphology**. As previously indicated, vascularization stops at the pulp-dentin interface. Odontoblastic cells are found as a layer between the pulp and the dentin (Fig. 1). These cells extend cytoplasmic processes through canaliculi (dentinal tubules) in the dentin. Odontoblasts are involved in secretory and exchange activities, such as deposition of collagen and minerals, which take place at all stages of dentinogenesis, including maturation and reorganization. In addition to these functions, evidence suggests that odontoblasts are involved in the perfusion mechanism necessary to maintain optimal dentinal function. Fenestration of pulpal capillaries allows rapid exchange between blood and odontoblasts lining the pulp. The density and cross-sectional area of dentinal tubules represent a fluid flow pathway compatible with the rapid movement of bulk flow.

II. **DFT**. The movement of fluid within the dentin has been reported by various investigators using different markers (methylene blue, trypan blue, fluorescent dyes, radiolabeled ions) and various animal species. We have used the rat model for the visualization of dentinal fluid movement. This is done by injecting a fluorescent dye, acriflavine HCl, intraperitoneally into anesthetized 4-week-old male rats and then decapitating at various times post-injection. Sagittal sections of teeth are prepared in the frozen state and observed by epifluorescence microscopy. A progressive appearance of fluorescence is observed initially in the pulp, then with time the dye migrates up to the dentinal canaliculi toward the enamel until they fluoresce their entire length. In rats fed Purina lab chow (a noncariogenic diet), this process takes place rapidly (within 30 minutes). The depth of dye penetration over a given length of time is indicative of basal DFT activity. In comparison, the DFT mechanism becomes severely depressed in rats fed a cariogenic diet (65% sucrose).

The direction of fluid flow within the tooth is centrifugal (moves in an outward direction). However, centrifugal dental fluid movement does not imply an equal flow through the entire tooth structure. The enamel capping the dentin acts restrictively on fluid flow because of its limited permeability. Enamel, as a dense structure, physically lacks open pathways. Therefore, in spite of its porosity, its permeability is limited when compared to dentin. We envision a 2-way fluid flow movement going up and down the tubules. This is in agreement with the observation that an extensive dentinal tubule side branching network exists at the level of the dentin-enamel junction, but is virtually nonexistent proximal to the pulp. If exchange of metabolites is to take place between dental tissue and the circulation, a 2-way flow process seems inevitable.

We theorize the following general process to account for dental fluid movement. Fluid derived from the circulation or the interstitial space, containing essential nutrients, is pumped up the dentinal tubules. Upon reaching the side-branching network, most of the fluid returns to the pulp (see above figure). In this proposed mechanism, the odontoblasts and their processes would play a determinant role either actively and/or passively as gate keepers and/or pumps. In addition, a fraction of the fluid permeates through the enamel due to differential hydrostatic pressure. The appearance of dentinal fluid on the surface of enamel has been observed in various animal species, including humans. Maintaining a hydrostatic pressure within teeth is important because it prevents the ingress of bacterial products, responsible for demineralization, into the tooth structure. The flow of fluid onto the enamel surface has a cleansing and neutralizing effect on the tooth surface.

The importance of maintaining hydrostatic pressure is shown by what happens after administration of bradykinin. Bradykinin is a hormone which acts as a potent vasodilator. The acute effect in response to bradykinin is a drop in blood pressure which results in a decrease in the perfusion pressure in body tissues. In teeth, the effect of bradykinin is dramatic. Because of the drop in hydrostatic pressure, centrifugal movement of dentinal fluid becomes impaired and a significant ingress of substances into the tooth structure occurs from the oral cavity extending down into the dentin. The reversal of dentinal fluid movement by bradykinin is detrimental to dental health because injecting rats 2x/week for 3 months caused a significant increase in dental caries, even though the rats were fed a noncariogenic diet.

III. **Hormonal Control of DFT.** Our contribution to the understanding of the significance of DFT in relation to dental health is the discovery of an endocrine mechanism which stimulates DFT. This discovery provides insight on the importance of systemic factors in maintaining optimal dental health. Tooth physiology is intimately related to a broad spectrum of physiological mechanism(s).

Under physiological conditions, a hormone is secreted by the parotid glands that stimulates the DFT mechanism in rat molar teeth. The secretion of parotid hormone (PH) is under the control of a hypothalamic releasing factor (PHRF), thus a hypothalamic-parotid gland endocrine axis (HPEA) has been identified. This endocrine system functions normally in rats fed a noncariogenic diet, however hormonal secretion becomes impaired when the diet is changed to a cariogenic diet (65% sucrose). As a result of ingesting a high-sucrose diet, a marked decrease occurs in basal hormonal secretion. However, the functional capability of the dentinal fluid movement mechanism does not become impaired. In sugar-suppressed rats, stimulation of DFT in molar teeth can be accomplished by infusing intravenous crude or purified parotid or hypothalamic tissue extract obtained from a variety of species. In addition, infusion of two closely related compounds, carbamyl phosphate and carbamyl DL-aspartic acid are capable of stimulating the DFT mechanism in rats fed the high-sucrose diet. In rats this capability has been exploited to inhibit caries formation 80-100% by supplementing the cariogenic diet with carbamyl phosphate and other co-factors. The cariostatic effect of these compounds is achieved by overcoming the suppressive effect of the cariogenic diet on the HPEA. We have shown in the sugar-suppressed rat that carbamyl-DL-aspartic acid stimulates the secretion of PHRF, which in turn stimulates PH secretion. PH then stimulates the DFT mechanism.

IV. **Dental Caries - Relationship Between the Oral Environment and Systemic Factors.** The current consensus is that acid from bacterial origin is a primary factor in the induction of dental caries. As a result, enamel, representing the interface with the destructive oral environment, is regarded as the primary determinant for either resistance of susceptibility to cariogenesis. Decay is assumed to be a reflection of the amount of acid which penetrates into the enamel, with more acid leading to more decay. The implication of systemic factors involved in resistance to dental caries arises from (1) the suppression of the HPEA as a consequence of ingesting a cariogenic diet, and (2) the in-depth development of the carious lesion, even before total destruction of the enamel.

To study the role of systemic factors on cariogenesis, we examined the role of pulpal function and the endocrine function of salivary glands. An association between pulpal malfunction and the incidence of dental caries can be deduced from the decrease in caries that occurs in endodontically treated teeth, both in humans and rats. It is also known that destruction of salivary glands, whether by surgical removal, irradiation, or disease, significantly increases the incidence of decay. Desalivation (removal or incapacitation of the salivary glands) not only eliminates saliva from the oral cavity, but also any endocrine function.

In the caries study, the role of pulpal and salivary gland function was examined in certain groups of rats by treating the upper left and lower right first molars endodontically. The opposing first molars were left vital. Total sialoadenectomy (removal of salivary glands) was performed in certain groups of rats. The animal groups were:

Group 1: Intact controls with regard to salivary glands and first molars
Group 2: Total sialoadenectomy, all first molars were intact (vital)
Group 3: Intact salivary glands but with upper left and lower right first molars treated endodontically
Group 4: Total sialoadenectomy with upper left and lower right first molars treated endodontically

Each group was then subdivided into 2 groups. Groups 1-4 were maintained on a 65% sucrose diet. Groups 5-8 were also fed the 65% sucrose diet, but it was supplemented with carbamyl phosphate along with other co-factors that stimulated DFT in the sugar-suppressed rats. The data from this experiment are summarized in the table below:_

TABLE I Body wt, diet consumption & caries score as affected by operative procedure & diet

			Operative Procedures		Caries	Statistical
Group	Body wt, g	Diet/day, g	Surgery	Teeth	score	significance
			UNSUPPLEMENTED DIET			
1	425	17.6	Intact	No endo	3.3	*
2	294	19.7	Desalivated	No endo	14.4	*
3	416	16.8	Intact	No endo	3.5	*
				Endo	0.5	*
4	322	18.3	Desalivated	No endo	15.7	*
				Endo	1.3	*
			SUPPLEMENTED DIET			
5	442	18.5	Intact	No endo	0.6	*
6	294	18.0	Desalivated	No endo	12.5	*
7	416	17.5	Intact	No endo	0.4	*
				Endo	0.4	*
8	313	18.0	Desalivated	No endo	13.7	*
				Endo	1.3	*

PURINA LAB CHOW

Group	Body wt, g	Diet/day, g	Operative Procedures		Caries score	Statistical significance
			Surgery	Teeth		
9	406	21.1	Intact	No endo	0.2	*

* All were p <.001

There are 3 control groups (Groups 1, 5 and 9), however Groups 1 and 5 must be referenced against Group 9. Group 9 reflects the spontaneous incidence of dental caries which occurs in rats fed Purina lab chow, a noncariogenic diet. The caries score in this group (0.2 ±0.2) is extremely low. Comparing Group 2 against 9 shows that the unsupplemented high sucrose diet is cariogenic, causing a 16-fold increase in the caries score for the vital first molars. The mechanism through which the high sugar diet is cariogenic is not apparent from this comparison. Further insight is gained when Group 2 is compared to Group 1. An additional 4-fold increase in caries score is noted after desalivation, or a 72-fold increase when compared to Group 9. This comparison suggests that in addition to the potentially destructive effect of sugar in the oral environment, the cariogenicity of the sugar diet can be enhanced by removal of the salivary glands. This comparison suggests that salivary glands through systemic mechanism(s), either saliva production and secretion and/or humoral mechanism(s), participate in cariostasis.

Group 3 shows the effect of endodontia in relation to susceptibility to caries. Endodontic treatment reduces the incidence of caries to the level found in Group 9. Since the oral environment surrounding the vital and endodontically treated teeth is the same, it becomes evident that the increased susceptibility of the vital teeth must be the result of an internal failure rather than effect of the external environment. Since endodontic teeth are pulpless, then pulpal malfunction becomes suspect.

Groups 2 and 3 identify two systemic components which markedly affect caries susceptibility: (1) loss of salivary gland function, and (2) pulpal malfunction.

In relation to salivary gland function, the data presented thus far does not distinguish which component of salivary gland function is more important, salivary or humoral. Group 4 provides some insight. In this group, the animals are both sialoadenectomized and endodontically treated. Group 4 differs from Group 3 in that there is no saliva in the oral cavity, yet comparison of the caries scores for the endodontically treated teeth between the 2 groups reveals no statistically significant difference. The absence of saliva in Group 4 did not enhance susceptibility to dental caries, therefore it is concluded that the role of saliva in cariostasis is minimal at best. Since the susceptibility of the vital teeth in Group 4 was markedly enhanced (similar to Group 20) the primary role of salivary glands in cariostasis appears to be humoral rather than salivary.

The essential points which can be deduced from Groups 1-4 and 9 are the following:

1. A high sucrose diet is cariogenic
2. The oral environment is destructive, but it is not the primary determinant for cariogenesis
3. Since removal of the pulp decreases cariogenesis, the internal dynamics within the teeth are more important than the oral environment
4. Salivary glands have an essential role in cariostasis, but it is not

mediated through their salivary function; most probably the function is hormonal

By examining the cariogenic response in Groups 5-8, we gain insight into what is alluded to in Groups 1-4 as pulpal malfunction and hormonal secretion from salivary glands. The rats in Groups 5-8 were fed the same high sucrose diet, but it was supplemented with carbamyl phosphate and other co-factors essential for maintaining the DFT mechanism functional in sugar-suppressed rats. Comparing the caries incidence in Group 5 to Groups 1 and 9, it becomes clearly evident that a significant inhibiton in cariogenesis has occurred even though the rats were fed a cariogenic diet. The incidence of decay was not significantly different from that observed in Group 9 fed a noncariogenic diet. However, when the supplemented high-sucrose diet was fed to desalivated rats (Group 6), the incidence of decay increased significantly and was no different than that observed in Group 2. This observation establishes an important point. The cariostatic effectiveness of the supplements is not mediated through an effect in the oral cavity, but through the salivary glands. The result obtained with Group 7 is of particular interest. Note that the caries score for both the vital and endodontically treated teeth are the same. This represents a significant departure from Group 3 where the marked increase in caries score for the vital teeth was attributed to pulpal malfunction. In Group 7, the supplements prevented the deleterious effect on pulpal function, consequently cariogenesis was significantly inhibited. Group 8 affirms what was stated for Group 4, that saliva does not appear to have a significant cariostatic function.

The essential points which can be derived from all 9 groups of rats in the above table are the following:

1. The oral environment is destructive, but it is not the primary determinant
2. A high-sucrose diet is cariogenic, but its cariogenicity is not mediated in the oral cavity but rather through systemic mechanism(s) which involve the salivary glands (exclusive of saliva), and pulpal function
3. Supplementation of a high-sucrose diet as described significantly decreases the cariogenic potential of the sugar diet
4. Optimal pulpal function and hormonal secretion appear to be essential components in system mechanism(s) directed towards preventing cariogenesis

The above evidence makes the following hypothesis plausible. Under optimal physiologic conditions dental health is maintained by a hormonal mechanism which maintains the DFT mechanism functional. At the pulp-dentin interface, fluid moves out of the capillaries into the interstitial space surrounding the odontoblasts. Under the influence of hormones from the HPEA, the odontoblasts move this fluid, containing essential nutrients and minerals, into the dentin. Most of the fluid returns to the capillaries, however a portion of the fluid moves through the enamel under hydrostatic pressure which prevents the ingress of bacterial products into the tooth structure. In acute studies, we have observed that the ingestion of a cariogenic diet suppresses the HPEA, which in turn depresses DFT. This suppressive effect on the HPEA and DFT can be reversed by supplementing the cariogenic diet with carbamyl phosphate and co-factors (see addendum about co-factors). These supplements stimulate secretion of HPEA hormones which in turn stimulate DFT, consequently pulpal function is maintained. We believe that this accounts for the significant reduction in caries in rats fed the supplemented diet because hormonal and pulpal-dentinal function is optimally maintained.

V. **Physiology of the HPEA.** All of our research on DFT has been done in the rat model and our work on the physiology of the HPEA has been done in pigs because it was necessary to obtain numerous blood samples to follow the changes in PH titer in the blood. We have isolated porcine parotid hormone in essentially pure form. We know that it has a molecular weight of approximately 8100 daltons and we also know approximately 3/4 of its amino acid sequence. In addition, we have developed a radio-immunoassay (RIA) for quantifying PH levels in the blood. Thus far, we have only been able to partially purify the hypothalamic-parotid hormone releasing factor (PHRF) which stimulates parotid hormone secretion.

The importance of the integrity of the HPEA is shown in Fig. 3A. When a fraction containing the releasing factor activity, porcine hypothalamus-thalamus tissue extract (PHTE), is infused intravenously into intact pigs, there is an almost immediate rise (within 5 min) in PH titer in the blood which peaks at about 10 min. The response is absent when the infusion is performed on parotidectomized pigs. Note that removal of the parotids drops the basal level of PH below the level observed when only saline is infused. The data in Fig 3B show that the change in hormone secretion is not due to a surgical effect. The sham operated pigs responded essentially the same as intact pigs. These data suggest that a more complete understanding of the etiology of dental caries has to recognize that functional failure within the CNS can lead to cariogenesis. There is clinical evidence which supports this concept.

Fig. 3 – Factors Affecting Secretion of Parotid Hormone

An appropriate physiological question to ask is, "What stimulates HPEA secretion to benefit the host in preventing cariogenesis?" Ideally hormonal secretion should occur when the microbe in the oral cavity is metabolically active. This occurs each time the host ingests food. Eating not only provides nutrients for the host, but it also provides metabolizable substrate for the microbe to produce acid. The most effective method for preventing decay is to deny the microbe metabolizable substrate. Carried to its logical conclusion, starvation prevents decay.

Our study in pigs shows that feeding is a potent stimulus for the secretion of the HPEA hormones. Fig. 4 shows that there is an almost immediate rise in hormone secretion in response to feeding. Within 10 minutes there is an 11-fold increase in the parotid hormone titer in the blood. The hormone is cleared rather slowly from blood over a 5-hour period. Providing a 2nd feeding 3 hrs after the 1st stimulates a second rise in hormone secretion.

Fig. 4 – Comparison of Responsiveness of Parotid Glands to Single and Double Feedings

After parotidectomy, the PH response to feeding was abolished. In contrast, the sham operation did not significantly alter the response (Fig. 5). This emphasizes the importance of maintaining the integrity of the HPEA if responsiveness to the feeding stimulus is expected.

Fig. 5– Immunoreactive Parotid Hormone Response in the Pig after Lab Chow Feeding

The effect of various stimuli on parotid hormone secretion is shown in Table 4. Chewing by itself is not particularly effective. Neither are visual and olfactory stimuli.

This is notable in view of the role of the CNS in preparation to eating. The most effective stimulus is feeding. Allowing a pig to eat for 15-60 seconds provides a sufficient neurogenic stimulus to cause a significant increase in parotid hormone secretion.

Table 4 – Effect of Various Stimuli Related to Feeding on Secretion of iPH in the Pig

Stimulus	Amount (gm)	iPH Titer Group number	Maximum response	N	Statistical Comparison	P
CHEWING VS. FEEDING						
None (fasting)		1	1.2	4		
Ice chewing		2	1.2	4	1 vs. 2	NS*
Feeding pig chow	1200	3	8.4	5	1 vs. 3	<0.01
VISUAL-OLFACTORY FEEDING						
None (fasting)		4	1.2	5		
Feed presentation		5	1.1	5	4 vs. 5	NS*
Feeding pig chow	1200	6	5.7	5	4 vs. 6	<0.01
VARIOUS AMOUNTS OF PIG CHOW						
None (fasting)		7	1.2	5		
15-sec feeding	32	8	2.0	5	7 vs. 8	<0.01**
1 min feeding	85	9	3.5	5		
5-min feeding	226	10	9.5	5		
Full meal	1200	11	10.2	5	10 vs. 11	NS

Values are means ± SE; N = no. of animals in the group. iPH = immunoreactive parotid hormone. *Significance was ascertained by Dunnett's test. ** Significance was ascertained by Student's t test for unequal variances.

In summary, we have physiological evidence that the secretion of HPEA hormones is linked to eating. In the rat, preliminary evidence shows that feeding stimulates DFT. In terms of tooth physiology, this is important. It means that we have linked hormonal secretion and DFT stimulation. The DFT mechanism is optimally functional when teeth are most vulnerable to microbial attack.

Article #83

The physiologic nature of caries susceptibility – Part I

Steinman RR. J Alabama Dent Assn. 66:20-23, 1982

Our knowledge of dental caries could be summarized by saying we know WHAT and HOW, but we don't know WHY. The major thrust of dental research has been directed toward the external environment of the teeth. It is well established that certain strains of bacteria are the infective agent in this disease, however there are no specific bacteria found only in those who have active caries and not found in those who are caries-free. Bacteria that have been shown to be related to caries are indigenous to both groups. Why do we find wide variations in the incidence of caries when both groups have the infective flora? This suggests the importance of resistance to caries as a possible explanation. Most theories of dental caries are concerned with what molecule destroys tooth structure, whether an acid, chelating agent, enzyme or whatever. The consensus is the destructive agent is an acid end product of bacterial metabolism, which may answer the question of *how* the tooth is destroyed. Rat saliva incubation studies have observed the production of acid on the external surface of a tooth may be essential for caries, but it does not predict how much caries will occur in relation to a given food, which is quite variable. Again the importance of resistance is suggested. In humans, teeth that are vital decay most readily. After endodontic treatment there is significantly less caries [refs]. The purpose of this paper is to examine *why* teeth may or may not develop caries in the presence of an obviously destructive oral environment.

Malfunction and Disease

The relation between malfunction and certain disease is well-recognized. When the blood vessels become partially obliterated in the heart, the patient develops heart disease. Restricted blood supply to any organ may encourage disease. Failure of endocrine glands may produce disease states, for example when the pancreas malfunctions the patient will probably develop diabetes. Malfunction of an endocrine gland usually causes disease in tissues it regulates. Is it possible that dental caries may also be related to a malfunction?

Fluid Exchange in Animals

Like the capillaries in the kidneys and the villi of the intestines, capillaries in the dental pulp adjacent to the odontoblasts are fenestrated [ref]. This special design encourages a rapid fluid exchange between the capillaries and the odontoblasts. The enamel is 2% mobile water by volume [ref]. The fluid connection between the pulp, dentin and enamel can be compared to a pipe with three sections open at both ends. The odontoblasts act as the gate keeper or director of traffic in this system. The direction of fluid movement depends on the forces applied. A normal healthy tooth has an outwardly mobile fluid movement [ref], which is regulated by the hypothalamic-parotid gland endocrine axis [refs], plus the hydrostatic pressure of the pulp [ref], which depends on normal blood flow through the tissue. If this complex biological system fails to function properly, the normal fluid movement tends to reverse. It flows inwardly through the enamel and dentin into the pulp [ref]. The tooth loses its resistance and caries ensues.

Influence of Blood Supply in Animals

As observed in other parts of the body, normal function requires an adequate blood supply. Ligating the major blood vessels to the teeth adversely affects their hydrodynamic system by reducing the amount of blood flow through the pulp. Ligation also reduces the supply of nutrients and hormones that regulate pulpal metabolism. Dental caries increases in teeth with restricted blood supplies [ref]. Further study revealed this surgery did not affect salivary gland function [ref]. It was caused by some unexplained alteration in the tooth pulp. Recent research [ref] showed increased caries in teeth with hindered vascularization compared to teeth with a normal blood flow in the same animals. It reported that “a positive correlation between caries score and the pulp inflammation grade was observed.” A reduced blood supply to the tooth pulp increased the incidence of dental caries.

Hormonal Influence in Animals

A malfunction of the pulp may be imposed by pharmacologic means. Intraperitoneal administration of the tissue hormone bradykinin caused an inward movement of material from the plaque through the enamel, dentin and into the pulp of molars in rats [ref]. When bradykinin was administered to young rats on a non-cariogenic diet, there was a highly significant increase in caries [ref]. Systemic administration of bradykinin has also been shown to decrease pulpal blood flow. Why the administration of bradykinin causes increased caries is not known, but its effect on pulpal blood flow could be a factor. The increase in caries may result from imposed adverse pulpal conditions.

Dietary Effect in Animals

Evidence shows that reduced fluid exchange in the dentin is associated with a high sucrose cariogenic diet in rats. In a study of the movement of acriflavine HCl, the fluorescent dye did not move toward the dentinoenamel junction as readily in the molars of rats on a high-sucrose cariogenic diet as in rats fed a noncariogenic diet [ref]. A malfunctioning dentin-pulp complex may be imposed by the diet with a concomitant increase in caries.

Human Teeth

Observation of human teeth also suggests that inward movement of fluid in the tooth structure is an important feature of this disease in humans. The presence of inflammatory cells in human pulps beneath early enamel caries suggests that an inward fluid movement is associated with the caries process [ref]. An increase in ninhydrin reaction beneath the caries process is also evidence of an inward movement of fluid (Figs. I, II, and III). This is further supported by the marked difference in the condition of pulps under erosion, which is a surface demineralization of tooth structure, and beneath true dental caries [ref]. If the vermiform process malfunctions resulting in appendicitis, the patient no longer has appendicitis after the offending appendix is removed. If malfunction of the pulp is related to dental caries, what effect does its removal have on the disease? Significantly less caries occurs in endodontically treated human teeth than in vital teeth in the same oral cavity [ref]. Similar observations have been made in experimental animal studies [refs]. Even in desalivated animals, endodontically treated teeth have less caries than vital teeth in the same mouth. The endodontic desalivation experiments separated the systemic effect of salivary gland hormones from the local effect of saliva. The increase in caries following desalivation appears to be caused by an absence of some hormonal factor of salivary gland origin rather than due to the absence of saliva in the oral cavity [ref]. **Endodontic treatment seals the hydraulic system of the tooth on one end and the fluid in the tooth is no longer free to move in either direction.**

Conclusion

Several experimental approaches to the question of dental caries susceptibility have been discussed. Restricting the blood supply to the pulp, systemically administering bradykinin, feeding a high sucrose cariogenic diet, and removing the pulp all affect the dentin-pulp complex. A malfunction of the dentin-pulp complex plays a major role in caries susceptibility. What is the basis of resistance? It is the normal biological system in the tooth. It can be manipulated to decrease caries in animals fed a high-sucrose cariogenic diet. In other words, if you restore normal function, you will reduce dental caries. Certain nutrients and hormones play a role in this phenomenon which will be discussed in Part II.

Article #84

The physiologic nature of caries susceptibility – Part II

(Interactions between plaque, bacteria and the tooth)

Steinman RR. J Alabama Dent Assn 67:51-53, 1983

The dictionary defines disease as "a disturbed or abnormal structure or physiological action in the living organism as a whole or in any of its parts; a morbid condition resulting from such disturbance." A disturbance in blood supply can cause disease in a tissue or organ, and conversely disease in a tissue or organ can cause a disturbance in blood supply. Failure of an endocrine gland can cause disease in the tissues it regulates. In Part I all three of these conditions were found to be associated with an increase in dental caries—an infectious disease. This suggests the oral cavity bacteria take advantage of a morbid condition in the teeth that prepares the way for a successful attack and invasion. Is the response of the teeth to bacterial invasion similar to that of other tissues, or are the teeth passive subjects to bacterial destruction?

Bacterial colonies are found in close proximity to many tissues of the body. This is particularly true of tissues covered with a mucous membrane or where moisture and food are available. What is unique about teeth is they are the only calcified tissue with bacterial colonies on their surfaces. All other calcified tissues are protected from a destructive environment by a soft tissue covering. Bacteria associated with the teeth have an ability to form plaque, which adheres to the smooth surfaces of the teeth as well as proliferates into the pits and fissures. The same food that nourishes the host also supplies nutrients to the bacteria. The presence of micronutrients is beneficial to both the host and the bacteria, as shown by saliva-food mixture studies [refs].

The consensus is that the decalcification of tooth structure is caused by acid—the end product of bacterial metabolism. **Also in the plaque are such toxic end products of bacterial metabolism as hydrogen sulfide, toxic amines and ammonia. If these chemicals penetrate into the tooth, they are capable of compromising the ability of the odontoblasts to function normally.** The bioelectrical potential of the plaque is thought to be a factor in the carious process. Consideration will be given first to the effect of bioelectrical phenomenon on calcified structures. This will be followed by observing the response of the teeth to bacterial invasion.

<u>Bioelectrical Phenomenon</u>

The fluid connection between the pulp, dentin and enamel during metabolism has been compared to a pipe of three sections which is open at both ends. This fluid, like other fluids in the body, is capable of conducting electrical currents that affect calcified tissues. An electrical potential applied to bone will cause demineralization at the positive electrode and calcification at the negative pole [refs]. Electric currents have been successfully applied to bone to increase the rate of healing of defects and fractures [refs]. Electric currents applied to tooth structure act to produce decalcification at the positive electrode and calcification at the negative electrode [ref].

Dental plaque can act as a fuel cell or battery, capable of generating an electrical potential well over 100 millivolts [ref]. **A dramatic increase in electrical potential occurs when the plaque is flushed with a sugar solution. It may go as high as 450 millivolts [ref]. Parker [ref], as well as Dickerson and Lenoir [ref], believe this electrical potential of the plaque may play a part in the decalcification of tooth structure associated with caries**.

Is the tooth defenseless against the applied electrical potential of the plaque? Bone and teeth maintain a resting electrical potential. Cellular activity regulates bioelectrical potential in bone and teeth, and when metabolism ceases the electrical potential also ceases [ref].

The enamel surface has an electrical potential of 0 to 20 positive millivolts in relation to the pulp's negative electrical potential. This is due to a difference in the ionic strength of saliva and of pulpal blood as well as to metabolism within the tooth. The average resting electrical potential of the enamel surface varies from 5 to 10 positive millivolts. Ion transport during metabolism is essential to maintain a resting electrical potential in the tooth. There is evidence that the resting electrical potential of the enamel surface is maintained by metabolism within the tooth. If acid is applied to the surface of a vital tooth, the surface electrical potential becomes 45-50 negative millivolts. However, it does not remain at that level but returns very rapidly to the resting electrical potential [ref]. Since the acid is not subject to change, it must be assumed that the movement of ions during metabolism within the tooth alters the difference in electrical potential. If the metabolism of the tooth is compromised, this can no longer be accomplished and the tooth mineral is in danger of electrolysis. Remember, it is the internal activity that maintains the resting electrical potential of the tooth.

Ca^{45} exchange studies in rat molars suggest that the exchange ratio is 8 for bone, 2 for dentin and 1 for enamel [ref]. The chemical composition of human enamel fluid has been partially characterized [ref]. Both calcium and potassium were found in measurable amounts. Of particular interest is that calcium in this fluid appears to be mobile, exchangeable, and can be influenced by an electrical field.

It appears that if the tooth is unable to restore the resting electrical potential due to a failure in metabolism within the tooth, calcium would tend to move from the deeper portions of the tooth to the negatively charged plaque on the surface. It is like applying a current to the tooth from a battery. If this movement of mineral occurs rapidly, the subsurface enamel tends to demineralize under the influence of the imposed positive electrical potential while the surface enamel tends to mineralize due to the negative electrical potential of the plaque [ref]. The plaque becomes dominant due to a failure of the tooth to maintain a resting electrical potential. Metabolic ion transport becomes a key factor in maintaining tooth structure against the electrical potential of plaque. This suggestion in no way reduces the importance of acid in the carious process.

Any surface mineral lost due to acid in early caries is replaced by the action of the negative electrical potential of the plaque. Thus, the observed intact enamel surface with a demineralized subsurface occurs. The mineral component of the tooth is influenced by the bioelectrical potentials operating in both the plaque and in the tooth. A disturbance in normal electrical potential may cause mineral exchange within the enamel.

Bacterial Invasion

It is well established that certain strains of bacteria are essential for the carious process. Other tissues subjected to bacterial invasion respond to the challenge. The body produces antibodies which move into the area in an effort to defend the body. There is an effort by the body to isolate or wall off the invading organisms. These defense reactions are not always successful and the bacteria may spread further into the body. What is the response of the tooth to bacterial invasion?

When the bacterial invasion reaches the dentinoenamel junction, immunoglobulins are "physiologically localized in the dentin in response to the destructive stimuli of caries" [ref]. These antibodies are arranged in a defensive formation to protect the pulp. The source of these antibodies is the blood supply to the pulp and they are apparently transported to their defensive position under the influence of the odontoblasts.

An additional response of the tooth to bacterial invasion concerns its mineral component. Hypercalcification may be found between the pulp and the area of invasion. This is an effort by nature to wall off the area of invasion. It is an effort by nature to wall off the area of infection from the rest of the body. Secondary dentin or reparative dentin is also formed to further protect the pulp from a direct invasion of bacteria. If these measures are not successful, the infection spreads to the pulp and to the rest of the body.

All activities of the body, whether calcification, nerve impulses, fluid transport, muscle contraction or brain function, require energy. This energy is supplied in the form of adenosine triphosphate (ATP). The more ATP present in a tissue, the greater its capacity for work. The ATP levels were measured in various layers of dentin beneath caries and beneath fillings placed in human teeth [ref]. Beneath caries confined to the enamel, there is a significant increase in ATP in the dentin. When the caries reaches the dentin or when a filling is placed, there is a 100% increase in ATP compared to the same areas when caries is confined to the enamel. There was increased phosphoesterase activity in the pre-pulpal dentin layer under incipient carious changes in the dentin [ref]. Apparently the dentin is already in the early stages of caries both anabolically and catabolically. The necessary energy for these defensive activites is supplied in the dentin.

The earliest evidence of demineralization of rat molars fed a cariogenic diet is often observed at the dentinoenamel junction. This will often remineralize if the animals are fed a noncariogenic diet. The addition of fluoride to the dietary regimen enhanced remineralization of these areas [refs]. A change in diet is essential to the remineralization of these teeth.

When the tooth's defense to bacterial attack fails, changes occur in the pulp. The most frequent changes observed are an impairment of the odontoblastic layer and an accumulation of exudate cells beneath the carious area due to toxic material from the plaque reaching the pulp of the tooth [refs]. This further compromises the ability of the pulp to function normally. Unless a filling is placed at this time, the tooth is doomed to destruction.

It should be obvious that the tooth is not an inert appendage in a destructive environment, but a vital organ capable of resistance when functioning normally. When these defenses fail, the tooth is left to bacterial invasion and destruction. As in any other organ with a number of biologic activities, different malfunctions can occur which adversely affect the health of the tooth. The problems are not amenable to one simple solution. Life is complex whether it concerns a tooth or the whole body.

Article #85

The physiologic nature of caries susceptibility – Part III

(Physiologic aspects of resistance to dental caries)

Steinman RR. J Alabama Dent Assn 67:46-49, 1983

"A healthy individual lives in harmony with his normal body flora, but his balance may be disturbed by disease" [ref]. The dictionary defines disease as "disturbed or abnormal structure or physiological action in the living organism as a whole or in any of its parts." Dental caries is an infectious disease caused by microbes that are members of the normal body flora, so freedom from caries is generally associated with normal physiologic function within the tooth. It has been previously suggested that susceptibility to caries is a reflection of malfunction. This concluding installment will consider how normal physiologic function is associated with resistance to dental caries and how this normal function may be improved.

The vital teeth of the young develop caries most readily, but not all young vital teeth become carious. This is a period of life when metabolic activity is greatest in the teeth. Has something gone wrong with the metabolic activity in those young teeth that decay? If no dental caries develops, may we conclude that normal activity is occurring? The experiments cited in this series of papers were conducted on young animals. If the findings are applicable to humans they would certainly apply to the young. The observations in human teeth referred to in these papers are also most frequently seen in the young.

FLUID TRANSPORT RATE IN DENTIN

What process in the teeth indicates normal or abnormal physiologic activity? Fundamental to metabolism in any tissue is the extravascular transport system at the cellular level. Animals fed Purina Laboratory Chow experienced little or no dental caries and demonstrated normal fluid transport in dentin while animals fed a high-sucrose cariogenic diet had a depressed fluid transport [refs]. If the rate of dentinal fluid transport can be used as an indication of normal physiological activity within the teeth, resistance to caries is associated with normal dentinal fluid transport.

The administration of a parasympathetic stimulant increased the rate of dentinal fluid transport in animals fed a high-sucrose cariogenic diet with a corresponding decrease in dental caries [refs]. The subcutaneous administration of urea also significantly increased the rate of dentinal fluid transport in animals fed a high-sucrose cariogenic diet and decreased caries [ref]. The restoration of a normal rate of dentinal fluid transport is associated with a reduction in dental caries. These observations suggest the essentiality of a normal dentinal fluid transport for dental health.

Intravenous administration of several compounds of the urea cycle has been found to stimulate the rate of fluid movement in the dentin of rats fed a high-sucrose cariogenic diet [ref]. When one of these compounds, carbamyl phosphate, was added in millimole amounts to a high-sucrose diet, a significant decrease in caries was observed [ref]. Again, when normal function was restored, a reduction in caries was observed. The addition of certain trace elements to this diet enhanced the effect of the carbamyl phosphate and further reduced the incidence of caries. **Resistance depends on normal dentinal fluid transport.**

Various organs and tissues are regulated by hormones and to a lesser extent by the parasympathetic system. **It is thought that compounds like carbamyl phosphate restore normal fluid transport in the teeth of animals fed a high-sucrose cariogenic diet by releasing hormones from the hypothalamic-parotid endocrine axis** [refs]. The hypothalamus produces a hormone that travels through the blood stream to the parotid salivary gland. The parotid salivary gland then releases the parotid hormone that travels to the pulp of the tooth and stimulates the fluid transport system in the dentin.

After one week of eating a high-sucrose cariogenic diet, demineralization is observed at the dentinoenamel junction. If the animals are then fed a noncariogenic diet, such as Purina laboratory chow, these areas of demineralization will often remineralize. The addition of fluoride to the dietary regimen has been found to enhance remineralization of these areas [refs]. **Caries was arrested when the malfunction was corrected by an improvement in the nutritional value of the diet. In addition to any**

local effect fluoride may have on the incidence of caries, it has been observed in our laboratory that it stimulates the fluid transport in dentin. This report has not been published. The restoration of normal physiological activity is associated with an arresting of dental caries.

A number of years ago Boyd and Drain, working in the Childrens Hospital of State University of Iowa with diabetic children, observed that when the diet of these children was corrected and the diabetes brought under control, the caries was arrested [refs]. At that time caries was thought to be a local problem and little notice was given to their work. Their findings agree with what was observed in the above-mentioned animal studies. Again, if the underlying problem of malfunction is corrected, dental caries may be arrested.

Diet

Food-saliva incubation studies suggest that the improvement of the diet in no way reduces the ability of the bacteria to produce acid [refs]. In fact, foods with micronutrients produced significantly more acid than an equal caloric amount of sucrose or glucose. Consumed foods nourish both the host and the bacteria. Excess of sucrose was found to inhibit the release of the parotid hormone which plays an important role in the health of teeth. The cariogenicity of foods may be a reflection of their deficiency in micronutrients, often produced by an excess of sucrose, and its effect on the host of suppressing the mechanisms of resistance. At least that is something to think about.

The components of the metabolic machinery found in teeth—ATP [ref], glycolysis [ref], collagen turnover [ref], cyclic AMP [ref]—are not unique to the teeth but are common in other tissues. The need of minerals for the gradual exchange [ref] through the years is not restricted to the teeth but is similar to calcified tissues in general, albeit at a slower rate. The need of hormones [refs] for metabolic regulation is common in all tissues. The need of energy for transport and physiologic activity is not unique to the teeth. It is required by many other tissues.

Where does the body get all these wonderful molecules? From what are they made? The body, including the teeth, gets the material for all its metabolic activity directly or indirectly from food. In addition to the calories food supplies, each calorie must be supplemented by vitamins, minerals and trace elements or it is useless to the body. For example, in order for the body to make ATP from carbohydrates it requires B_1, B_2, niacin, pantothenic acid, magnesium, phosphorus, iron, copper, zinc and manganese.

It is not my purpose, nor is it possible within the confines of this article, to review all of the experiments concerning various nutrients and their effect on dental caries. Since saliva-food incubation studies show that acid production by bacteria is enhanced in food with a micronutrient content, in contrast with the small amount of acid produced in sucrose, glucose or starch [ref] alone, and since the parotid hormone is important in maintaining dental health, this article will be confined to the effect of nutrients on the production, suppression and release of the parotid hormone.

Protein

The parotid hormone is a polypeptide [ref]. The building blocks to make this hormone are found in the protein segment of the diet. No doubt, certain vitamins, minerals and trace elements are also required.

Compounds like urea, carbamyl phosphate and citrulline are of protein origin. These compounds stimulate the dentinal fluid transport by their effect on the hypothalamic-parotid endocrine axis [ref]. The administration of these compounds also reduced the incidence of caries in animals fed a high-sucrose cariogenic diet [refs]. The importance of protein in the diet for physiologic activity within the tooth, which seems to be related to dental caries resistance, is obvious. **A number of studies have shown that an increase in dental caries may be associated with a deficiency of protein in the diet.**

<u>Sucrose</u>

A high-sucrose diet causes a significant increase in dental caries compared to Purina laboratory chow. There is a suppressed rate of fluid transport in the dentin of rats fed a high-sucrose diet [refs].

The addition of carbamyl phosphate in millimole amounts stimulates fluid transport in dentin and reduces dental caries in animals fed a high-sucrose diet [ref]. This increase in the dentinal fluid transport is thought to be caused by the release of the parotid hormone into the blood stream and its subsequent stimulation of the pulp-dentin complex in the teeth.

<u>Trace Elements</u>

The enrichment of a high-sucrose diet with Zn, Mo, Cr and eggshell meal enhanced the stimulating effect of the carbamyl phosphate and further reduced caries.

The desalivation endodontic study, using both a high-sucrose cariogenic diet and an enriched high-sucrose diet, separated the systemic effect from the local oral cavity effect of these two diets. It was concluded that for enrichment to be effective in reducing caries, the enriched diet must be given to animals with vital tooth pulps. In other words, it reduced caries by some systemic means. Furthermore, the increase in caries associated with desalivation was largely due to the absence of some hormonal factor of salivary gland origin [ref]. Whatever local effect sucrose may have in increasing caries, it also suppresses the release of the parotid hormone which is an important determinant in maintaining dental health.

By means of a radioimmunoassay of the parotid hormone in a live pig, a series of studies were done to determine the effect of various foods on the release of the parotid hormone, which will be published later. Sufficient for our discussion is that immediately upon eating the pig chow, a very rapid increase in blood level of the parotid hormone is observed which reaches a maximum in 20 to 30 minutes. When the pig is fed a high-sucrose cariogenic diet, there is no release of the parotid hormone into the blood stream. If the pig chow and sucrose are combined, the release of the parotid hormone is significantly reduced from that observed when only pig chow is fed.

<u>CLINICAL IMPLICATIONS</u>

What about the sugary between-meal snack? It will not cause the release of the parotid hormone that stimulates a defense mechanism in the teeth and is nature's way of defending the teeth against caries. It will give the plaque organisms nutrients to produce acid and any other destructive material in their arsenal. And it will do this at a time when the teeth are defenseless.

What about sugar at meal time? There is some stimulating effect on the release of the parotid hormone, the amount depending on the amount of sugar, the amount of micronutrients in the meal and the response of the host, which can vary among individuals.

Since milk and milk products are usually associated with less caries, what about the bottle-fed caries syndrome? I would suggest there is probably a depressed release of parotid hormone influenced by the amount of sugar in the formula and by less hormone being released during sleep [ref].

Normal function of the teeth prevents caries. The answer to the problem is not likely to be found in a prescription which can be given to all, but, since the problem is as complex as life, everything that affects the health and welfare of the body may affect the health of the teeth.

Perhaps no better recommendation can be made than the *Dietary Goals for the United States,* prepared by the staff of the Senate Select Committee on Nutrition and Human Needs [ref]. **They recommend that we reduce the added sucrose in the diet by 40% (I would suggest 80%),** increase the use of fruit and vegetables and replace the refined cereal products with corresponding whole grain products. What would this do for the teeth? It would reduce the amount of sucrose and increase the amount of micronutrients in the diet, which are so essential for the health of the teeth and the body. The basis of resistance is normal function.

What does all of this have to do with the validity of the chemico-parasitic theory of dental caries? Most theories of dental caries are concerned with what destroys the teeth, what is the decalcifying agent. This article says nothing about what destroys teeth, but rather why the active agent destroys teeth. **The chemico-parasitic theory stands unchallenged by this material. What this paper does is explain why the theory may be valid and why the teeth are susceptible.**

Article #86

Biologic activity in the tooth in health and disease

Steinman RR. Comp Contin Educ Dent 9:722-728, 1984

Disease and malfunction in the hydraulic system

A reduction in the blood supply to a tissue may be associated with disease. A disturbance of fluid transport in a tissue may result in edema. The failure of endocrine glands is often associated with an increase in susceptibility to disease. Could any of these conditions adversely affect the health and physiologic activity of the teeth?

In fact the hydraulic system of the tooth could be affected by these conditions. This system can be compared to a pipe that consists of two sections—dentin and enamel—and which is open at both ends. It is filled with fluid which can move in either direction or not move at all. The dentin end is in contact with pulpal fluid. In this system, the odontoblasts act as gatekeepers or directors of traffic flow. Whether there is fluid movement in this imaginary pipe depends largely on the enamel. The enamel is porous. The pore size of the enamel is 5 nanometers [ref] which is large enough to permit the passage of molecules the size of methylene blue [ref] or acriflavine hydrochloride [ref] dye materials. Two percent by volume of the enamel is mobile water [ref]. This water is not bound but rather is free to move in either direction, depending upon the forces applied to it. Normally, the enamel fluid moves from the dentinoenamel junction toward the surface of the tooth [refs].

The normal hydraulic system of the tooth is important because the dentin requires an active transport, without which its rate of metabolism would not be possible [ref]. The pulp is designed to support this hydraulic system. **The rate of blood flow in the pulp of the tooth is four times the rate of blood flow in resting muscle** [ref]. **The capillaries**

adjacent to the odontoblasts are fenestrated [ref]. Such capillaries are found in areas of rapid exchange, such as the kidney or the villi of the intestines. It is obvious that the teeth are designed to facilitate a rapid exchange between the blood vessels and the adjacent tooth structure.

Restriction of the Blood Supply to the Teeth

Ligating the major blood vessels to the teeth could adversely affect the hydraulics, the nutrient supply, and the availability of hormones for pulpal regulation. This observation stems from an experiment which resulted in a significant increase in the amount of caries in the teeth of rats whose blood supply was restricted [ref]. Further study revealed that the associated surgery did not adversely affect salivary gland function [ref]. This increase in caries could be explained most logically as resulting from some effect upon the pulp or adjacent tissue of the tooth.

A recent report showed that, when the pulp vascularization of hamsters had been hindered, there was an increased incidence of caries compared to that of teeth with normal blood flow in the same animal. It stated further that "a positive correlation between caries score and the pulp inflammation grade was observed" [ref].

Alteration in Fluid Transport in the Dentin and Associated Increase in Caries

A malfunction in the hydraulics of the tooth can be imposed by an intraperitoneal administration of bradykinin, a tissue hormone. When administered to rats, it was found to cause an inward movement of fluid—from the plaque, through the enamel, through the dentin, and into the pulps of molars [ref] (Figs 1A and 1B). When administered regularly to young rats fed a noncariogenic diet, the imposed disturbance was associated with a highly significant increase in caries [refs]. It was also demonstrated that the administration of bradykinin caused a decrease in pulpal blood flow [ref].

Another technique that produced a malfunction in the hydraulics of the tooth, with a reversal in the normal direction of fluid transport, was the administration of hydrogen peroxide to rats by stomach tube [ref]. With this procedure, dye placed in the oral cavity penetrated through the tips of the cusps of molars. The tips of the cusps of rat molars have no enamel protection (Fig's 2A and 2B). Although bacteria are present on this surface and there is occasional invasion of the tubules, usually no caries is present [ref]. However, when the administration of hydrogen peroxide was continued regularly to young rats, it was associated with dental caries in the tips of the cusps, the area of penetration [ref]. Logically, it could be assumed that the caries was due to the inward movement of fluid. The authors suggest that the absence of caries normally is the result of the fluid transport in the dentin. Thus, reversal in the normal direction of fluid through the teeth is associated with a dramatic increase in caries, strongly suggesting the role of fluid transport in the health of the teeth.

Effect of a High-Sucrose Cariogenic Diet on the Hydraulics of the Teeth

A study of the movement in dentin of acriflavine hydrochloride, a fluorescent dye, showed that the dye did not move to the dentinoenamel junction as readily in the molars of rats fed a high-sucrose cariogenic diet as it did in animals fed a noncariogenic diet [refs] (Fig's 3A and 3B). This was true in both germ-free animals and those with the conventional oral flora [ref].

The accumulation of trypan blue in the dentin of rat molars following the intraperitoneal injection of the dye was also less in the teeth of rats fed the high-sucrose cariogenic diet than in the teeth of rats fed the noncariogenic diet. This was true in both crowned and uncrowned teeth [ref]. Thus, malfunction of the pulp-dentin hydraulic complex can be imposed through alteration in diet. There is also, of course, a concomitant increase in the incidence of dental caries with the high-sucrose cariogenic diet.

Stasis of the hydraulic system of the teeth is found in endodontically treated teeth. There is no inward fluid movement beneath the plaque, which may help to explain why endodontically treated teeth have a lower incidence of caries than intact teeth in the same oral cavity [refs]. Passive diffusion would be the mode of penetration beneath the plaque into these teeth.

The Effect of a Reduced Rate of Fluid Transport in Teeth on Their External Environment

Concomitant with reduced dentinal fluid movement is a movement from outside the tooth beneath the plaque into the tooth. This is a reversal in the normal direction of fluid transport in the tooth. It is demonstrated by the movement of methylene blue from the oral cavity beneath the plaque through the enamel into the dentin [ref] (Fig's 4A and 4B), compared with little or no inward movement of dye into animal teeth that are caries-free.

The presence of inflammatory cells in the pulps of human teeth beneath early caries would suggest that an inward movement of fluid is occurring with the carious process [ref]. The marked increase in ninhydrin reaction beneath the carious process in human teeth also may be evidence of this inward movement [ref] (Fig's 5A and 5B). The lack of ninhydrin reaction beneath erosion would suggest that no inward movement is associated with erosion (Fig 5C).

The suppressed rate of fluid transport in the dentin of animals fed the high-sucrose cariogenic diet is thought to be due to the suppression of the hypothalamic-parotid gland endocrine axis. The hypothalamus releases into the blood stream a factor which stimulates the parotid gland, in turn, to release into the blood stream the parotid hormone. This hormone stimulates the transport system in the dentin of the teeth [refs]. Thus, the removal of the salivary glands may adversely affect the health of the teeth, both through the absence of saliva on the external surfaces of the teeth and through the absence of hormonal stimulation of the fluid transport within the teeth [ref].

Stimulating the Rate of Fluid Transport

Can the suppressed rate of dentinal fluid transport be stimulated in animals fed the high-sucrose cariogenic diet? How would this procedure affect the incidence of caries? The administration of a parasympathetic stimulant was found to increase the rate of dentinal fluid transport in the teeth of animals fed the high-sucrose cariogenic diet. There was also a corresponding decrease in the incidence of dental caries [refs]. The subcutaneous administration of urea also was found to significantly increase the rate of dentinal fluid transport in the teeth of animals fed the cariogenic diet. Again there was a corresponding decrease in caries [ref].

When infused intravenously, several compounds of the urea cycle have been found to stimulate the rate of fluid movement in the dentin of rats fed the high-sucrose cariogenic diet [ref]. When one of these compounds, carbamyl phosphate, was added to the cariogenic diet in millimole amounts, a significant decrease in caries was observed [ref]. Thus, when normal function of the hydraulic system was restored, a reduction in caries was observed. Furthermore, the addition of certain trace elements to this diet was found to enhance the effect of carbamyl phosphate and result in a further reduction in the incidence of caries. However, enriching the diet was only effective in reducing the incidence of caries in intact teeth of intact animals [ref].

It is thought that compounds like carbamyl phosphate restore normal fluid transport in the teeth of animals fed the high-sucrose cariogenic diet by releasing hormones of the hypothalamic-parotid gland endocrine axis [refs]. The restoration of the normal rate of fluid transport in turn restores normal function in the pulp-dentin complex, thus resulting in a reduction in the incidence of dental caries. The oral flora are still eating the high-sucrose diet, although the caries rate has been reduced.

Reversing Induced Malfunctions

If one malfunction has been induced in the teeth of young animals, can it be reversed, and what would be the result of such reversal?

After one week of eating the high-sucrose cariogenic diet, young animals often demonstrate demineralization at the dentinoenamel junction. If the animals are then fed a noncariogenic diet, these areas often will remineralize [refs]. In addition, the caries process is arrested when the malfunction is corrected by an improvement in the nutritional value of the diet.

A number of years ago, Boyd and Drain, working with diabetic children in the Childrens' Hospital of the State University of Iowa, observed that when the diets of these children were corrected and the diabetes brought under control the caries was arrested [ref]. Again, if the underlying problem of malfunction is corrected, caries may be arrested.

What is the Response of the Tooth to Bacterial Invasion?

When the bacterial invasion reaches the dentinoenamel junction, immunoglobulins are "physiologically localized in the dentin in response to the destructive stimuli of caries" [ref] (Fig 6). These antibodies are arranged in the dentin in a defensive formation. The source of these antibodies is the blood supply of the pulp. They are apparently transported to their defensive position under the influence of the odontoblasts.

Another response of the tooth to bacterial invasion involves the mineral component. **Hypercalcification may be found between the pulp and the area of invasion. Also, secondary dentin is formed to further protect the pulp from a direct invasion of bacteria (Fig 7). This process is an effort by nature to wall off the area of infection from the rest of the tooth. If these measures are not successful, the infection may spread to the pulp** and to the rest of the body.

All activities of the body, whether calcification, nerve impulses, fluid transport, muscle contraction, or brain function, require energy. This **energy usually is supplied in the form of adenosine triphosphate (ATP). The more ATP in a tissue, the greater that tissue's capacity for work. In one study, the ATP levels were measured in various layers of dentin beneath both caries and fillings in human teeth [ref]. Beneath caries confined to the enamel, there was a significant increase in ATP in the dentin. When the caries reached the dentin or when a filling was placed, there was a 100% increase in ATP compared with the same areas when the caries was confined to the enamel. While these changes in ATP content were occurring in the dentin no significant differences in ATP levels in the pulp were observed** [ref].

Also reported was **increased phosphoesterase activity in the pre-pulpal dentin layer under incipient carious changes in the dentin** [ref]. Apparently the dentin is already responding both anabolically and catabolically in the early stages of caries.

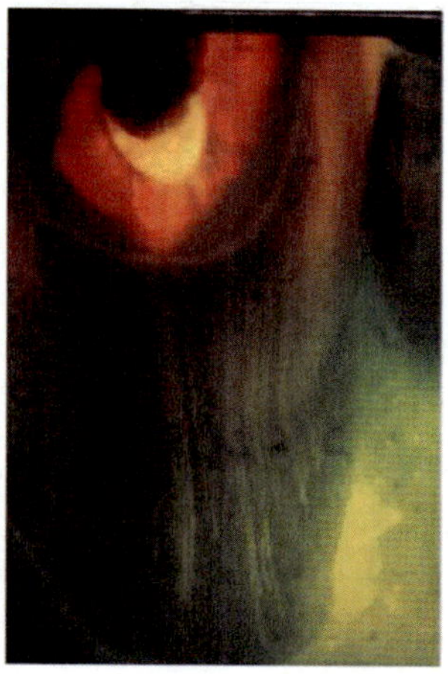

1A - Normal rat molar

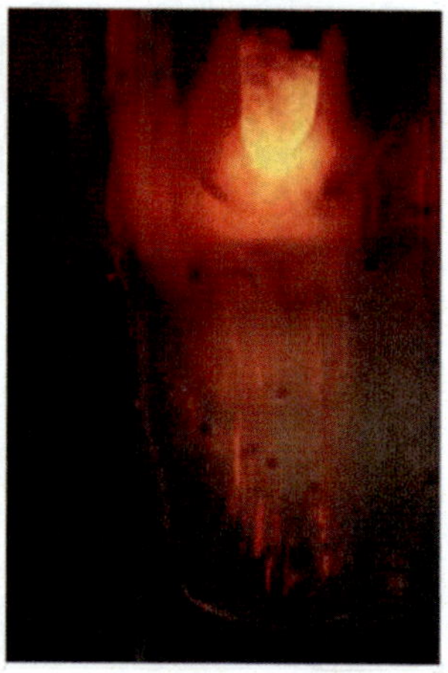

1B - Bradykinin causes red material beneath the plaque to penetrate the tooth structure as far as the pulp.

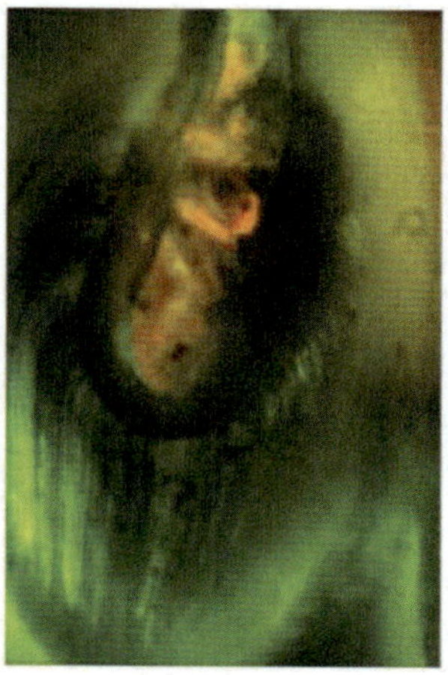

3A - Normal fluid movement in dentin beneath the occlusal groove.

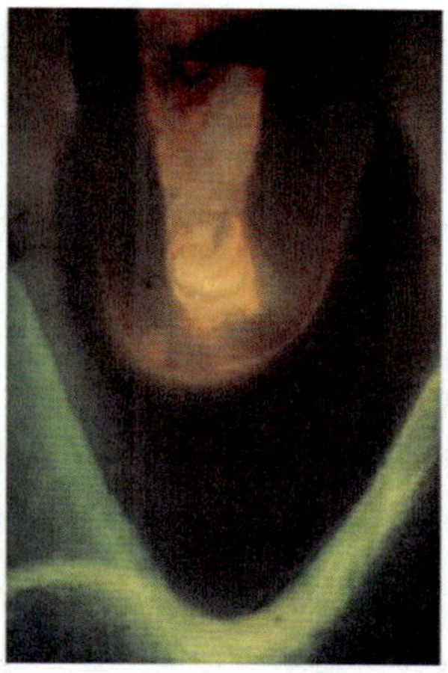

3B - Fluid movement suppressed by high sucrose diet; yellow material from plaque penetrates dentin.

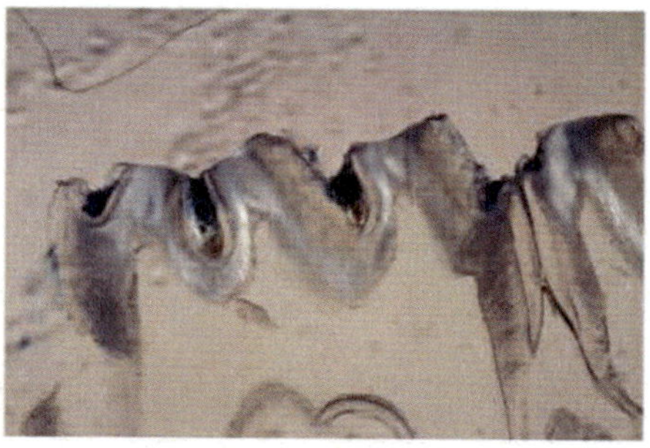

4A - Methylene blue in teeth on non-carious diet. No movement of the dye is seen.

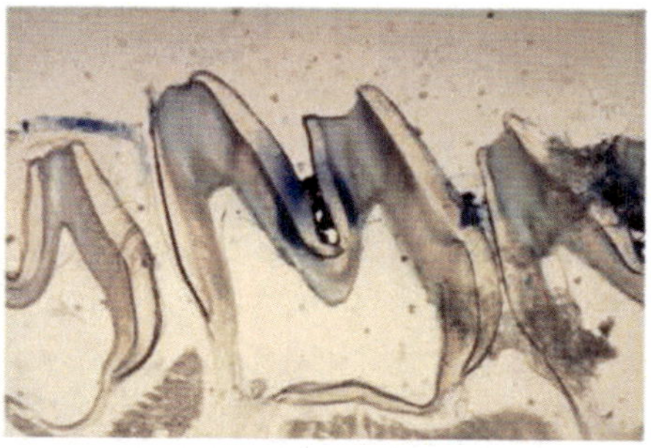

4B - Penetration of methylene blue beneath plaque in teeth on a cariogenic diet.

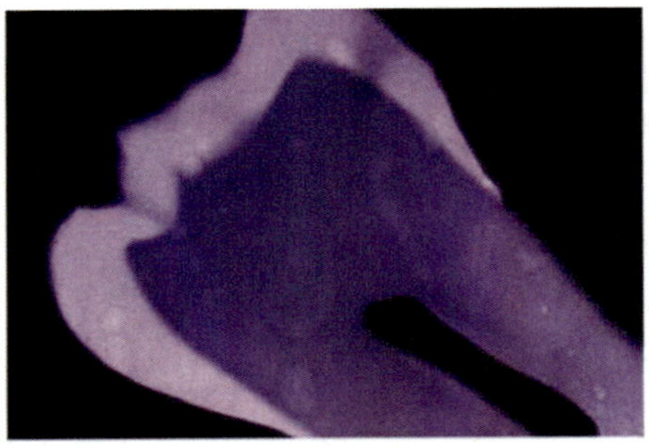

5A - Radiograph of tooth

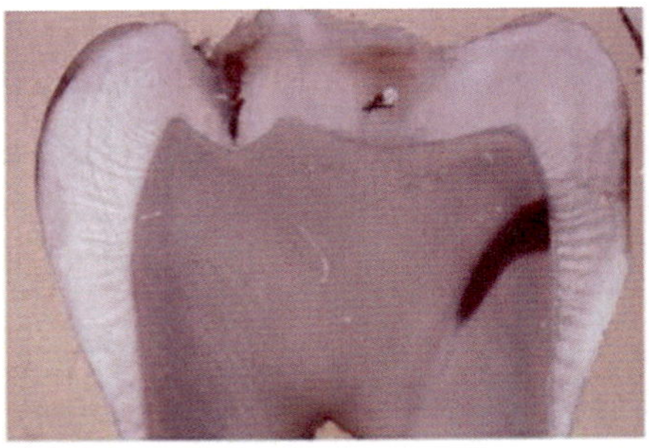

5B - Section of same tooth treated with ninhydrin, showing penetration of the distal surface beneath plaque.

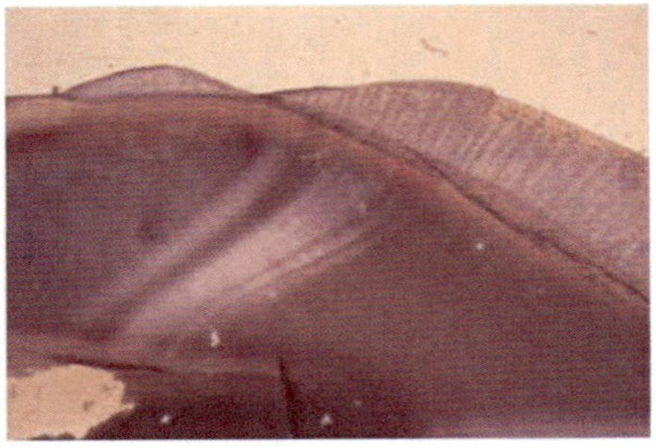

5C - No ninhydrin reaction occurs in a section of a tooth with erosion.

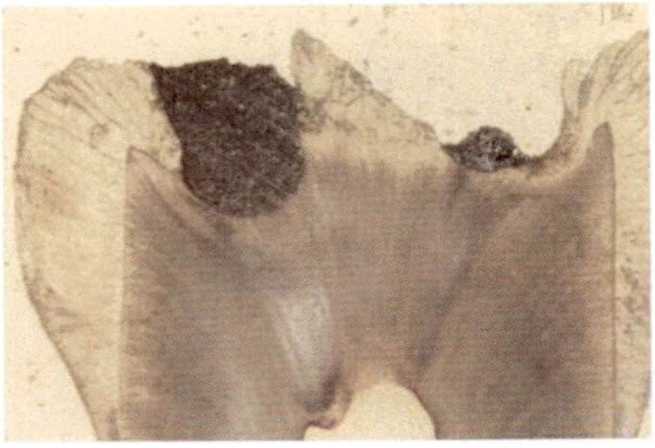

7 - Another defensive reaction of the tooth is secondary dentin formation and hypercalcification

What Happens If the Tooth Fails to Prevent the Ingress of Noxious Material from the Plaque?

The pulp of the tooth also is adversely affected by the carious process. Changes were observed in the pulp beneath white spots of the enamel before cavitation. The most common changes were an impairment of the odontoblastic layer and an accumulation of exudate cells [ref]. Thus, **the entire thickness of the tooth—the pulp, the dentin, and the enamel—is affected by the carious attack.**

Summary

It should be clear from all that has been presented in this paper that the tooth is not a helpless appendage in a destructive environment; rather, it is a living, vital organ capable of resistance, repair, and a vital response to attack. In order to maintain its integrity, it is necessary that it be supplied with the correct nutrients and that its physiologic processes be supported, not suppressed. **The tooth is a vital part of the body, and what affects the body for good or ill may also affect the teeth to a greater or lesser degree. If the patient has a mouth full of caries, there is probably more wrong with the patient than holes in his or her teeth!** The patient may need more than having cavities filled or purchasing a new tooth brush. In order to restore the tooth to health, the dentist may have to consider more than the surface of the tooth. **Unless the underlying malfunction is corrected, the restoration may fail.**

Article #87

<u>The carious process as it may be influenced by the physiology of the tooth</u>

Steinman RR. Unpublished syllabus, 1984

A major feature of dental caries is demineralization. However, an increased solubility of the enamel alone is not related to susceptibility. As observed by several investigators, the demineralization associated with caries occurs in depth and not only that but there is an intact surface of the enamel beneath which the earliest demineralization is evident.

Bacteria are essential for the caries process. It also appears that caries does not occur in the absence of plaque. Consensus says that acid is produced in the plaque which causes demineralization to occur. It is also evident that plaque may be present on the tooth surface without caries resulting. Even though it is true that those bacteria associated with caries produce acid, not all bacteria that produce acid produce caries when introduced into germ-free caries-susceptible animals being fed a cariogenic diet.

Normally, there is found on the surface of the enamel in the oral cavity a layer of protein or organic polymers. This is weakly bound to the apatite crystals and is thought to protect the surface apatite crystals from the action of acid produced by the plaque. Since the surface enamel remains intact during the initial stage of decalcification, it may be assumed that this may be partially due to the protective organic material on the surface of the tooth. **A question of importance is how does the decalcifying material move through the protective coating and react with the subsurface enamel? It is our thinking that this is brought about by the reversal of the normal direction of fluid movement in tooth structure. The hydraulic system of the tooth normally moves in a direction from inside the tooth to the surface. The tooth becomes susceptible when this direction is reversed. Now the plaque fluid is moved through the protecting coat deep into the structure of the enamel. As this process continues, the pore size of the enamel is increased allowing ever more and larger molecules to penetrate into the tooth structure.**

Another force that is acting upon the enamel beneath the plaque is bioelectrical. The plaque has been shown to be electronegative. It has also been shown that the electronegative area is associated with the deposition of mineral in calcified structure. Further support for this is shown by the movement of mineral from the deeper portions of the tooth being deposited in the surface mineral structure (Caries Res 11(Suppl 1) 59-84, 1977).

<u>Some reports on bacteria and caries</u>

"The clear interstrain difference in dental caries level maintained under both conditions, shows that caries activity was hereditable and not dependent on the type of oral microflora harbored by the two strains [of rats]" (Caries Res 14:434-440, 1980).

Concerning the immunity concept in dental caries "Negative results are always disappointing, but, in summary, they show that if antibodies specific for cariogenic bacteria are present in the saliva at all, they are in very low concentration and, even if the amount of antibody were greatly increased, there is no evidence that they would in any way modify the progress of dental caries." (Oral Surg 34:69-86, 1972) Antibodies would find it very difficult to survive in the oral environment.

The sequence of physiological events in the carious process

In a previous section material was presented that attempted to show what susceptibility to dental caries is not, and also what it is. From the evidence presented, susceptibility appears to be a manifestation of a malfunctioning pulp. **From the late 1940s to the present time, a number of authors have suggested that a malfunctioning pulp is indeed the central problem. Bodecker (1960) gave as evidence that the pulp was the problem by the absence of caries in central incisors with calcified pulp chambers compared to caries in the adjacent tooth which had a pulp. Sharpenak (1972) deduced that the pulp was malfunctioning by observing differences in the movement of dye in teeth relative to caries. He also surmised that this malfunction was in some way related to the salivary glands.** ***DeVries (1949) in his study of carious human teeth outlined the problem as being the result of a failure of metabolism brought about by a failure of fluid transport in specific areas of the tooth and that this brought about bionecrosis. This bionecrosis opened the tooth to microbial activity which finished destroying the tooth.***

Article #88

Physiologic activity of the pulp-dentin complex

Steinman RR. Quintessence Int 10:723-726, 1985

The integrity of any tissue depends upon metabolic stability and physiologic activity. Disease is often the result of adversely altered metabolic activity. If bacteria are present, the tissue with the disturbed metabolism may be invaded. Might this also be true of the teeth?

In this paper the term *Base Decay Rate* is applied to caries in endodontically treated teeth, which are influenced by the external environment, plaque, food residue, oral hygiene, and saliva. The term *Combined Decay Rate* refers to caries found in intact vital teeth. Both the external and the internal influences in the vital pulp may alter the incidence of dental caries.

Ethical restraints make it impossible to conduct experiments on humans. In such cases animal experimentation is utilized. Fortunately animal caries is similar to that found in humans, making comparisons relevant.

It is the purpose of this paper to (1) compare the incidence of caries in internally inactive, endodontically treated teeth with caries in vital teeth in the same oral cavity, and (2) consider the effect that biologic activity in the pulp-dentin complex has upon the incidence of dental caries.

Base decay rate

Teeth are usually treated endodontically because of the ravages of dental caries. After treatment, the remaining structures of these teeth appear to be less caries-susceptible than intact teeth in the same oral cavity [refs].

The incidence of caries in rats varies from very little to rampant, depending on the experimental conditions imposed. The incidence of caries in the endodontically treated teeth of rats is compared to the incidence of caries in vital teeth in the same oral cavity. **Any difference in decay rate between these two groups could be assumed to be the result of influences imposed by the pulps of the teeth.** Fig. 1 illustrates the findings of three studies comparing the Base Decay Rate to the Combined Decay Rate in rats under varying conditions [refs]. **As susceptibility increases, the Combined Decay Rate varies only slightly. This suggests that the pulp is playing a major role in**

susceptibility variations and the external environmental factors remain comparatively constant. The major difference in the incidence of dental caries between these two groups is probably due to variations in physiologic activity within the pulp-dentin complex. Variations between studies may be due to differences in rats, diet, and laboratory technique.

Physiologic difference

Fluid transport is essential for the health of any tissue. The relationship between the Combined Decay Rate and fluid transport through the dentin is shown graphically in Fig. 2. Animals with suppressed fluid transport in the dentin have a high rate of dental caries. Yet, those animals with a normal rate of fluid transport in the dentin have little or no caries. This is true whether or not the animals are fed a high-sucrose diet. Consequently, the essential feature for a low Combined Decay Rate is an adequate rate of dentinal fluid transport [refs].

Hormones

In restoring normal fluid transport to the dentin of animals fed a high-sucrose cariogenic diet, it is thought that the effect of compounds such as carbamyl phosphate is the release of hormones from the hypothalamic-parotid gland endocrine axis [refs]. The hypothalamus produces a hormone which is released into the blood stream and travels to the parotid salivary gland. The parotid releases the parotid hormone into the blood which travels to the pulps of the teeth where it stimulates the dentinal fluid transport (Fig. 3). The stimulation of suppressed fluid transport in the teeth of rats fed a high-sucrose cariogenic diet was associated with a reduction in the Combined Decay Rate (Fig. 2).

Biologic activity in human teeth

The fluids in the various compartments of the body, including the teeth, are in communication with each other. This communication in human teeth is suggested by the movement of fluid from inside the tooth to the surface of the enamel (Fig. 4) [refs], and by the movement of antibodies into the dentin in a defensive position beneath caries that has reached the dentinoenamel junction [ref]. Similar to other tissues, human teeth actively respond to the attack of external bacteria. **This response requires a transport system in tooth structure and is supported by a healthy life-style.**

Conclusions

Animal and human studies show that the physiologic activity of the tooth's pulp-dentin complex has a significant effect upon its health. An essential element of this physiologic activity is the dentinal fluid transport which is controlled by the pulp. When this fluid transport is suppressed there is a significant increase in the Combined Decay Rate. A normal rate of fluid transport is associated with little or no caries.

Teeth are a biologic entity and should be given the same support as any other vital tissue of the body. All parts of the body are interconnected, including the teeth. Consequently, whatever affects the health of the body may, to a greater or lesser degree, affect the health of the teeth.

Article #89

Nutrition of the teeth and dental caries

Steinman RR. J Appl Nutr 39(1):42-50, 1987

Abstract: **Numerous animal studies have shown that high-sucrose diets tend to be cariogenic. Enriching these diets with nutrients, however, significantly diminishes**

the incidence of dental caries, suggesting that resistance to caries may involve systemic effects of nutrition. Separating the systemic effect from the external effect in the oral cavity has been approached in several ways. Restricting the normal flow of blood to the teeth increases caries. Endodontic treatment involving removal of the dental pulp reduces caries. Systemic administration of specific nutrients also reduces the incidence of caries. Thus, a nutritionally or physiologically compromised pulp-dentin complex reduces resistance to caries. In this light, recommendations to reduce dietary sucrose and increase consumption of whole grains, fresh fruits and vegetables take on added importance. Key Words = Nutrition, Resistance to dental caries, Sucrose, Dental pulp.

It is generally assumed that ingested foods affect the incidence of dental caries solely through their local action in the oral cavity. In this simple view carbohydrates in food provide nourishment for oral microorganisms which metabolize the carbohydrates to acids. These acids then dissolve the dental hard tissues—enamel and dentin—to produce the carious lesions.

This theory of dental caries pathogenesis, however, may be incomplete and inadequate for several reasons. The solubility of enamel in acid has not been shown to be an indication of susceptibility to dental caries [refs]. The acidogenic potential of foods also fails to show a relationship to caries when these foods are fed to experimental animals [refs]. The restricted local view of dental caries further fails to consider the metabolic activity observed in teeth [refs] and the hormones which influence this activity (5 refs). **All of this suggests that factors other than the local environment of teeth may be important for their health**.

The purpose of this paper is to review the evidence that nutrition may have an effect on the health of the teeth internally through the pulp-dentin complex, in addition to any local effect these foods may have in the oral cavity. If this biological approach to dental caries is valid, it may well have important implications for the prevention and treatment of caries in humans.

Evidence for systemic factors

The nutritional state of any tissue depends upon an adequate blood supply. Restriction of the blood supply to the teeth of rats and hamsters significantly increases the incidence of caries compared to other teeth in the same oral cavity having a normal blood supply [refs] (Table 1). This restriction of circulation to the pulp-dentin complex of the teeth probably impairs the nutritional state and may produce a disturbed physiologic activity within the teeth.

The high-sucrose cariogenic diet used by Sognnaes [ref] in 1949 to induce caries in rats has been used by many investigators through the years. The diet contained casein, sucrose, corn oil, liver powder, salt mixture, and vitamin mix. When the salt mixture was replaced with ashed Purina laboratory chow, significant reduction in the incidence of dental caries was observed [ref] (Table 2). Enrichment of a similar high-sucrose diet with carbamyl phosphate (1.56 mg/kg of diet), Zn 250 ppm, Mo 10 ppm, Cr 8 ppm, and eggshell meal 2% also caused a highly significant reduction in caries [refs] (Table 2). Note: No fluoride was found in the eggshell meal.

Separation of local and systemic effects

Whether these reductions in caries were due to systemic or to local effects, or to a combination of both, cannot be determined from these reports. To resolve this uncertainty, the effect on the external surface of the teeth must be separated from the systemic effect. This separation can be accomplished by suitable endodontic treatment of selected teeth (molars) in each oral cavity. In this procedure the metabolically active pulp tissue is removed and the resulting space within the molars is filled with an inert material. This treatment effectively eliminates any internal biological activity, either beneficial or detrimental, from the teeth. Because dental caries rarely occurs on the mesial surface of molars under these conditions, endodontic treatment is performed there to avoid biasing the outcome.

Any caries occurring in these endodontically-treated teeth is thus due solely to the external influences of plaque, food residue and saliva. The number of caries in treated teeth is compared with the number of caries found in untreated, vital teeth in the same oral cavity which is influenced by both the internal and the external conditions of those teeth. Any difference in the incidence of caries between these two groups of teeth is assumed to represent the influence of the intact pulps of the untreated vital teeth in the same oral cavity, since both groups of teeth are exposed to the same destructive environment of the oral cavity. The incidence of caries in the vital teeth of animals fed the high-sucrose diet turns out to be much higher than in the endodontically treated teeth in the same oral cavity [refs] (Table 3). This shows that a high-sucrose diet has a major detrimental effect on the pulp-dentin complex of intact teeth in addition to its local cariogenic effect.

When this same experiment was conducted using the enriched high-sucrose diet, caries incidence declined as expected, but much more so in the untreated teeth. This result shows that the added enrichment benefited both the external and the internal condition of the teeth (Table 3).

No difference in dental caries was observed between endodontically treated teeth and vital untreated teeth in the same oral cavity of rats (Table 3). This suggests that the enriched high-sucrose diet adequately nourished the pulp-dentin complex of the vital teeth.

In a study of the effect of cooked human foods on the incidence of caries in rats, it was found that the inclusion of desserts caused an increase in caries [ref]. **When rats fed the same diet minus desserts were given intraperitoneal injections of glucose and fructose, a significant increase in the incidence of caries was observed** [ref] (Table 4). **This finding also indicated that an important part of the cariogenic effects of sugars is not due to their local effects during oral ingestion.**

Other possible systemic effects

Animals fed an L-lysine-deficient diet were found to have an increase in the incidence of dental caries above that found in animals receiving adequate L-lysine. When L-lysine was given to the deficient rats by intubation in adequate amounts, the incidence of dental caries was significantly reduced (Table 5). Hence, L-lysine helps teeth resist decay, but its protective effect is systemic, not local. At least the protection is not *directly* local. It may operate, at least in part, by changing the composition of the saliva, which in turn could promote caries resistance by a local effect. Endodontics experiments such as previously described would be required to demonstrate whether L-lysine and other dietary deficiencies increase caries susceptibility by impairing the physiological function of the tooth pulp.

Human teeth

Ethical constraints make it impossible to perform similar experiments on humans. For this reason, we usually must depend upon animal experiments to study dental caries. Although the relevance of animal experiments to the human situation cannot be assured, encouraging evidence is available. A few observations have been made of caries in endodontically treated human teeth. As in the animal experiments with the high-sucrose diet, the vulnerable areas of treated teeth were found to be less subject to dental caries than corresponding areas of intact teeth in the same oral cavity [refs].

Other reports of human caries experience are consistent with the concept that systemic nutritional factors affect caries incidence in humans. Examples include the relationship between good physical status and low incidence of dental caries [refs], the high incidence of dental caries found in young diabetics [refs], the poor teeth of individuals with sickle cell anemia [ref] and the increase in caries found in individuals under undue stress [ref]. More directly related to the subject of this paper is the reduction in caries following the supplementation of pyridoxine to pregnant women [ref]. However, unlike the observations on endodontically treated animal and human teeth, these findings do not exclude the possibility that the "systemic" effects are mediated, partially or wholly, through the local, external environment of the teeth.

Results*:*

TABLE 1. Effect of Restricting Blood Flow to the Dental Pulp on Subsequent Dental Caries

Animal	Treatment	Molar Lesions	Difference	p
Rat	Restricted blood flow, right side	5.4	69% increase	<0.001
	Normal blood flow, left side	3.2		
Rat	Restricted blood flow	10.7	43% increase	<0.01
	Normal blood flow	7.5		
Hamster	Restricted blood flow	12.2	618% increase	<0.01
	Normal blood flow	1.7		

TABLE 2. Effect of Enriching a High Sucrose Cariogenic Diet on Subsequent Caries

Animal	Treatment	Molar Lesions	Difference	p
Rat	High sucrose diet	6.2	343% increase	...
	Enriched sucrose diet	1.4		
Rat	High sucrose diet	9.2		0.001
	Enriched sucrose diet	0.0		
Rat	High sucrose diet	3.3	450% increase	0.001
	Enriched sucrose diet	0.6		

TABLE 3. Effect of Removing the Dental Pulp on Subsequent Dental Caries

Animal	Treatment	Molar Lesions	Difference	p
		High Sucrose Cariogenic Diet		
Rat	None	1.5	88% increase	<0.001
	Pulp removed	0.8		
Rat	None	3.5	600% increase	<0.001
	Pulp removed	0.5		
Rat	None	5.0	317% increase	<0.001
	Pulp removed	1.2		
		Enriched High Sucrose Cariogenic Diet		
Rat	None	5.0	317% increase	<0.001
	Pulp removed	1.2		

TABLE 4. Effect of Intraperitoneal Injections of Sugar on Subsequent Dental Caries

Animal	Treatment	Molar Lesions	Difference	p
Rat	Normal diet plus i.p. sugar	10.9	18% increase	<0.01
	Normal diet alone	3.8		

TABLE 5. Effect of Intubated Lysine on Subsequent Dental Caries Experience

Animal	Treatment	Molar Lesions	Difference	p
Rat	L-lysine deficient diet	4.6	130-165% increase	<0.01
	L-lysine deficient diet + water by intubation (control)	5.3		
	L-lysine deficient diet + L-lysine by intubation	2.0		

[Note: Ref's for each study above are included in original paper]

Discussion

When food is eaten, both the oral microorganisms and the host are nourished. Several experimental approaches indicate that the nutrition of the pulp-dentin complex is important for the health of the teeth. These experiments include a reduction in blood supply to the pulp, endodontic treatment of the teeth, and systemic administration of specific nutrients.

Because endodontic removal of the pulp eliminates internal blood flow in teeth, one might expect that endodontic treatment would increase--not decrease--tooth decay, just as in the experiments which restricted blood flow (Table 1). However, the effect of endodontic treatment depends on the diet used and the resulting physiological conditions within the tooth [ref]. With the high-sucrose cariogenic diet, pulp removal protects against high rates of decay. With the same diet enriched with minerals (not including fluoride), the decay rate is low and endodontic treatment has no discernible effect (Table 3).

The effect of endodontic elimination of internal blood flow on caries susceptibility depends at least in part on the direction of fluid flow through the surface of the teeth. Even in tooth enamel there is about 2% mobile water [ref]. If this fluid flows abnormally inward from the surface of the tooth [ref], as observed with the high-sucrose unsupplemented diets, it promotes decay [ref], and blocking the flow by pulp removal reduces caries. If the fluid flow is normal (outward) [ref], it protects the tooth from the external destructive environment. Restricting or reversing this normal flow may increase caries [refs].

This poorly appreciated complexity of caries susceptibility can help explain the facts mentioned in the introduction that decay does not correlate well with the acidogenic potential of foods or with the solubility of enamel in acid. Sucrose and other cariogenic foods cause decay not only because of the unfavorable external environment they produce in the mouth. Such foods may also disturb the physiological resistance of teeth to decay, including the normal outward flow of fluid through the teeth [ref].

Like the bones, the teeth are sensitive to deficiencies of minerals and trace elements imposed either by a direct deficiency in the diet or by a relative deficiency due to an excess of refined foods in the diet, particularly sucrose. The biological activity of the teeth requires an adequate quantity of all essential nutrients.

Because the potential nutritional problems of teeth are similar to those of other tissues with special emphasis on minerals and trace elements, perhaps no better dietary recommendation can be made than those contained in the Dietary Goals for the United

States [ref]. Of special importance for the health of the teeth are the recommendations for less sucrose in the diet, more whole grain products and more fresh fruits and vegetables.

The well-known chemo-parasitic theory of dental caries is concerned only with the external environment of the teeth. It is valid as far as it goes. Some proponents go so far as to say, "There is no evidence that nutrition in the post-developmental period has any influence on caries" [refs]. However, this view seems inadequate and incomplete because it fails to account for evidence that the nutritional and physiological state of the teeth also has a significant effect on the incidence of dental caries. **The chemico-parasitic theory should be reexamined and tested further, and if necessary altered to state that caries is caused by acids produced by microorganisms of the oral cavity acting upon *physiologically compromised* teeth.** According to evidence reviewed here, teeth may be physiologically compromised by restricted blood flow or by poor nutrition.

Article #90

Physiological factors affecting secretion of parotid hormone

Leonora J, Tièche JM, Celestin, J. Am J Physiol 252 (Endocrinol. Metab. 15):E477-E484, 1987

The concept of the existence of a hypothalamic-parotid gland endocrine axis originated from studies attempting to identify the physiological factors that regulate a dentinal fluid transport (DFT) mechanism in teeth [ref]. The parotid glands secrete a hormone that stimulates this mechanism in rat teeth whereby dental lymph is pumped through the dentin and onto the surface of the enamel. Because dentinal tissue is avascular, it appears that a DFT mechanism is essential for the fulfillment of its metabolic requirements. Parotid hormone (PH) was isolated from porcine parotid glands and partially characterized [ref]. From other studies we deduced that PH is under the control of a hypothalamic-parotid hormone-releasing factor [refs].

Our studies on cariogenesis in rats show an inverse relationship between the incidence of dental caries and the functioning of the DFT mechanism [ref]. By maintaining the DFT mechanism in a functional state with dietary supplements, cariogenesis can be significantly inhibited even though rats are fed a cariogenic diet. We postulated that the optimal operation of this fluid flow may provide a systemic defensive mechanism against cariogenesis [refs].

The development of a radioimmunoassay for quantitating PH in biological fluids [ref] enabled us to investigate under various conditions the secretion pattern of PH in the pig. To establish the physiological basis for the endocrine control of the DFT mechanism through the hypothalamic-parotid gland endocrine axis, we examined a variety of factors that affect the secretion of PH. We linked the DFT stimulation effect of a hypothalamic PH-releasing activity in rats to its effect on the secretion of PH in the pig, and we demonstrated that feeding is a potent stimulus for PH secretion.

STUDY:

The Duroc-Hampshire castrated pigs in this study were anesthetized for bilateral parotidectomy, a difficult procedure requiring 5-7 h. The traumatic effect of surgery on PH secretion was evaluated by performing sham parotidectomies on control animals involving total parotid exposure before suturing of the wound site.

Isolation of a parotid hormone-releasing factor (PHRF):

Hypothalamus-thalamic tissue samples average 4.37 g were dissected from pigs weighing 85-100 kg. and frozen on dry ice within 30 min of the animals' death. Batches of 400 pieces (1,750 g) were extracted, thawed and homogenized in an acetone mixture. After 2 h of mixing, this solution was centrifuged and the supernatant decanted through glass wool. The residue was sequentially collected and similarly processed twice more with acetone evaporated under vacuum at 45°C for 30 min each time. The resulting extracts were pooled, pH neutralized, passed through membrane filters and freeze-dried. The purified fraction was labeled porcine hypothalamus-thalamic tissue extract PM-10 filtrate (PHTE PM-10 filt).

PH radioimmunoassay (RIA):

The titer of plasma immunoreactive PH (iPH) was determined using a double-antibody RIA. Reduction and statistical analysis of the RIA data were done according to Rodbard [ref]. The precision of the iPH determination for pig plasma was assessed by measuring the "within assay" and the "between assay" coefficients of variation of iPH titer estimates from plasma pools of low, medium, and high titer.

Biological assay of DFT-stimulating activity:

Male Sprague-Dawley rats were used in the DFT bioassay procedure in which half were parotidectomized and the other half experienced sham surgery. After anesthesia with pentobarbital sodium, a fluorescent dye (acriflavine hydrochloride) was injected intraperitoneally. A bolus dose of PHTE PM-10 filt.was administered into the subclavian vein of intact and parotidectomized rats. Control intact and parotidectomized rats received saline. The presence of fluorescent dye in the dentinal tubules was observed by fluorescence microscopy. A fluid movement ratio (FMR) value was ascribed to each animal [ref].

Fasting level of iPH in pigs:

Plasma fasting titers of iPH were observed in 22 pigs monitored over periods of time ranging from 1 to 9 wks. An estimate of the fasting titer of the pig population was calculated and expressed as overall mean, SD, and coefficient of variance (CV) between animals.

General experimental protocol:

Pre-treatment fasting blood samples were taken at -10, -5, and 0 min. At *time 0* the experimental procedure started and blood samples were drawn at specified intervals. Plasma iPH titers were determined in all samples by RIA.

Results:

The effect of visual and olfactory stimuli in comparison to feeding is shown in Table 4.

TABLE 4 – Effect of Various Stimuli Related to Feeding on Secretion of iPH in the Pig

Stimulus	Amount (gm)	Group number	iPH Titer maximum response	N	Statistical comparison	P
		CHEWING VS. FEEDING				
None (fasting)		1	1.2	4		
Ice chewing		2	1.2	4	1 vs. 2	NS*
Feeding pig chow	1200	3	8.4	5	1 vs. 3	<0.01
		VISUAL-OLFACTORY FEEDING				
None (fasting)		4	1.2	5		
Feed presentation		5	1.1	5	4 vs. 5	NS*
Feeding pig chow	1200	6	5.7	5	4 vs. 6	<0.01

VARIOUS AMOUNTS OF PIG CHOW

Stimulus	Amount (gm)	Group number	iPH Titer maximum response	n	Statistical compari-son	P
None (fasting)		7	1.2	5		
15-sec feeding	32	8	2.0	5	7 vs. 8	<0.01**
1 min feeding	85	9	3.5	5		
5-min feeding	226	10	9.5	5		
Full meal	1200	11	10.2	5	10 vs. 11	NS

Values are means ± SE; N =no. of animals in the group. iPH = immunoreactive parotid hormone. *Significance was ascertained by Dunnett's test. ** Significance was ascertained by Student's t test for unequal variances.

iPH RIA – iPH in pig plasma contains PH with binding and displacement characteristics similar to pure PH.

Fasting level of iPH – Ranged between 22 and 99% coefficient of variation.

Effect of PHTE infusion on rat DFT activity – PHTE PM-10 filtrate at a dose of 6.25 x 10^{-4} p eq stimulated DFT activity in sham-operated rats. This same dose or greater was without significant effect in parotidectomized animals.

Effect of PHTE infusion on iPH secretion in intact, parotidectomized, and sham-operated pigs - The mean maximum response in four pigs from infusion of 15 p eq of PHTE PM-1- filt reflected a five-fold increase over the basal iPH level. After parotidectomy, the basal pretreatment iPH titer decreased to ¼ the original value and the response to PHTE infusion was totally abolished. The sham operation did not significantly change the responsiveness of the animals to PHTE infusion.

Effect of feeding on iPH secretion in pigs – Feeding 1,200 g of pig chow to intact pigs was an effective stimulus for iPH secretion, increasing rapidly to an 11-fold increase over the fasting titer within 10-20 min, then decreasing slowly over the next 2 h. After parotidectomy, the iPH response to feeding was abolished, however the sham operation, in contrast, did not significantly alter the response.

The sight and smell of feed elicited an immediate state of excitement accompanied by profuse salivation. This reaction lasted for 30 min with no significant increase in iPH observed until the animals actually began feeding. Mastication of a non-nutritive substance, crushed ice, proved ineffective in stimulating iPH secretion. In contrast, feeding that took place immediately after crunching the ice caused a significant increase in iPH. iPH increased with the amount of feed ingested or the feeding duration. Feeding for 15 sec was sufficient to significantly increase the iPH titer from the fasting level and a maximum response was attained within 5 min of feeding. Feeding itself brought about an immediate rise in iPH whereas PHTE infusion involved a 3-min delay before rising.

Discussion:

The importance of an intact hypothalamic-parotid gland endocrine axis is emphasized by the failure of both DFT stimulation and the secretion of iPH to occur in parotidectomized rats or pigs, respectively. Furthermore, because PH and PHRF are both capable of stimulating DFT in the intact rat, and because PHRF stimulates iPH secretion in the intact pig, we conclude that iPH originates in the parotid glands and is likely to be the same chemical entity as the PH, which we have previously isolated from porcine parotid glands [ref].

We have established, in a preliminary fashion, the physiological context within which the hypothalamic parotid gland endocrine axis functions by studying the effect of feeding on the secretion of iPH. Feeding serves as a potent stimulus for the secretion of iPH. A detectable increase in plasma iPH is observed within 1 min of the onset of feeding, and peak titer reached within 10-20 min. Failure to observe an increase in iPH in fed parotidectomized pigs adds support to the hypothesis that the parotid glands are the primary source for iPH.

A direct relationship between feeding duration and/or amount ingested, and the magnitude of the iPH response that suggests that this endocrine system is capable of modulating its hormonal output. However beyond a certain point the strength of the stimulus no longer appears to have a decisive effect on hormonal response.

It is generally accepted that the sight of food, particularly when hungry, generates a variety of neural signals in anticipation of eating. In pigs, profuse salivation begins when they hear feed containers being opened and then see and smell the feed as their troughs are filled. This study demonstrates that the arousal of auditory, visual, and olfactory stimuli related to feeding that cause profuse salivation is ineffective in stimulating iPH secretion. Neural stimuli from chewing non-nutritive crushed ice are essentially ineffective. The almost immediate secretion of iPH in response to feeding suggests the involvement of a neural pathway in the release mechanism and may involve recruitment of other unidentified neural and/or hormonal factors. The possibility exists that the PH secretory mechanism is analogous to the neural, hormonal, and substrate factors that optimize the secretion of insulin in response to feeding.

We postulated earlier the existence of a systemic mechanism by which resistance to cariogenesis may be achieved [refs]. Linking the immediate secretion of iPH in response to feeding and the stimulation of the DFT mechanism by PH provides evidence for the existence of a physiologically controlled defensive mechanism against dental caries. The general consensus is that dental caries is the result of a bacterial assault on tooth structure through the production of acidic metabolites in the presence of substrate. In previous publications we demonstrated that the cariogenicity of a high-sucrose diet can be significantly inhibited (85-100%) with the addition of dietary supplements that stimulate DFT in intact rats but are ineffective in sialoadenectomized animals [refs]. From these results we concluded that these supplements exercise their cariostatic effect through systemic mechanisms(s) involving salivary glands. In addition, it was shown that the incidence of dental caries in vital teeth is significantly higher than in endodontically treated teeth within the same animal [ref]. We hypothesized that teeth become susceptible to decay primarily as a result of systemic failure as reflected in part by the inverse relationship between DFT activity and dental caries. By maintaining the operation of the DFT mechanism, the microbial assault is countered by the flushing and neutralizing effects of dental lymph as it moves through the dental structure onto the surface of the tooth. The immediate release of PH in response to eating could ensure the optimal function of the DFT mechanism at a critical time when the acidogenic potential of the microbe is maximum.

Article #91

Evidence for insulinotropic effect from rat parotid glands

Leonora J, Tièche JM, Cook, DS. Diabetes (April) 37:441-445, 1988

The physiologic role of parotid glands is more complex than their recognized salivary function. Various investigators have suggested an endocrine relationship between the parotids and the pancreas. Asymptomatic bilateral enlargement of the parotid glands has been associated with diabetes mellitus in 61% of cases in North American Pima Indians [ref], interpreted as compensatory hyperplasia in response to decreased insulin secretion [refs]. Parotidectomy caused a transient decrease in blood glucose which was reversed to hyperglycemia by administration of parotid gland extract [refs]. Some investigators found that the parotid protein, parotin, increased glucose tolerance [ref]. The purpose of this study was to observe the chronic effect of sialoadenectomy on the secretion of insulin in response to intra-arterial infusion of glucose in experimental rodents.

STUDY:

Male Sprague-Dawley rats were anesthetized by cannulation of their left common carotid arteries.

Glucose tolerance test (GTT):

A baseline blood sample was drawn from rats which had been fasting for 24 h. Subsequent samples were taken at 6 and 10 min following an infusion of 78 μmol glucose/100 g body wt. Plasma immunoreactive insulin (IRI) was determined by radioimmunoassay (RIA). Glucose levels were determined by the glucose oxidase method [ref].

Plasma insulin RIA:

We used a modified double-antibody procedure derived from the Novo RIA kit. Rat insulin (NOVO) was used as the standard. Each sample determination was done in triplicate and analyzed statistically according to Rodbard [ref].

Sialoadenectomy and sham operation:

The parotid or submandibular glands were removed by blunt dissection and the animals given 5% glucose drinking water for 5 days. Glands of sham controls were mildly manipulated with blunt forceps and left intact.

Effect of parotidectomy on the β-cell response:

Adult 300-g rats were chronically arterially catheterized and divided into 4 groups.

Between days 15 and 0 (day 0 = day of surgery), 5 GTTs were done at 3-day intervals to determine IRI titer and plasma glucose levels before glucose infusion and at 2-, 6-, and 10 min post-infusion.

On day 0, each group of rats was either parotidectomized, submandibularectomized, totally sialoadenectomized, or had sham operations. The GTT was repeated in each rat on postoperative days 5, 8, 2, 15, 19, 22, 26, 29, and 33.

Effect of age and parotidectomy on IRI and glucose responses after GTT:

The effect of parotidectomy on the β-cell response to a glucose load was assessed in weanling (21-day-old) and adult (~80-day-old) rats compared to sham controls. β-cell responsiveness to glucose was tested on days 85, 89, 92, 96, and 100. Data from several tests were averaged and mean values computed per rat. Statistical differences were assessed by Student's t test for unpaired data.

Results:

There were no significant long-term effects of parotidectomy on either body weight or daily food consumption in both immature and adult rats. **Parotidectomized rats within each age group had a significantly lower insulin response than did the intact rats. Concomitantly the blood glucose titers remained significantly higher at all times in the parotidectomized rats compared with intact controls.**

Discussion:

This study indicates that parotidectomy chronically decreases the responsiveness of the β-cells to an acute change in blood glucose concentration. It suggests that parotidectomy deprives the β-cells of a parotid signal that appears to be essential for optimizing the immediate insulin response to a glucose challenge. We hypothesize that a humoral principle secreted by the parotid glands affects the pancreatic function as it modulates the sensitivity of the β-cells to blood glucose and/or the insulin reserve. This insulinotropic effect appears to reside primarily with the parotids, and the role of the submandibular glands seems to be permissive at best.

Several investigators have demonstrated the presence of immunoreactive and bioactive insulin-like material in various tissues, including the parotid and submandibular glands [refs]. Biosynthesis of insulin was demonstrated in these glands [refs]. From this perspective, the researcher may conclude that the decrease in circulating IRI after parotidectomy is a consequence of the removal of parotid insulin. For several reasons, we believe that this position is not tenable. First, the collective tissue concentration of extra-pancreatic insulin is low, and its concentration in the parotids is estimated to be 1/7000 of that in the pancreas [ref]. Second, attempts to stimulate secretion of IRI from extra-pancreatic sources in eviscerated rats with either arginine or glucose have been unsuccessful [ref]. Third, if several extra-pancreatic sources of insulin exist and are significant in glucose homeostasis, the removal of one of them should trigger compensatory secretion from remaining sources. For example, in our study the submandibular glands, which have been claimed to be a possible source of insulin [ref], did not show any appreciable effect on the IRI secretion, as indicated by their removal. In our opinion the physiologic role of extra-pancreatic insulin in glucose homeostasis remains to be established. The 45% decrease in circulating IRI after parotidectomy observed in this study represents a significant departure from the normal response and suggests an impairment of β-cell function.

In conclusion, the parotids appear to be the source of an insulinotropic principle that may be significant in maintaining the sensitivity of β-cells to circulating glucose. We have isolated a parotid hormone (PH) from porcine glands, the function of which is critical for maintaining a systemic resistance mechanism against dental decay through the activation of a dentinal fluid transport. This PH-mediated mechanism can be suppressed by a cariogenic, high-sucrose diet [refs]. Other studies have shown that poorly controlled, insulin-dependent diabetic humans and diabetic rats have a higher incidence of dental caries, which can be corrected in the rat with insulin therapy [refs]. From a systemic point of view, cariogenesis, diabetes, and PH secretion have a common denominator, glucose intolerance. Such a coincidental dependence suggests that PH may be involved in a parotid-β-cell relationship.

Article #92

Biological and chemical evidence for the existence of a porcine hypothalamic parotid hormone-releasing factor

Tièche JM, Leonora J. Biochem Biophys Res Commun. March 159(3):899-906, 1989

The existence of a hypothalamus-parotid gland endocrine axis was deduced from studies on the dynamic nature of a dentinal fluid transport mechanism present in teeth [ref]. The parotid glands secrete a hormone that activates a centrifugal dentinal fluid transport mechanism in rat molar teeth; in addition, secretion of this hormone was found to be under the control of a releasing factor from the hypothalamus. Existence of a dentinal fluid transport mechanism has been observed and reported by various investigators over the past 75 years (see review refs), but its relevance to dental health has not been widely recognized. Rat studies have demonstrated that an inverse relationship exists between the rate of dentinal fluid transport activity and dental decay, and that a significant reduction in decay can be achieved by maintaining the hypothalamus-parotid gland endocrine axis functional in spite of a cariogenic oral environment [refs]. It was suggested that the physiologic significance of the hypothalamus-parotid gland endocrine axis resides in its ability to regulate the dentinal fluid transport mechanism. The latter enables the avascular dentin to maintain its metabolic requirements and simultaneously provides a systemic defense mechanism against decay. In 1980 we reported the isolation from porcine parotid glands of an essentially pure polypeptide (8,100 molecular weight) capable of stimulating dentinal fluid transport in rats at picogram (pg) levels. This polypeptide was named parotid hormone (PH) [ref]. Recently, other investigators have purified a dentinal fluid transport-stimulating protein and peptide from bovine and rat parotid glands, respectively [refs].

The physiological context within which the hypothalamus-parotid gland endocrine axis functions was indicated by the observation in pigs that the plasma titer of immunoreactive PH (iPH) increases immediately following the onset of feeding, and that the responsiveness of this endocrine system is directly related to the duration of the stimulus. However, it was also demonstratred that iPH response to feeding is completely blunted after parotidectomy [ref]. Furthermore, evidence has been presented showing that this endocrine function of the parotid glands is dissociated from its exocrine function [ref].

The concept of a hypothalamus-parotid gland endocrine axis implies the existence of two secretory components. PH, secreted by the parotid glands, has been identified [ref]; and we are now presenting further evidence of the reality of the hypothalamic component—parotid hormone-releasing factor (PHRF)—thus confirming the coherence of the hypothalamus-parotid gland endocrine axis.

STUDY:

Purification of crude porcine hypothalamus-thalamus tissue extract (pHTE) was accomplished as previously described in Leonora, Tièche and Celestin, 1987. PHRF present in pHTE-PM10 filtrate) was further purified by size-exclusion chromatography. PH-releasing activity of the pHTE ultrafiltrate was assessed by the dentinal fluid transport stimulation assay in intact and parotidectomized rats and by the *in vivo* PH stimulation assay in the pig. Briefly the assay consists of infusing a test solution into a chronically catheterized pig and measuring by RIA changes in iPH titer in blood samples collected in the awake state at set time intervals for 30 min. Release of PH from the parotid glands was indicated by an increase in plasma iPH titer 3 to 5 min post-infusion, which peaked between 10 and 15 min. PHRF assays were conducted in intact and parotidectomized pigs. The iPH dose-response effect was examined using increasing amounts of pHTE in intact pigs. Results were analyzed statistically by Student's t-test for paired data when done in the same animals and by the same test for unpaired observations when not all control and experimental infusion data were available from the same animal. Analysis of variance followed by the multiple comparison test of Dunnett for iPH dose response were used when multiple levels of comparison were sought.

Results:

Of the four experimental animal species assessed for PHRF extractability from hypothalamic tissues, the pig animal model represented the highest dentinal fluid transport stimulating activity per piece of tissue equivalent as shown in Table 1.

TABLE 1. PHRF activity potency of crude hypothalamic tissue extracts from 4 animal species by the *in vivo* DFT stimulation assay in the rat and expressed as the least effective dose

Animal Source of Hypothalamic Tissue	DFT Response Dose[a]	(FMR)[b]	p
Rabbit	0.125	0.37± .03 (14)[c]	<0.001[d]
(Control)	Saline	0.36±.03 (12)	
Pig	**0.003**	**0.32± .04 (10)**	**<0.002[d]**
(Control)	**Saline**	**0.17± .03 (10)**	
Sheep	0.0075	0.24± .05 (5)	<0.014[d]
(Control)	Saline	0.10± .03 (7)	
Rat	0.10	0.28± .05 (5)	<0.002[d]
(Control)	Saline	0.10± .03 (7)	

a, dose = hypothalamic piece-equivalent/rat; b, dentinal fluid movement ratio (FMR) mean ± SE; c, number of animals; d, compared with saline control

Infusion of the pHTE-PM10 filtrate fraction not only caused a rise in iPH titer but also a drooling and frothing around the mouth. Increased agitation and retching were also observed. It was ineffective in parotidectomized pigs. The same extract was also capable of stimulating the dentinal fluid transport mechanism in intact rats but failed in parotidectomized animals. The biological activity data of the PHRF fractions at each step of purification are summarized in Table 2.

TABLE 2. Summary of biological activity and yield of the different PHRF fractions at each stage of purification, and effect of protease treatment, as measured by the *in vivo* PH stimulation assay in the pig

Fraction	Amount tested (g eq fresh tissue)	iPH response[a] (ng/ml)	Yield (g protein)	Specific Activity[b]
Fresh tissue	-	-	1[c]	
pHTE	-	-	2.3×10^{-3}	
pHTE	65	79 ± 12 (4)[d]	1.4×10^{-3}	11
Saline	0	3 ± 1 (4)e	-	
pHTE-P2 active fraction	80	102 ± 21 (6)	2.7×10^{-4}	45
Saline	0	2 ± 1 (6)[e]	-	
pHTE-RP8 active fraction	180	71 ± 17 (3)	5×10^{-6}	1111
Untreated pHTE-P2 active fraction	80	106 ± 19 (3)		
pHTE-P2 active fraction treated with pronase	80	4 ± 1 (3)[e]		
Saline	0	2 ± 1 (3)NS		

a, maximum plasma iPH increase following infusion in the pig; **b**, expressed as number of effective doses for pigs/g protein; **c**, fresh tissue weight in g; **d**, mean increase ± SE of the number of pigs in parenthesis; **e**, p <0.01 compared to the previous group; **f**, p <0.02 compared to the previous group; **NS**, not significant.

Discussion:

Porcine hypothalamus-thalamus tissue was selected for isolating PHRF because it displayed the highest potency per piece of tissue. We also surveyed other porcine tissues for PH-releasing activity. No activity was found in cerebral cortex, cerebellum, anterior and posterior pituitary, pancreas and kidney tissues. Tissue samples from the cerebral peduncles, pons, and medulla did demonstrate a weaker and less sustained iPH response.

PH-releasing activity of the pHTE-P2 fraction was destroyed by incubation *in vivo* with pronase E suggesting the peptidic nature of PHRF. As a releasing factor, PHRF represents a significant departure from hypophysiotropic hormones. Because of the proximity of the anterior pituitary to the hypothalamus, the concentration of hypophysiotropic hormones reaching the pituitary is effectively maintained against the dilution and enzymatic degradation that would become serious problems if these hormones entered the systemic circulation. In contrast, PHRF remains biologically active even after entering the systemic circulation. This survivability suggests (1) PHRF must have a peptidic structure that is resistant to serum endopeptidases, (2) its transport may be associated with a carrier protein, and/or (3) the quantity of PHRF released into the circulation is sufficient to compensate for degradation.

The activity present in pHTE demonstrated characteristics consistent with the putative hypothalamic component of the hypothalamus-parotid gland endocrine axis. Using two independent assays, pHTE stimulated the release of iPH in the pig and the dentinal fluid transport mechanism in the rat, but it was ineffective after parotidectomy. These results confirm the requirement of an intact hypothalamus-parotid gland endocrine axis for PHRF to express itself because pHTE alone does not display PH activity (dentinal fluid transport stimulation). In addition, the graded iPH response to infusion of increasing amounts of pHTE-P2 active fraction suggests that the porcine parotid gland is capable of modulating its PH output as a function of circulating PHRF.

In conclusion, biological evidence confirms the existence in porcine hypothalamus-thalamus of an extractable peptidic factor capable of regulating the secretion of PH from the parotid glands. This strengthens the concept of a hypothalamus-parotid gland endocrine axis which has been presented as a physiologic determinant in the regulation of a dental health-promoting mechanism of dentinal fluid transport.

Article #93

The effect of dietary factors on intradentinal dye penetration in the rat

Leonora J, Tièche JM, Steinman RR. Arch Oral Biol 37:733-741, 1992

The possibility of a circulation of dental fluid within dentinal tubules was suggested by Fish (1927) and supported experimentally by others (Bodecker and Lefkowitz, 1937; Lefkowitz, 1943). **Although dentinal fluid flow has not been observed directly *in vivo* due to technicalities involving hard dental tissues, evidence has accumulated for the existence in the pulp-dentin complex of structures and pathways that could support fluid flow (for review, see Thomas, 1985: Holland, 1985).* The physical variables controlling the hydraulic conductance of dentin have been defined in *in vitro* and *in vivo* models (Reeder et al., 1978; Pashley, 1989; Maita et al., 1991), thus laying the foundation for the existence of a mechanism for dentinal fluid flow. The physiological significance of fluid flow across the dentin was first suggested by Gysi (1900)* in an attempt to explain dentinal sensitivity. Later, the concept of dentinal hydrodynamics linked to dentin sensitivity was developed by Brännström and others (see Pashley 1990* for review on dentin sensitivity). That the dentinal hydraulic system could be in continuity with the systemic circulation became apparent when Fish (1927) showed accumulation of dye in the dentin of dogs 30 min after its subcutaneous injection. The passage of radioisotopes from the circulation to the dentin has been demonstrated in monkey [refs] and in dogs [refs]. Movement of markers in the reverse direction was also shown in dogs (Pashley et al 1981a,b, 1983). By using a "push-pull" perfusion device fixed to the incisor dentin of rats, Litovsky and Arancibia (1988) showed that colchicine or ouabain could inhibit the flux kinetics of a radiotracer through the dentin, indicating the existence of active mechanisms regulating movement of dentinal fluid *in vivo.***

Passage of the fluorescent dye, acriflavine, from the circulation through dentinal tubules and to the dentin-enamel junction was demonstrated with histological and fluorescence microscopic techniques (Steinman 1967, 1968; Steinman and Leonora 1975a). This intradentinal dye penetration was believed to reflect bulk fluid flow between capillaries and dentinal tubules; hence, it was termed "dentinal fluid movement." It was suggested that perfusion of the avascular dentin by a process of fluid flow could be a determinant in maintaining the integrity of dental tissue. Also, preliminary observation indicated that dye penetration into dentinal tubules was faster in rats maintained on a noncariogenic diet than in rats fed a cariogenic diet (Steinman 1967).

In 1968, Leonora and Steinman observed that crude extracts of parotid gland and hypothalamic tissue infused into rats by intravenous injection stimulated

intradentinal dye penetration. They suggested that dentinal fluid flow could be under hormonal control, and postulated the existence of a hypothalamus-parotid gland endocrine axis. According to this notion, the hypothalamus secretes a parotid hormone-releasing factor that triggers the release of a parotid hormone; the latter stimulates intradental dye penetration (Leonora and Steinman 1968). Factors stimulating intradentinal dye penetration have been isolated in pure form from porcine (Tièche, Leonora and Steinman 1980), and rat (Yamamoto, Kobayashi and Kobayashi 1986b) parotid gland extracts.

The preliminary qualitative observation that a high-sucrose diet could affect the rate of this dye penetration compelled us to investigate the issue in more detail. In addition, and because this penetration seems to be controlled by a parotid factor, we now examined the possibility that dietary factors might affect it through changes in parotid function.

STUDY:

Intradentinal dye penetration measurement:

Sprague-Dawley male 21-day-old rats were maintained for 1 wk on high-sucrose or Purina rat chow diets, after which they were injected intraperitoneally with acriflavine dye. At various times following injection, their jaws were immediately frozen and prepared for microscopic observation. A microtome slice 50-80 μm was obtained parallel to the dentinal tubules and as near to the greatest depth of the occlusal grooves as possible. The presence of fluorescent dye was observed in dentinal tubules at the base of the occlusal grooves. Microscopic viewing areas were carefully oriented in a standardized fashion for maximum accuracy of comparative scoring. Tubules fluorescing brilliant green the entire length from pulp to enamel within the delineated area received a positive rating. Fluorescence not reaching the DEJ was scored zero. 1/3 increments were counted in between.

Parotidectomy:

Parotid ducts were tied in 22-day-old rats and bilateral parotidectomies performed 3 days later. Sham-parotidectomized control animals had their parotid ducts ligated without removal of their glands. Normal food intake occurred within 24 hr.

Preparation of hormonally active plasma:

Blood was obtained by heart puncture from several animals and pooled according to the rats' diet category, then centrifuged, and the plasma frozen until needed for infusion.

Stimulation test for intradentinal dye penetration:

IDDP was determined in rat molar teeth after the infusion of plasma, 55 min after injection of the dye. Acriflavine dye was administered i.p. 10 min before plasma was infused gradually over a 35-min period via the subclavian vein. 10 min after plasma administration, jaws were removed, frozen and prepared as previously.

Specific experiments:

Experiment 1 – Dye penetration of dentinal tubules was evaluated from rats fed either a high-sucrose diet or Purina rat chow. Also it was measured in each diet group in the unanesthetized or aneasthetized states. All 4 groups received an injection of dye i.p. and their teeth scored for dye penetration.

Experiment 2 – Dye concentrations in blood circulation were assessed at 10, 35, 60 and 90 min times post-dye-injection from small, diluted blood samples analyzed with a fluorimeter.

Experiment 3 – Rat teeth were analyzed at the 55-min basal level for IDDP following 1 wk on the two diets.

Group 1– High-sucrose diet, intact
Group 2– High-sucrose, parotidectomized
Group 3– Purina chow-fed, intact
Group 4– Purina chow-fed, parotidectomized
Group 5– Purina chow-fed, sham (controls)

Experiment 4– To test the hypothesis that diets may either stimulate or inhibit IDDP (Steinman 1967), plasma obtained from intact rats maintained for 1 wk either on Purina chow or high-sucrose diet was infused i.v. into parotidectomized rats fed Purina chow and intact rats fed high-sucrose diet. As a control, saline was infused into the two recipient groups of rats.

Data analysis:

IDDP was expressed as a ratio of the number of dentinal areas where positive fluorescence was observed/total number of areas for each animal and these values were tabulated.

Results:

Experiment 1 – FIG. 1 demonstrates various patterns. Intradentinal dye penetration was slower in anesthetized rats than in unanaesthetized. Feeding the high-sucrose diet for 1 wk resulted in significant depression of dye penetration compared to 1 wk on the Purina chow. In unanesthetized rats on Purina chow IDDP was rapid, peaking at 30 min. Unanesthetized rats on the high-sucrose diet displayed a lower, slower rise in the number of fluorescing tubules, peaking at 45 min, and a lower level of maximum tubule fluorescence.

Experiment 2 – Plasma dye concentrations at 10 min were 630 ± 50 and 750 ± 30 ng/ml in the Purina chow and high-sucrose anesthetized rats, respectively. At 35 min the levels were 860 ± 40 and 830 ± 40 ng/ml, respectively. At 60 and 90 min dye levels remained elevated with no significant difference between groups.

Experiment 3 – The effect of changing diet from Purina chow to the HSD was a significant drop in the dye penetration score (Fig. 2). Parotidectomized Purina-fed rats resulted in significantly lower scores despite the nonsuppressive diet. Sham surgery showed no suppressive effect, neither did parotidectomized rats on a high-sucrose diet. The saline controls showed no significant effect on intradentinal dye penetration in any group.

Experiment 4 – Plasma infusion from Purina-fed rats significantly increased IDDP in parotidectomized animals, whereas 2 ml plasma from HSD-fed rats proved ineffective (Fig. 3). 2 ml plasma from Purina-fed rats infused into intact high-sucrose animals resulted in significant increase in dye penetration, while no elevation was observed after infusion of plasma from HSD-fed rats. IDDP-stimulating factor was present in plasma from Purina-fed rats whereas no detectable activity was demonstrated in plasma from HSD-fed rats

Discussion:

The acriflavine dye technique enables us to present physiological evidence that dietary factors affect dentinal fluid movement, presumably through an endocrine mechanism. This approach involved no operative dental procedures that could potentially disrupt the internal environment and lead to inaccurate conclusions. Our experience has shown that dye movement within dentinal tubules does not occur synchronously in all dentinal areas within the same animal, however it is relatively uniform in single areas such as the dentin beneath occlusal grooves.

Dye penetration should be understood as a dynamic process with time and magnitude of response related. Dye penetration is intrinsically time-dependent. The rate of dye passage from pulpal circulation through odontoblasts and up the tubules is related to the status of the host animal (Fig. 1**). A rapid rate was associated with feeding non-cariogenic Purina rat chow whereas decreased rate was noted with feeding a cariogenic high-sucrose diet which was further enhanced by anesthesia** (Fig. 1).

It is not known if mechanisms driving DFT are cyclical in nature, in which case extending the experiment longer would have given different results. Anesthesia and dietary quality could affect both the rate and kinetics of dye penetration as well as the periodicity of the activity, which would influence height of the dye penetration peak. This might explain the lower peak level in anesthetized Purina-fed rats compared with their sucrose-fed counterparts, whereas the pattern was reversed in the unanesthetized state. The important feature here was relative dye penetration rate per treatment rather than absolute peak magnitude.

Acriflavine toxicity should be considered as a possible artifactual factor in dye penetration in the descending part of the time-curve because it was being administered at 20% lethal dose levels. Centrifugal flow cessation could cause flow direction reversal, since its bi-directionality has already been reported earlier [refs]. Centripetal flow toward the pulp would draw fluid out of the tubules leaving them vacuous in which case they would appear empty. With increase in flow rate, toxicity would be a function of increased acriflavine uptake affecting susceptible tissue. In this context, the meaningful part of the time-curves (Fig. 1) would be limited to the ascending portion.

We chose a decapitation time of 55 mins because it was the most favorable considering (1) the basal intradentinal dye penetration was low in sucrose-fed and high in Purina-fed animals (Fig. 2) and at the same time, the stimulated animal would have an elevated dye penetration score when compared to the unstimulated control. It is difficult to conceive that parotidectomy depressed the basal rate of dye penetration because dentinal fluid could still be stimulated in these animals by infusing plasma from Purina-fed rats (Fig. 3). **Within the time-frame of our experiments, the responsiveness and/or vitality of the pulp-dentin complex was maintained in spite of diet or surgical treatments. It appears that the sucrose diet effect was directed at a control mechanism rather than at the fluid transport process.**

Recent hemodynamic studies have indicated a direct relationship between systemic vascular pressure and pulpal interstitial pressure [refs] that could influence DFT. We have observed in 180+ g rats that the tail systolic BP was 123 ± 7 and 120 ± 6 mm Hg in 90-g sham-operated and parotidectomized rats respectively, which indicates no significant difference. To our knowledge feeding of a high-sucrose diet also has no appreciable effect.

Because potential vascular changes do not seem to affect i IDDP, **we speculate that a parotid endocrine factor uniquely affected a pulpal vascular factor or some cellular process at the level of the odontoblastic cell layer resulting in increased DFT.**

Dye transfer from general circulation to the DEJ may involve at least 3 steps. The dye (1) crosses the pulpal capillary wall to the odontoblastic cell layer, (2) crosses the odontoblastic barrier and enters the odontoblastic peritubular space or into the odontoblast, and (3) travels via odontoblastic processes within dentinal tubules to reach the DEJ. Consequently, it is conceivable that this transport may involve more than one mechanism. **Passive diffusion is unlikely because of the rapidity (15 min) with which the dye appeared within the tubules of Purina-fed unanesthetized animals (Fig. 1A). Also Litovsky and Arancibia (1988) showed that ouabain or colchicine agents significantly reduced rate of tracer ion appearances on exposed dentin surfaces.**

We theorize that a controlled mechanism of fluid flow exists between pulpal capillaries and dentinal tubules. Maita [ref] suggested a differential hydrostatic pressure between pulpal tissue and dentinal tubule spaces might be sufficient to produce a bulk fluid flow. **We postulate a process occurring at the level of odontoblasts that under activation by various factors allows passage of pulpal fluid to the DEJ. This may or may not involve gap junctions but occurs through changes in pulpal capillary and odontoblastic intercellular permeability and/or pressure [ref]. Possibly a pumping mechanism exerted by odontoblasts and their cytoplasmic extensions could be involved [ref]. It would seem that fluid reaching the DEJ must leave at a rate equal to that of its influx in order to maintain a dynamic flow.**

Enamel is generally viewed as a dense, glassy material. However, it is porous and exhibits relative permeability to small molecules such as shown by a variety of dyes and radioactive tracers [refs]. In addition, an accumulation of enamel fluid on the surface of human teeth was observed [ref]. Methylene blue on the surface of rat molars showed penetration into the dentin with time. **It appears that enamel in general is a porous material that behaves like a semipermeable membrane** [ref], **therefore a fraction of dentinal fluid can permeate the enamel to its outer surfaces**, however it isn't possible to estimate that fraction as a ratio to the dentinal flux fraction.

There exists an extensive side-branching of dentinal tubules that appear to anastomose and form a series of lateral channels close to the pre-dentin and DEJ [refs]. This system could provide pathways for lateral movement over significant distances. Perhaps if combined with odontoblastic cell-to-cell contact, a synchronization of activity could take place between groups of tubules coordinated such that some would channel fluid up while others would move it back down. This mechanism would involve an active pumping process by the odontoblasts to overcome hydrostatic pressure. Returned fluid could then be taken up by lymphatics, the existence of which has been suggested by Heyeraas (1989).

A substantial transfer of proteins and minerals occurs between odontoblastic processes and dentin during dentinogenesis and later tissue remodeling. Endocrine or other regulatory mechanisms may be important to optimize this function in developing as well as in erupted teeth.

Dietary considerations affect parotid endocrine secretion as suggested in studies with pigs, but not when pigs had undergone parotidectomy procedures [ref]. It appears that ingestion of food has an acute effect on the secretion of parotid hormone that presumably controls DFT. Could this serve to maximize a protective mechanism for the teeth at times when they are subjected to greater destructive potentials?

Young Purina-fed rats were shown to exhibit higher levels of dye penetrance activity (Figs. 1, 2) and fewer dental lesions at a mature age [refs]. In contrast, young sucrose-fed rats showed a lower level of dye penetrance activity (Figs. 1, 2) and higher incidence of dental lesions at maturity [refs]. Similarly, carbamyl-DL-aspartic acid and carbamyl phosphate, which acutely stimulated intradentinal dye penetration, can, as dietary additives to a high-sucrose diet, significantly reduce dental decay [refs]. These observations suggest that the activity associated with maintenance of dye penetrance may be significant in preserving the integrity of dental structures.

Earlier work suggested that secretion of parotid hormone (PH) is under the control of a hypothalamic releasing factor (HRF); these two hormonal components would then constitute the hypothalamus-parotid gland endocrine (HPGE) axis [refs]. It is conceivable that the effect of diet on IDDP may actually involve both components of the endocrine axis.

Article #94

<u>Stimulation of intradentinal dye penetration by feeding in the rat</u>

Leonora J, Tièche JM, Steinman RR. Arch Oral Biol 38:763-767, 1993

Markers have demonstrated the flow of fluids/solutes from general circulation to dentinal tubules *in vivo* in several animal species. Fish (1927) showed dye in the dentin of dogs 30 min after its subcutaneous injection. Von Kreudenstein measured amounts of penicillin, tetracycline, and glucose in dentinal fluid from intravenous infusion in dogs. Glucose was timed 10 min after infusion, similar to Potts who timed radioactivity in dentinal fluid 10-15 min from i.v. injection of tritiated water. Also, radioactive iodine was collected from incisor dentin 15-30 min after infusion (Litovsky & Arancibia 1988). Steinman observed that fluorescent dye injected intraperitoneally reached dentinal tubules by 10 min and the DEJ by 20 min in young rats. Furthermore, these studies indicated the rate of appearance was alterable by changes in the animals' diet or by injection of bethanecholchloride, a parasympathetic stimulant. These observations led investigators to the possibility that dye penetration could be controlled by systemic factors.

Leonora and Steinman (1968) observed in young rats that infusion of crude extracts of parotid glands or hypothalamic tissue stimulated intradentinal dye penetration (IDDP), which caused them to postulate involvement of an endocrine system regulator. In 1980 an intradentinal dye penetration-stimulating factor was isolated from porcine parotid tissue by Tièche, Leonora and Steinman and termed parotid hormone (PH).

Independently, IDDP stimulating factors were also isolated from bovine and rat parotid glands in Japan in 1986. Immunoreactive PH was measured at normal levels and found to be higher in the pig circulation following i.v. infusion of hypothalamus-thalamus tissue extract (Leonora, Tièche and Celestin 1987). The physiological reality of PH was demonstrated in pigs, in which feeding proved to be a potent stimulus for iPH secretion: 2 min after the onset of feeding an increase in circulating iPH titer was detected, which peaked in 10-20 min to a level 10 times higher than before feeding, and then decreased slowly over the next 2 h. Furthermore, the iPH response was totally abolished when the pigs were parotidectomized (Leonora et al 1987).

Stimulation of IDDP in response to infusion of parotid hormone or hypothalamic tissue extract in rats, and the secretion of iPH after the onset of feeding in pigs, supports the concept of a parotid endocrine function that seems to be physiologically implicated in the control of IDDP. If this proposition is true, feeding should trigger both secretion of parotid hormone and activation of IDDP. Since, for technical reasons, simultaneous measurement of iPH and IDDP cannot be done in the same animal, this study tested the hypothesis that feeding physiologically stimulates IDDP through a parotid function using a rat model.

STUDY:

Male 21-day-old Sprague-Dawley rats were maintained for 1 wk on pelleted Purina rat chow. Then, after fasting 18 h they were offered Purina chow. Once eating began, which usually took 1-2 min, timing was started and the rats were allowed to eat for exactly 15 min at which time they were anesthetized and injected with acriflavine fluorescent dye intraperitoneally. Jaws were quickly removed and frozen on dry ice from animals decapitated at time intervals of 20, 23, 28, 33 or 38 min after dye injection. Frozen sections 80-100 μm were prepared for microscopic analysis of dye penetration as previously described. Intradentinal dye penetration (IDDP) was expressed for each animal as a ratio of the number of areas of fluorescence to the total number of areas examined.

IDDP and feeding: Effect of sialoadenectomy

To test the possible effect of surgery on feeding-stimulated IDDP, the rats underwent 4 surgical procedures (1) bilateral parotidectomy, (2) submandibular and sublingual glandectomies, (3) total sialoadenectomy that included all three glands, and (4) a sham operation. As a control, a 5th group was left intact. All animals were maintained on Purina rat chow for the next 6 days. Following a similar fasting procedure, these animals were again fed Purina chow for 15 min then dye-injected and killed 33 min later for IDDP examination.

Results:

TABLE 1. Effect of partial or total sialoadenectomy on IDDP in rats fasted or fed for 15 min

Group No.	Status	IDDP ratio	(N)	Statistical comparison between groups
1	Intact fasted	0.106	(10)	...
2	Intact fed	0.418	(10)	1 vs. 2, $p < 0.001$
3	Sham fasted	0.100	(5)	...
4	Sham fed	0.525	(4)	3 vs. 4, $p < 0.01$
5	Parotidectomized fed	0.066	(5)	4 vs. 5, $p < 0.01$
6	Submandibularectomized fed	0.487	(5)	4 vs. 6, NS
7	Total sialoadenectomized fed	0.176	(3)	3 vs. 7, NS

IDDP in rats fed for 15 min was significantly more extensive than in the unfed group. This increase was observed starting at 23 min and lasting beyond 38 min after the end of the 15-min meal (Fig. 1). A high IDDP response was measured 33 min after feeding in the intact-fed, sham-fed and fed animals whose submandibular and sublingual glands had been removed. However, the IDDP level was significantly lower in parotidectomized or totally sialoadenectomized groups. The parotidectomized group showed an IDDP level similar to fasted (non-fed) animals.

Discussion:

Considering the chemical nature of the dye, the fast rate of appearance of dye in the tubules does not necessarily support the concept of movement via a passive bulk fluid flow from transcapillary permeation of plasma ultrafiltrate into the pulpal interstitial space. **The present findings indicate that the rate or magnitude of IDDP changed significantly after food ingestion. This suggests that physiological changes, triggered by feeding, occurred within the pulp-dentin compartment resulting in IDDP activation.** Several hypothetical mechanisms may be advanced to explain this. Among these are changes in capillary permeability and changes in the odontoblastic layer. **Increased interstitial fluid pressure as observed in experimentally induced pulpitis (Tønder and Kvinnsland 2983, Heyeraas 1989, Maita et al 1991) supports the concept of pulpal fluid extravasation from increased capillary pressure and permeability.**

Studies indicate that pulpal blood flow is affected by sympathetic adrenergic nerve fibers (Kim, Dorscher-Kim and Liu 1989); **furthermore, neuropeptides and vasoactive agents have been identified in the pulp and/or shown to cause changes in pulpal blood flow when infused or applied topically. These agents include: bradykinin, acetylcholine, histamine, substance P, serotonin, vasoactive intestinal peptide, noradrenaline, neuropeptide Y, somatostatin, prostaglandin E_2** (Todoki 1988, Narhi 1989, Olgart, Edwall and Gazelius 1989, Liu et al 1990, Kim 1990, Casasco et al 1991).

It is possible that feeding could stimulate oral sensory receptors through a neural pathway ending in the pulp, where vasoactive factor(s) could be released. These factors might trigger tissue reactions, leading to an increase in permeability of the capillaries and/or of the odontoblastic cell layer. Also, neural pathways could entail pulpal or dentinal sensors to feeding (mechanical receptors), which under stimulation would signal the release of vasoactive factor(s) from nerve endings. **Analogous physiological arrangements have been suggested in cat teeth [ref] in which deformation of dentin resulted in instant dilation of the pulpal capillaries. However, changes in vascular permeability and/or the permeability of the odontoblastic layer have to occur for fluid and solutes to increase their rate of dentinal penetration.**

A relation of causality between secretion of parotid hormone and stimulation of IDDP appears plausible and would explain changes in intradentinal dye penetration activity associated with feeding. The iPH data in pigs indirectly support the possible endocrine role of parotid hormone in feed-stimulated activation of intradentinal dye penetration.

That stimulation of IDDP by feeding is mediated through activation of a parotid function was further suggested by the results of surgical treatment on IDDP (Table 1). Removal of salivary glands abolished the feeding-stimulated IDDP response only when the parotid glands were involved. The results suggest the importance of the integrity of the parotids in activation of IDDP.

A tentative schema may be presented: Feeding may stimulate oral receptors whose afferents would relay neural message(s) to the hypothalamus, which could respond by releasing into the circulation a parotid hormone-releasing factor (PHRF), which upon reaching the pulpal capillary-odontoblast space, would activate passage of fluid from the circulation into the dentinal tubules. In addition

to an expected hormone-tissue receptor type of activation, the process could possibly also involve pulpal neurotransmitter(s) as secondary messages or cofactors.

The significance of a pulpal process regulating IDDP is a puzzling but intriguing question. Two assumptions can be made. (1) The movement of fluorescent dye is likely to follow that of fluid originating from transcapillary permeation or bulk fluid flow. (2) As in all living tissue, there must be fluid continuity throughout the various levels of dental tissues—between capillary spaces and dentin. It would follow that fluid in amounts equal to that entering the dentin space must also leave that space following a pressure gradient generated at the entry site, and imposed by the incompressibility of dentin. **Fluid has been reported permeating dog dentin at atmospheric pressure** [refs]. The observations suggest that fluid flow up the dentinal tubules may continue, at least partially, by permeating through the enamel.

The essential function of the teeth is in eating. Remarkably, the ingestion of food threatens the teeth because it provides substrates for bacterial byproducts that are potentially injurious to tooth structure. We postulate that as the passage of dye and fluid across the dentin increases in response to feeding, there is a build-up of hydrostatic pressure, which causes the permeation of minute amounts of fluid through the enamel. Such outward flux through the enamel would oppose the ingress of injurious bacterial substances and provide a physiological defense mechanism at a time when the integrity of dental tissue is at high risk.
[Bar graph in Fig. 1 shows dramatic increases in IDDP ratios between fed and unfed rats]

Article #95

Further evidence for a hypothalamus-parotid gland endocrine axis in the rat

Leonora J, Tièche JM, Steinman RR. Arch Oral Biol 38:911-916, 1993

Both centrifugal and centripetal fluid flow within dentinal tubules have been demonstrated (for review, see Leonora et al 1992). Histological methods and fluorescence microscopy have demonstrated passage of fluorescent dye from the circulation to the pulp and through the dentinal tubules of rat molar teeth. **We interpret intradentinal dye penetration to be a reflection of bulk fluid flow through the dentinal tubules** (Leonora et al 1992). Vongasavan and Matthews (1992) directly measured the outward flow of fluid permeating through exposed dentin at the tips of fractured cat canine teeth.

In 1968 Leonora and Steinman reported an increased rate of IDDP elicited by infusion of crude extracts of parotid gland or hypothalamic tissue. Since it appeared to be under hormonal control, the concept of a hypothalamus-parotid gland endocrine axis was then advanced: The parotid glands secrete PH that stimulates IDDP, and that secretion is under the control of PHRF from the hypothalamus (Leonora & Steinman 1968). Subsequently, IDDP factors have been isolated in pure form from porcine, rat, and bovine parotid tissues, and a PHRF was partially purified from porcine hypothalamus tissue. This PHRF stimulated IDDP only when infused into intact rats and triggered the release of plasma immunoreactive PH after infusion into intact pigs. Parotidectomy blocked this response [refs].

The parotid IDDP-stimulating polypeptide and a hypothalamic parotid hormone-releasing activity supports the hypothalamus-parotid endocrine axis, the physiological existence of this axis has not been firmly established. **At present, modulation of**

intradentinal dye penetration is the only documented effect of the putative secretions of this axis. Earlier work (Steinman and Leonora 1975a) indicated that carbamyl aspartic acid, a compound of the ornithine-urea cycle is capable of IDDP. **This study sought to use CAA's IDDP-stimulating effect to ascertain existence of endocrine factors.**

STUDY:

IDDP was determined in 28-day old male rats on a high-sucrose diet for 1 wk. Fluorescent dye was administered as previously described and the jaws frozen and sectioned for observation.

Parotidectomy: 25-day-old rats underwent bilateral parotidectomy under anesthesia.

I.V. and I.A. infusion: i.v. infusion was done via subclavian vein, i.a. infusion via internal carotid artery, with 2 ml gradually over 35 min's.

Plasma collection: CAA was infused i.a. then after 45 min exsanguinated by cardiac puncture. 3 pooled samples of plasma were obtained: (1) from 100 intact rats infused with CAA, (2) from 25 intact control rats after saline infusion, and (3) from 30 parotidectomized rats that received CAA.

Experiment 1 – intact and parotidectomized rats on a HSD received i.a. CAA in various doses to determine the IDDP response.

Experiment 2 – blood was collected from intact or parotidectomized rats after CAA i.v. infusion to elucidate the mechanism of action of CAA in stimulating IDDP.

Experiment 3 – hypothalamic lesions were electrolytically produced in rats with electrodes. Sham-operated animals had electrodes placed but no current applied. This was to show how much IDDP occurred in the absence of a functioning hypothalamus.

Results:

Experiment 1 - CAA infusion stimulated IDDP in a dose-related fashion (Fig. 1). CAA infused i.a. into parotidectomized rats proved ineffective, however.

Experiment 2 – Saline-treated intact controls and parotidectomized rats showed ineffective IDDP. In contrast, CAA-treated intact rats did show IDDP stimulation. A similar effect was obtained from 1 and 2 ml of the same plasma into parotidectomized animals. This indicates the presence of parotid glands was optional for IDDP stimulation. However, plasma from parotidectomized rats treated with CAA was effective for IDDP in intact but not in parotidectomized rats (Fig. 3).

Experiment 3 – Plasma from intact or sham-operated CAA-infused rats was equally effective in stimulating IDDP. However, plasma from rats with hypothalamic lesions was ineffective.

Discussion:

This study showed the ability to stimulate *in vivo* dentinal fluid flow by CAA infusion and indirectly established an endocrine link between stimulus and effect. It appears that irrespective of whether dye movement within dentinal tubules takes place intracellularly or through the peritubular space, and whether it follows bulk fluid flow and/or involves some active transport, the rate of transfer can be modified. This implies a regulatory control mechanism that we postulate has an endocrine component.

CAA had no direct IDDP-stimulating effect on teeth (Fig. 1) but instead required the parotid glands for expression. In experiment 2 when plasma from unstimulated (saline-infused) rats was infused into intact animals, no increase in

IDDP was observed. However, plasma from CAA-treated rats was capable of stimulating IDDP in recipient animals whether they were intact or parotidectomized (Fig. 2). Therefore, a parotid signal implicated in IDDP stimulation was absent in parotidectomized rats of Experiment 1 but present in plasma from CAA-treated intact rats of Experiment 2. This suggests a parotid factor release into circulation following CAA infusion. In all probability, this parotid endocrine factor and the IDDP-stimulating factor are one and the same.

It appears that IDDP stimulation in intact rats with plasma from parotidectomized CAA-stimulated rats involved primarily an endogenous, non-parotid circulating factor released under CAA stimulation and present in the infused plasma.

The striking functional similarities between the previously purified parotid hormone-releasing factor and the second IDDP-stimulating factor of this study strongly suggest that they represent the same hormonal entity. IDDP is believed to reflect dentinal fluid movement.

The physiological relevance of a hypothalamus-parotid endocrine axis may be best understood in conjunction with the earlier observation that changes in composition of the diet affect negatively the basal rate of IDDP, presumably through stasis in parotid function (Leonora et al 1992). Teleologically, that dietary factors could modulate the secretions of the hypothalamus-parotid axis and thereby affect dentinal fluid flow may be indicative of the potential importance of this physiological function.

It would appear that the specific modulation of a dentinal fluid flow mechanism by an endocrine system may serve a discrete purpose. Because of the avascular nature of dental tissues, maintenance of tissue perfusion by a controlled mechanism could be of more significance than anticipated. Centrifugal dentinal fluid flow could carry with it substances contributing to the formation of reparative dentin and also prevent the inward diffusion of potentially harmful solutes from the outside.

Article #96

<u>High-sucrose diet inhibits basal secretion of intradentinal dye penetration-stimulating parotid hormone in pigs</u>

Tièche JM, Leonora J, Steinman RR. J Appl Physiol 76:218-222, 1994

Evidence for dentin permeability or hydraulic conductance through dentinal tubules has been available for >50 years. Although studies have shown that dentinal fluid movement can occur either outward or inward from the pulp, depending on experimental conditions [refs], normal movement is considered to take place centrifugally from pulp to enamel [refs].

Dentinal fluid movement may play a role in dentin sensitivity [ref] and may represent a physiological means by which integrity of the avascular dental tissues is maintained despite the ingressive diffusion of bacterial of bacterial cytotoxic products from the oral environment [refs]. Caries studies in rats showed an inverse relationship between cariogenicity of certain dietary factors and pharmacological agents and the ability of the latter to stimulate centrifugal IDDP under acute administration [refs].

Furthermore, it appears that intradentinal dye penetration in the rat is regulated by an endocrine system—the hypothalamus-parotid gland endocrine axis (HPEA). The parotid glands secrete an IDDP-stimulating hormone, parotid hormone (PH), which appears to be under the control of a hypothalamic-releasing factor [refs]. A PH that stimulates intradentinal dye penetration in rat molars was isolated from porcine parotids [ref], and similarly active factors have been isolated from bovine and rat parotid tissue [refs]. Also a PH-releasing factor was partially purified from porcine thalamus-hypothalamus tissue [ref].

Excessive sucrose consumption has been closely linked to a high incidence of human dental caries [ref] and animals [ref]. We observed a significant reduction in IDDP in rats fed a cariogenic HSD compared with those fed standard Purina lab chow [refs]. At the same time, plasma from HSD-fed rats had low IDDP-stimulating activity when infused into other rats compared with the plasma from standard chow-fed animals [ref].

Presently immunoreactive PH (iPH) can be determined by radioimmunoassay (RIA) in pig plasma [ref]. Because PH affects IDDP, which can be inhibited by HSD ingestion, the question arises whether the dietary effect could be mediated through changes in PH secretion. Therefore, using the pig model, we propose to test the hypothesis that chronic ingestion of a HSD affects the basal iPH secretory function.

STUDY:

Since depressed IDDP has been found to occur after 1 wk on a HSD, we wanted to ascertain these findings after 3 wks. Male Sprague-Dawley rats were maintained on the HSD or standard Purina chow until 28, 35, or 42 days of age and tested for intraperitoneally-introduced acriflavine dye penetration into the dentinal tubules as previously described.

Chronic effect of HSD on Plasma iPH in fasting pigs:

Three-month-old castrated pigs weighing ~20 kg were housed in raised pens controlled for light-dark cycle and for temperature, and fed twice daily to satiety. After 1 wk the jugular veins were catheterized to leave valve portions accessible for i.v. antibiotics t.i.d.

Group 1 – 5 pigs 18-28 kg were given standard pig chow, chronically catheterized, and allowed 5 days for recovery. For the following 21 days they were fed standard pig chow, then switched to HSD for 60 days.

Group 2 – 4 control pigs were given standard pig chow continuously for 70 days, with their fasting iPH determined regularly.

The iPH was quantitated by a double-antibody RIA. Plasma glucose concentration was determined by the glucose oxidase method. Data computation and statistical analysis were performed using SPSS computer software.

Results:

TABLE 1 – Chronic effect of standard pig chow or HSD on fasting pig plasma iPH

Time period (days)	Diet	N	Fasting iPH % of baseline	p (vs. Baseline)
1-21 (baseline)	Standard	5	100	
22-39	HSD	5	74	NS
40-59	HSD	5	27	<0.05
60-82	HSD	5	30	<0.05
83-90	Standard	5	3	NS

TABLE 2 – Fasting iPH in pigs maintained on standard pig chow for 70 days

Time period (days)	Diet	N	Fasting iPH % of baseline	p (vs. Baseline)
1-21 (baseline)	Standard	4	100	
22-39	Standard	4	99	NS
40-70	Standard	4	92	NS

TABLE 3 – Fasting blood glucose in pigs fed standard pig chow for 21 days then maintained on pig HSD for 61 days

Time period (days)	Diet	N	Fasting iPH % of baseline	p (vs. Baseline)
1-21 (baseline)	Standard	4	94	
22-39	HSD	4	82	NS
40-59	HSD	4	84	NS
60-82	HSD	4	86	NS

Mean fasting iPH plasma titers varied widely from 2.4 to 36 ng/ml at the beginning. Rats fed HSD had significantly lower intrinsic basal IDDP scores than Purina-fed controls (Fig. 1) and iPH decreased progressively from 22 to 39 wks where it stabilized for the rest of the study. When the diet was reverted to standard pig chow, each surviving animal experienced a rebound in fasting iPH titer (Fig 3). However, when the diet was returned to standard pig chow, fasting iPH titer increased within 3-4 days, surpassing the original level. After the diet was changed to HSD, fasting plasma glucose values were insignificantly lower than before the diet change (Table 3).

Discussion:

When the diet was changed from standard pig chow to the HSD, each animal experienced a progressive and significant decrease in iPH titer, irrespective of the original level. Chronic inhibition of the basal iPH secretion appears to be related to dietary change. Substitution of non-purified simple and complex carbohydrates for a large quantity of sucrose was the major difference between the 2 diets and is likely to be responsible for the hormonal change. The complex source of proteins was replaced by a single source, soybean meal. The energy value for the HSD was 25% higher than for the standard diet.

Parotid salivary function has been shown to be dependent on diet texture. Standard pig chow was pelletized, whereas the HSD was granulated and therefore required less chewing.

Endocrine secretion of the parotid glands does not seem to parallel salivation. The sight and smell of food triggered salivation without release of iPH [ref], indicating a separate control mechanism.

Ingestion of large quantities of sucrose from the HSD could have resulted in elevated postprandial glycemia compared with standard pig chow. Preliminary work in our lab indicated that peak postprandial glycemia was 50% higher in pigs fed the HSD than regular chow. It is possible that glycemia could act as a signal to the hypothalamic glucostat center.

After 60 days on the HSD, the pigs were returned to standard pig chow, which allowed fasting iPH to return to normal in 3-4 days. Because the inhibition was revoked within this short a time, it appears the endocrine control signal must have been maintained, and suggests that inhibition of iPH basal secretion was likely directed at the endocrine control mechanisms.

PH has one known function or effect—to stimulate dentinal penetration presumably by activating IDDP [refs]. The possible existence of a direct relationship between PH secretion and IDDP appears even more promising because it has been observed that feeding causes an immediate release of iPH in the pig circulation [ref] and an increase in IDDP in rats [ref]. Furthermore, infusion of

purified tissue extract from hypothalamus-thalamus tissue generated increased IDDP in rats and iPH release in pigs [ref]. These effects only occurred when parotid glands were present. A more definitive understanding will be possible only when iPH and DFT can be measured in the same animal.

We hypothesize that if DFT, as evidenced by IDDP, is physiologically under the regulation of PH, inhibition of that endocrine function by dietary factors, such as sucrose, could render dental tissues more susceptible to the carious process. [Note: It is important to view graphs (Fig's 1-4 in original text) to show the dramatic differences.]

Article #97

Acute secretion of immunoreactive parotid hormone in response to different diets in the pig

Tièche JM, Leonora J. Arch Oral Biol 40(6):559-565, 1995

The exocrine salivary function of the parotid glands is generally considered to be its major physiological role. However, experimental evidence has been presented for the existence of a parotid endocrine function that regulates fluid flow within dental tissue [refs]. A parotid hormone isolated from parotid glands stimulates the penetration and movement of systemically administered fluorescent dye from the pulp, throughout the dentine and extending to the dentine-enamel junction of rat molar teeth [ref]. Parotid hormone appears to be part of a larger endocrine system, the hypothalamus parotid gland endocrine axis in which the hypothalamus secretes a releasing factor which causes the parotid glands to release the hormone into the systemic circulation, resulting in stimulation of intradentinal dye penetration [refs].

Porcine parotid hormone is a proline- and glycine-rich small glycoprotein of 8100 mol. wt. [ref].

Feeding is a potent stimulus to the secretion of immunoreactive parotid hormone. In pigs the plasma titer rises within 1 min of the onset of feeding and peaks between 10-20 min before decreasing progressively over the next 3-4 h. Ingestion of a high-sucrose diet chronically induces a significant reduction in intradentinal dye penetration in rats [refs] and in pigs is followed by a lower basal plasma titer of immunoreactive parotid hormone [ref].

STUDY:

The acute secretory response of iPH to the feeding of three different test diets was measured repeatedly in young pigs over prolonged periods of time, during which the maintenance diet was switched from standard to high sucrose. After an adaptation period of 7-10 days, a Teflon monitoring catheter was introduced into the superior vena cava. Four pigs, weighing between 18 and 28 kg were maintained on standard pig chow and catheterized. The experiment started five days later by feeding standard pig chow. On the 24th day, this maintenance diet was changed to pig high-sucrose diet for 65 days. During the 89 days of the study, at 1-5 day intervals the pigs were fasted 15-16 h then fed three test diets: pelleted standard pig chow, crushed standard pig chow or granulated high-sucrose diet. Baseline blood samples were obtained through the catheter at time intervals of 5, 10, 15, and 20 min while the pig was eating, and again after the food was taken away at 30, 45 and 60 min. Blood samples were centrifuged immediately after collection and the plasma was separated and refrigerated for radioimmunoassay of immunoreactive parotid hormone.

Diets: Standard pig chow was a pelleted commercial non-purified swine chow used as the control diet. Crushed standard pig chow was the same except ground into a coarse meal. High-sucrose diet was basically purified and granulated soybean meal with 620 g sucrose/kg. The entire study was arbitrarily divided into 4 time periods: T1 = 24 days before day 0 in which the pigs were maintained on standard chow, T2 = days 1-21, T3 = days 22-39, and T4 = days 40-65.

Results:

Feeding triggered an acute release of iPH. Pelleted standard chow elicited a high response, crushed chow a low response, and high-sucrose diet a very weak response. Chronically, when the maintenance diet was changed from standard chow to high sucrose there was a significant decrease in the fasting plasma titer. There was no statistical difference between the maximum response to feeding the crushed standard chow test diet before and after the change in maintenance diet. There was a significant decrease in the maximum response to the high-sucrose test diet between T2 and T3 or T4. The maximum response within each time period was significantly different between all 3 test diets.

Discussion:

The critical factors governing the magnitude of the hormonal response seem to rest with the quality and texture of the diet. The nutritional quality of the test diet appears unlikely to be the stimulus for the initial (5 min) secretion of iPH because absorption of nutrients has not significantly begun. Food taste could be a significant component in the stimulatory process. Sensory inputs elicited by food texture may also be important. A possible pathway leading to feeding-related secretion of iPH could include sensory receptors in the oropharyngeal cavity leading to efferent signals to the hypothalamus to trigger secretion of PHRF, and ultimately stimulate PH secretion.

No evidence of a second secretory phase for iPH has yet been demonstrated, and the sight and smell of food without actual ingestion do not trigger a response even though the pigs are in a state of excitement and salivate profusely. This suggests a stimulus-secretion mechanism parallel to that of cephalic-phase secretions. It is postulated that discrete oropharyngeal signals may be at the origin of the reflex secretion of iPH.

A liquid diet induces a reversible decrease in saliva flow and protein content. **In rabbits and man, parotid salivation can be acutely stimulated by chewing, and periodontal mechanoreceptors appear to be involved in the control loop.**

Parotid hormone has no known digestive function. Its only known effect in the rat is the stimulation of dye and fluid movement from the circulation through the dentinal tubules of molar teeth [refs]. Steinman, Leonora, Vongsavan and Pashley have suggested that maintenance of a centrifugal dentinal fluid flow could have a protective role by preventing inward diffusion of oral cytotoxic bacterial products. The synchrony of feeding and iPH secretion, although each was observed in a different animal species, might possibly suggest the existence of a biological defense mechanism against destructive bacterial assault on dental tissues.

Further studies are needed to determine the relation among parotid hormone secretion, food and meal composition and eating pattern, and dental status.

Article #98

Parotid gland function and dentin apposition in rat molars

Leonora J, Tjäderhane L, Tièche JM. J Dent Res 81(4):259-264, 2002

Observations of decreased dentinogenic function and of decreased parotid function that result from ingesting a high-sucrose diet raised the possibility that the parotid glands may have a role in regulating dentinogenesis. The latter function may be down-regulated in response to ingestion of a high-sucrose diet.

The objective of this study was to provide evidence for the existence of a regulatory link between parotid gland function and dentin formation.

STUDY 1:

Dentin apposition:

Partial desalivation and standard rat diet

Sprague-Dawley 21-day-old male rats were assigned to 4 groups

Group 1- Control, intact

Group 2- Control, sham-operated (sham)

Group 3- Parotidectomized (Px)

Group 4- Submandibular/sublingual glands removed (Smx/Slx).

Oxytetracycline injection at the beginning of the experiment served as a time marker for dentin apposition. Rats were fed powdered standard rat chow for 5 wks. Body wt. and food consumption were monitored twice a week throughout the experiment. On day 56 the food was removed and 1-2 hours later their salivary glands removed and weighed. 1st and 2nd molars from each mandible were sectioned sagittally for planimetric measurement of dentin formation beneath the main central transverse fissure of each molar.

STUDY 2:

Dentin apposition Partial desalivation and high-sucrose diet: The effect of partial desalivation on HSD-fed rats

Group 1 – Control; sham-operated and fed the standard rat diet

Group 2 – High-sucrose diet (HSD); sham-operated

Group 3 - High-sucrose diet (HSD); parotidectomized

Group 4 – High-sucrose diet (HSD); submaxillary/sublingual glands removed

The HSD was a powdered diet containing 50% sucrose. After 5 wks, dentin formation was measured in mandibular molars by the sagittal planimetric method

STUDY 3:

Dentin apposition and diet: Composition vs. texture:

To create a similar solid consistency between the standard rat diet and the HSD, we mixed each powder diet with water and extruded it through a meat grinder to create irregular hard pellets after drying. Dentin apposition in mandibular molars was measured after 5 wks of treatment.

Results:

Parotidectomy was associated with significant reduced dentin apposition, 21% and 16% respectively, in 1st and 2nd molars. In HSD rats, parotidectomy was accompanied by a 41% reduction in 1st molar dentin apposition. In contrast, removal of the submandibular/sublingual glands had no significant effect. Parotidectomy was followed by a significant increase in submandibular/sublingual gland weight relative to sham-operated rats fed the standard diet.

Within each diet, texture did not affect parotid gland weight. The critical factor proved to be diet composition. However, the submandibular/sublingual glands were affected by diet texture.

To our knowledge, there is no evidence that has been published showing that parotin affects apposition.

Discussion:

In 1st and 2nd molars of sham-operated animals fed the sucrose diet, a respective 42% and 47% decrease in dentin apposition was noted. Parotidectomized animals fed the standard diet experienced a 21% decrease in dentin apposition relative to sham controls. By comparison, the high-sucrose-fed rats that had already experienced a 421% reduction, when compared with animals fed the standard rat diet, sustained a further 4% diminution in dentin apposition after parotidectomy. Thus a 66% reduction in dentin apposition between sham-operated rats fed the standard diet and parotidectomized rats fed the HSD resulted from the combination of feeding the sucrose diet and parotidectomy.

When the reductive effect of high sucrose intake (42%) in intact animals is subtracted from the combined sucrose-parotidectomy effect (66%), the remaining 24% is attributable to the effect of parotidectomy. This is essentially the level of reduction (21%) in dentin apposition observed in rats fed the standard rat diet following parotidectomy. This suggests the possibility of a parotid control mechanism working independently of that affected by diet composition.

This observation does not support our premise that the deleterious sucrose effect on dentin apposition is solely the consequence of a sucrose-induced depression of a parotid function, as may be the case for the intradentinal dye penetration process [refs].

It appears that removal of parotid function(s) resulted in down-regulation of dentin apposition. In biological systems, control mechanisms imply some type of signaling process(es) between the moderator and the target tissues--in this case, the parotid gland and the pulp-dentin tissues. If parotid hormone is implicated in the control of intradentinal dye penetration, we may envision the control of dentinogenesis by parotid hormone as either a direct systemic effect upon the dentinogenic functions of odontoblasts, or as activation of dentinal fluid movement, which would facilitate the extracellular transport.

Conclusions:

We found that the primary determinant affecting dentin apposition was the composition of the diet. In contrast, the same conversion from pellet to powder form caused a significant increase in the weight of the submandibular/sublingual glands. These data suggest parotid control of dentinogenesis may work through function(s) other than the secretion of saliva.

Parotid glands appear to have a positive effect on primary dentin apposition in rat molars. We propose that if a parotid factor exists which is involved in the control of dentin apposition, this factor may not be related to salivary function, but rather it could be derived from a parotid endocrine function.

Article #99

Effect of dietary carbamyl phosphate on dentine apposition in rat molars

Leonora J, Tjäderhane L, Tièche JM. Arch Oral Biol 47:147-153, 2002

High concentrations of dietary sucrose have profoundly deleterious effects on the teeth and also impair odontoblastic function by reducing dentin apposition during primary dentinogenesis [refs]. Mechanism(s) by which a high-sucrose diet down-regulates the dentinogenic function of odontoblasts remains largely unknown. Earlier work showed that the high-sucrose diet negatively affects intradentinal dye penetration which apparently regulates solute movement within dentinal tissue. This function appears to be under the control of a putative endocrine system, the hypothalamus-parotid gland axis [ref]. Several compounds of the ornithine-urea and pyrimidine metabolic pathways, particularly carbamyl aspartate and carbamyl phosphate, can significantly reverse high-sucrose diet-induced cariogenesis and stimulate high-sucrose diet-depressed intradentinal dye penetration [refs]. Stimulation of dye penetration appears to require the integrity of parotid gland function(s) [ref]. Thus, the susceptibility to a high-sucrose diet of three co-localized processes—dentin apposition, intradentinal dye penetration and cariogenesis—could also have a beneficial effect on dentin apposition in the presence of a high-sucrose intake.

On the basis of our previous studies, our objective now was to determine whether dietary carbamyl phosphate could overcome the high-sucrose diet-induced reduction in dentin apposition, possibly through a similar mechanism involving parotid functions.

STUDY 1:

21-day-old Sprague-Dawley rats were divided into (1) control—powdered standard rat diet, (2) Powdered 50% high-sucrose diet (HSD), (3) Powdered 50% high-sucrose diet supplemented with carbamyl phosphate, (4) Powdered 50% high-sucrose diet supplemented with carbamyl phosphate at 6.2 mmol/kg.

Animals received an i.p. injection of oxytetracycline-HCL to mark the beginning of experimental dentin formation. Body wt. and food consumption were measured twice a week for 5 wks. On day 56 the animals were sacrificed. Their body wts. and parotid gland wts. were obtained. Their jaws were preserved and coded for further processing without investigator awareness of previous treatment. 1st and 2nd molars of each mandible were sectioned sagitally and dentin apposition measured planimetrically beneath the main central transverse fissure.

STUDY 2:

21-day-old Sprague-Dawley rats were subjected to 2 surgical treatments. 2 groups were parotidectomized and 1 group parotidectomized, under general anesthesia. They were maintained for 5 wks in the following 3 groups: (1) Sham-operated, standard diet, (2) Parotidectomized, standard diet, and (3) Parotidectomized, standard diet supplemented with 6.2 mmol carbamyl phosphate/kg diet. Completeness of parotidectomy was assessed before decapitation and 2 rats were discarded when it was found that incompletely removed parotid tags remained.

Dentin apposition between 1 and 56 days was measured in 1st and 2nd molars and averaged per molar between the right and left mandible.

<u>Results</u>:

Compared to controls, dentin apposition in molars of HSD-fed rats was significantly lower (38 and 42% respectively for 1st and 2nd molars). In 1st molars, supplementation of the HSD with carbamyl phosphate (CAP) was accompanied by an increase in dentin apposition compared with effects from the HSD alone. This was especially seen in 1st molars of the .2 mmol/kg CAP group, but was still less than that in rats fed the standard diet.

Parotidectomized standard-diet rats experienced a significant 18% reduction in 1st molar dentin apposition. Addition of CAP to the diet produced no significant change.

HSD rats experienced a significant decrease in parotid gland weight. Addition of CAP to the HSD prevented that decrease. The HSD + CAP group showed a significant decrease in body weight. This was also found in parotidectomized animals fed the standard diet supplemented with the same amount of CAP.

Discussion:

The finding that dentin apposition decreased 38-42% in HSD rats was in agreement with previous studies which found between 21 and 47% decrease [Tjaderhane et al 1994, Autio et al 1997].

Here, to our knowledge, for the first time we found that CAP (6.2 mmol/kg) added to a HSD can significantly reduce the negative effect of sucrose on dentin apposition in 1st molars by 53%. It appears to do this in a dose-related manner. Higher amounts of CAP could possibly further reduce the effect of the HSD. The actual mechanism of how CAP lessens the down-regulation of dentin apposition is not clear. It may result from direct control of odontoblastic function or indirectly by an unknown mechanism.

Carbamyl phosphate and carbamyl aspartic acid were found similarly effective, a result that could be anticipated because of the close association of the two compounds in the pyrimidine metabolic pathways [ref].

The present observation that increased intradentinal dye penetration (IDDP) occurs only when the parotids are intact and the HSD-reduced dentin apposition similarly requires intact parotids suggests that both effects may well be under a common control mechanism. Under this premise, 2 possibilities may be proposed (1) the parotid endocrine factor could induce odontoblastic up-regulation of dentin apposition in addition to stimulating IDDP or (2) activation of dentinal fluid movement (as measured by IDDP) could facilitate the extracellular transport of dentinal matrix proteins and thus enhance dentin apposition.

Whether a HSD can impair genetic control mechanisms needs to be established. The finding that on HSDs both dentin apposition and parotid gland weight were reduced along with the observation that CAP was ineffective in parotidectomized rats, strengthens the possibility that the effect of CAP may be at least partly mediated by parotid gland function.

Summary:

We have presented evidence that dietary CAP supplementation can substantially prevent the HSD-induced reduction in dentin apposition in rat first molars. Circumstantial evidence suggests that a parotid regulatory function may be involved.

Article #100

Cloning and functional study of porcine parotid hormone, a novel proline-rich protein

Zhang Q, Szalay AA, Tièche J-M, Kyeyune-Nyombi Eru, Sands JF, Oberg KC, Leonora J

J Biol Chem 250(23):22233-22244, 2005

Department of Biochemistry, Department of Physiology and Pharmacology,
Department of Human Anatomy and Pathology, Department of Internal Medicine,
School of Medicine, Loma Linda University, Loma Linda California 92350

Abstract/ Summary:

A parotid gland hormone that stimulates intradentinal fluid movement is believed to play a significant role in maintaining the vitality of dentin. This hormone had been purified from porcine parotid glands and partially sequenced in our previous study (Tièche, J.M., Leonora, J., and Steinman, R.R. (1980) *Endocrinology* 106, 1994-2005). We now report the cloning and functional study of porcine cDNA that code for this hormone and its complete amino acid sequence. Three cDNA clones were isolated from a porcine parotid cDNA library. The last 30 amino acids encoded by two of the cDNAs agreed with the amino acid sequence of the isolated parotid hormone. *In situ* hybridization and immunohistochemical staining demonstrated that the acinar cells of the parotid glands were the primary location for both parotid hormone related mRNAs and the translation products. A 216-bp fragment of the cDNA that contains the coding sequence for the porcine hormone was subcloned into an expression vector, and the protein expression was detected by immunoblot analysis and quantified by enzyme-linked immunosorbent assay (ELISA). In addition, the 30-amino acid parotid hormone was synthesized. Both the expressed and the synthetic proteins were biologically active in that they enhanced intradentinal fluid movement as measured by intradentinal dye penetration (IDDP).

....

A new insight into the fundamental basis of resistance to cariogenesis is provided by research in dentinal ultrastructure and internal dynamics. Odontoblastic cells at the pulp-dentin junction have cytoplasmic extensions extending within canaliculi that stretch from the pulp-predentin area to the dentin-enamel junction. The canaliculi are filled with dentinal fluid. The inward diffusive passage of bacterial cytotoxic products is opposed by a continuous outward flow of dentinal fluid that normally is maintained by an elevated hydrostatic pressure within the tooth. This movement may represent a physiological means by which the integrity of avascular dental tissues is maintained despite the potential for ingressive diffusion of exogenous substances (refs). Therefore, natural resistance of teeth to decay may involve maintaining adequate endogenous centrifugal dentinal fluid movement (DFM). DFM can be visualized with an intradentinal dye penetration (IDDP) assay in which a fluorescent dye, acriflavine hydrochloride, is injected intraperitoneally into rats, and the magnitude of dye penetration into the dentinal tubules is evaluated in sectioned molar teeth.

The significance of DFM in relation to dental health is suggested by caries studies done in rats that show an inverse relationship between the cariogenicity of a high sucrose diet and certain dietary supplements that stimulate DFM (ref). The observation that the supplements are ineffective in stimulating DFM in

parotidectomized animals (refs) implies that they exercise their cariostatic effect through mechanism(s) involving the parotid glands. A factor in parotid glands that stimulates DFM when infused into rats has been purified from porcine parotid tissue and its partial amino acid sequence was determined (ref). This factor, designated the parotid hormone (PH), is a moderately basic, small glycoprotein. Its amino acid composition and partial sequence indicate a molecule particularly rich in proline and glycine (ref).

Parotid glands secrete a number of salivary proline-rich proteins (PRPs) that represent a unique family of molecules, classified either as acidic or basic on the basis of their charge (ref). Typically, these proteins contain 25-40% proline. **Sequences of human, rat and mouse PRP genes exhibit a high degree of similarity (refs). This high conservation of sequence and structure of PRP genes and PRPs argues for specific biological functions for these unusual proteins.** Functions such as calcium binding, hydroxyapatite binding, and formation of the dental acquired pellicle have been attributed to acidic PRPs (refs) whereas antiviral activity has been demonstrated with basic PRPs (refs). **There are reports of a decrease in PRPs, including basic PRPs, under several conditions (refs), each of which is associated with increased caries susceptibility (refs).**

A comparison with reported PRPs suggests that porcine PH is unique in its amino acid sequence and that its amino acid composition hints at a possible linkage with basic PRPs. Further characterization of porcine PH is needed.

We now report (1) the isolation and sequence of several full-length cDNAs related to porcine PH, (2) the tissue distribution of the PH mRNA and proteins, and (3) the expression of the PH-encoding cDNAs in transfected COS-7 cells. PH was also commercially synthesized. The functions of the expressed proteins and the synthetic protein were assessed with the intradentinal dye penetration (IDDP) assay and the degree of stimulation was compared with that induced by feeding, a potent physiological stimulus for endogenous PH secretion (ref).

<u>Materials and methods</u>:

STUDY 1: <u>Tissue collection</u> – Tissue samples of salivary glands, pancreas, liver, small intestine, kidney, trachea, lung, skeletal muscle hypothalamus and pituitary gland were dissected from 3-month-old male pigs. Tissues were frozen in liquid nitrogen and stored at -80 C. Also, rat salivary glands removed from Sprague-Dawley rats were similarly frozen and stored.

Amino acid sequence determination of porcine PH – **Only a partial amino acid sequence for porcine PH had been published earlier; we now determined the complete sequence.** Ten μg of purified porcine PH were sequenced with an Applied Biosystems sequencer. The phenyl-thiohydantoin (PTH) amino acids were identified by automated high-performance liquid chromatography using an Applied Biosystems PTH amino acid analyzer. A porcine parotid cDNA library was constructed using 3 μg of mRNA extracted from total RNA purified with the Oligotex spin column.

DNA sequencing of positive cDNA clones – The cDNA inserts of positive clones were sequenced from both directions and partial sequences analyzed for locations of sites complementary to PHiA. Three full-length cDNAs, D_2A, TP_{23} and SL_{44-1}, were taken through the process of progressive unidirectional deletions with the Erase-a-Base system (Promega) to obtain a series of overlapping clones (each overlap was at least 50-100 nucleotides in length). Representative clones containing appropriate truncations were sequenced and these sequences compiled to obtain the complete sequence of the original clone.

PCR cloning of the cDNA for porcine PH – A deletion clone of TP_{23} was used as the PCR template, which had been obtained previously during the process of generating progressive unidirectional deletions with the Erase-a Base system. The PCR products were purified and ligated with the pCR-Blunt vector (Invitrogen) and introduced into $DH_{5\alpha}$ cells. The presence of the PH cDNA insert in plasmid pCR-D_{15} was confirmed by DNA sequencing.

Coupled in vitro transcription/translation of the PH-encoding cDNAs – The cDNA insert of TP_{23} was subcloned into the vector pET-28a(+). The fusion was determined to be in-frame with the His tag by DNA sequencing. Plasmid pET-28a(+)-TP_{23} was then subjected to the TNT quick-coupled transcription/translation system. Translation products were analyzed using electrophoresis in 12% SDS-polyacrylamide gel and Western blotting. Translated products were separated in SDS-polyacrylamide gel and transferred to a nitrocellulose membrane. Detection was performed using PH-Ab, horseradish peroxidase-conjugated goat-anti-rabbit antibody, and an Immun-Star substrate with enhancer. The membrane was exposed to x-ray film for 30 s to 2 min, which was then processed and analyzed.

Quantifying porcine PH expression in the cell lysate with ELISA – A direct competitive enzyme-linked immunosorbent assay (ELISA) was developed with a polyclonal antibody, PH-Ab. Porcine PH that had been used for amino acid sequence determination served as immobilized tracer and standard. PH-Ab rabbit antibody was the primary antibody and goat anti-rabbit IgG-peroxidase conjugate was the secondary antibody. The optical density of each well was read at 450 nm after developing indicative color with enzyme substrate *o*-phenylenediamine.

Functional determination of the expressed and synthetic PH with an IDDP assay in rats – Rats were divided into 4 groups with at least 6 animals per group as follows: Group 1, fasting only (- control); Group 2, fed only (+ control), Group 3, fasting plus intravenous infusion with cell lysate obtained from $pCEP_4$-transfected COS-7 cells; and group 4, fasting plus intravenous infusion of the cell lysate obtained from $pCEP_4$-His-D_{15}-transfected COS-7 cells. All experiments were conducted on the rats' 28th day after 2 weeks of adaptation to their environment.

STUDY 2: In a separate study, **the activity of synthetic PH was also assessed. The 30-amino acid peptide of PH was commercially synthesized and purified by means of high-performance liquid chromatography. The retention time for the synthetic PH peaked at 10.82 min** and the **molecular weight by electrospray mass spectrometry analysis was 2,858.** The synthetic PH was tested at the dose of 0.5 ng, consistent with the upper range of the original PH isolation study dose-response curve (ref).

Two groups of male Sprague-Dawley rats were housed similarly and after fasting overnight Group 5 rats were anesthetized and injected with acriflavine dye whereas those in Group 6 received 0.5 ng synthetic PH. Rat jaws were collected after 30 min. Dye penetration within dentinal tubules was measured by fluorescence microscopy within a strictly defined area beneath the bottom of each occlusal groove. Scoring was measured from digital photos recording the extent of dye penetration.

Data analysis – The IDDP score was calculated as a ratio of the number of occlusal grooves exhibiting fluorescence divided by the total number of occlusal grooves. [Notable color representation of IDDP is shown in Fig. 6 of the original text.]

Results:

The complete amino acid sequence for parotid hormone isolated and purified from porcine parotid glands was found to be 30 amino acids in length and consisted of NH_2-Ala-Pro-Pro-Gly-Ala-Arg-Pro-Pro-Pro-Gly-Pro-Pro-Pro-Pro-Pro- Pro-Gly-Pro-Ser-Pro-Pro-Arg-Pro-Pro-Pro-Gly-Pro-Pro-Pro-Gln-COOH.

To identify the cDNA sequence encoding PH, a porcine parotid cDNA library was constructed and screened with the ^{32}P-labeled oligonucleotide probe PHiA, which corresponded to the N-terminal sequence of the isolated porcine PH.

The nucleotide sequences of D_2A and TP_{23} contained open reading frames encoding polypeptides of 511 and 566 amino acids respectively. The complete nucleotide and the deduced amino acid sequences for these two cDNAs are presented in Fig. 1, A and B [extensively occupying three pages in the original text, not duplicated here]. The last 30 amino acids encoded by the cDNA insert of both TP_{23} and SL_{44-1} were identical to the amino acid sequence of the isolated porcine PH.

Tissue-specific expression of PH genes was determined by examining the RNA and protein expression patterns of the TP_{23} cDNA. *In situ* hybridization of parotid gland slices with the riboprobe showed a high density of silver grains over acinar cell cytoplasm. No significant silver grains were seen in other porcine tissues such as liver, pancreas, small intestine, trachea, lungs, kidney, hypothalamus, pituitary, and skeletal muscles. None were seen in the submandibular glands.

Immunohistochemical staining of parotid gland slices with PH-Ab was most intense over acinar tissue. Some of the serous cells from the sublingual glands were also stained, correlating with results from the above *in situ* hybridization. [Various salivary gland tissue sections showing localization of PH gene transcripts are shown in Fig. 2 of original text.]

The expressed PH and its related products in the cell lysate were quantified with ELISA. ELISA displacement curves for the PH standard and for serial dilutions of the $pCEP_4$-His-D_{15}-transfected cell lysate showed parallel linear regression curves [Fig. 5 of original text]. The dentinal fluid-stimulating activity of the expressed and synthetic PH was assessed with the IDDP assay in rats. **Consistent with previous studies (ref), IDDP in the molar teeth of rats fed for 15 min was significantly greater than that in fasting animals.** The difference between dye penetration scores in fasting animals and animals injected with the cell lysate from COS-7 cells transfected with vector alone was not statistically significant.

Synthetic PH was also active in stimulating IDDP. Infusing 0.5 ng synthetic PH resulted in an impressive IDDP ratio of 0.52, comparable with that obtained from rats infused with the expressed PH and from rats stimulated by feeding.

Discussion:

Screening of the porcine parotid cDNA library resulted in the identification of numerous full-length cDNAs. These porcine proteins are particularly rich in proline (52-61%). Relatively high amounts of arginine and lysine (5.6-7.4%) suggest that they are basic proline-rich proteins (PRPs). Similar to human PRPs, these porcine PRPs contain 21-amino acid repeats, but with the prototype sequence PPPGPPPPGPPPPGPAPPGAR.

The IDDP assay was performed on 28-day-old male Sprague-Dawley rats, divided into six groups of number N. Statistical comparisons were made by analysis of variance and multiple comparisons were performed with a Bonferroni test with p values as presented below:

TABLE I - Effects of feeding and infusion of synthetic, expressed and isolated porcine parotid hormones on intradentinal dye penetration in rat molar teeth

Group	Dietary state	PH source	Dose (ng)	IDDP ratio	N	P
1	Fasting			0.187± 0.056	6	1 vs. 2; p=0.015
2	Fed	Endogenous secretion		0.567±0.088	9	2 vs. 3; p=0.004
3	Fasting	Mock-expressed cell lysate		0.135±0.040	6	3 vs. 4; p=0.001
4	Fasting	cDNA-expressed cell lysate	10	0.660± 0.097	6	4 vs. 5; p=0.004
5	Fasting	Saline		0.219±0.095	6	5 vs. 6; p=0.007
6	Fasting	Synthetic peptide	0.50	0.524± 0.063	6	
7	Fasting	Saline		0.163±0.026	16	7 vs. 8; p=0.001
8	Fasting	Porcine parotid glands	0.54	0.378±0.030	17	

As indicated by an increase in IDDP, the infusion of a PH-containing protein extract produced from pCEP$_4$-His-D$_{15}$-transfected COS-7 cells stimulated DFM in rats comparable to the natural stimulus of feeding. The fact that the synthetic peptide was active in stimulating IDDP suggests that at least the last 30 amino acid sequence derived from pCEP$_4$-His-D$_{15}$ was responsible. This implies a systemically-mediated response mechanism and strengthens the concept of the endocrine nature of PH. These data suggest that, besides salivary function, parotid acinar cells also possess an endocrine function by secreting PH involved in inhibiting cariogenesis. To our knowledge, this finding is the first evidence among major salivary glands that intracellular mechanism(s) regulate two important complex functions, exocrine and endocrine (ref). Studies indicate parotid glands are capable of secreting transgene-encoded proteins into serum as well as saliva (refs), which implies at least two transport mechanisms directing the distribution of molecules associated with each function. Salivary PRPs appear to be directed toward the apical end of the acinar cells and PH toward their basal portion for direct secretion into the blood stream.

Conclusions:

We have identified the cDNAs from porcine parotid glands that encode the amino acid sequence of a protein previously isolated from porcine parotid glands that possess DFM-stimulating activity. Our present data provide further confirmation that the parotid glands, in addition to their salivary function, possess an endocrine function that participates in systemic mechanism(s) directed toward preventing cariogenesis. This may likely further involve integration of a mechanism(s) associated with nutrient homeostasis since secretion of PH is initiated with the onset of nutrient intake (ref).

[ED. NOTE: These research results convincingly close the loop on Steinman's and Leonora's theory of dentinal fluid transport (movement) as a hormonally-influenced systemic adjunct to an active mechanism of caries resistance. This implies that especially during and after feeding a positive hydrostatic pressure of dentinal fluid is exerted from the inside to the outside of teeth. This continual action serves the moisturization, nourishment, antibiotic, and buffering needs of the dentin and enamel structures, and ultimately resists the ingress of harmful external cytotoxic products.]

APPENDIX A

TOOTHSOME DESSERTS

The Elusive Answer...

Cavities, appointments, dental bills—a never-ending cycle, it seems. You've found that miracle toothpastes don't perform in their advertised way, even when used more than once a day. What *is* the missing ingredient for healthy teeth?

It is my belief that it isn't heredity or frequent brushing, but *diet*. The record of our family has satisfactorily demonstrated this. Our children are careless about oral hygiene, yet all three have never had a decayed tooth. We thank a wholesome, sensible diet, for at our home we have three rules:

No between-meal snacks
Whole grain bread and cereals exclusively
Desserts not more than once a week

The snack tide-over so common today is very high in sugar and low in vitamins, minerals, and protein—poor food at any time, and more so *entire* meals. To avoid the periodic hunger bout, we eat a good breakfast, long and supple, of cereal, milk, toast, eggs, or even nuts—any good solid food that will stay with the active person all morning.

No cornflakes, white bread, or macaroni are invited to our table. Instead, the bulk whole grain breads and cereals rich in vitamins and minerals are honored.

The desserts our family eats include fruits and melons and are of the simple, low-sugar variety—not the type that is high in sugar and low in vitamins and minerals. Whereas the usual dessert has 5 to 16 teaspoonfuls of added sugar per serving, our desserts do not have over 2 teaspoonfuls. Even this amount of sugar would not be good to eat every day. So we serve desserts once a week.

Featured in this booklet are desserts such as are found on our table. There is a stated price for everything in this world. We think the price of healthy teeth is a unique diet. The investment has been paying us dividends for more than fifteen years.

Ralph R. Steinman, DDS, MS

[To bring his research findings down to practical, everyday level, Dr. Steinman developed the following recipes designed to be as low in sucrose (table sugar) as possible. Use of today's artificial sweeteners might further reduce or even totally eliminate sucrose in some of these recipes.]

Fruit Desserts

Baked Apples

Choose good baking apples such as Rome Beauty, Jonathan, or Pippins. Wash and core, being careful not to break through the blossom end. Fill with nuts and raisins, dates and peanut butter, coconut and honey, or 1 tsp. brown sugar. Place apples in baking dish with half inch of water. Bake at 350° for 30-45 minutes or until tender when pierced with fork.

Baked Bananas

1 ripe banana | **1 t. honey**

Slit banana, peel once, its full length. Dribble honey into slit and press edges together. Bake at 425° for 10-12 minutes. Serve hot (1 serving).

Chilly-Night Dessert

Halve a grapefruit, top with chopped prunes, dribble with honey, and heat in the broiler.

Fruit Compote

- **1 lb. prunes, cooked**
- **2 cans (11 oz) mandarin orange sections, drained**
- **2 t. sugar**
- **1 c. orange juice**
- **1 t. grated orange rind**
- **2 large bananas, sliced**

Pit prunes. Combine with orange sections, sugar, and orange juice. Let stand in refrigerator 30 minutes, mixing several times. Just before serving, add bananas. Makes 8-10 servings.

Fruity Chews

- **1 lb. dried figs**
- **1 lb. dried apricots**
- **1 lb. dates**
- **1-1/2 c. shredded coconut**
- **1/2 c. nut meats**
- **Sprinkle of salt**

Grind the dried fruits and the nuts together. Add the coconut and a sprinkle of salt. Moisten with honey to a consistency that will form easily. Press into a shallow pan, cut into small bars, and chill. Wrap in waxed paper. Keep refrigerated.

Lazy Gal Dessert

- **1 c. fresh pineapple cut in small pieces**
- **3/4 c. chopped dates**
- **1/3 c. chopped walnuts**

Combine all ingredients. Chill for several hours. Serve with low fat topping.

Melon Ball Rainbow

Using the melon-ball maker, prepare balls from cantaloupe, Crenshaw, Persian melon, casaba, watermelon, etc. Serve one kind, or a combination, in any fruit fuice. Always have melon balls and juice chilled. Garnish simply with a mint sprig or a grape leaf. This dessert is most attractive when served in clear glass or crystal.

Melon balls combined with other fruits (strawberries, grapes, etc.) also make attractive and delicious desserts.

Southern Ambrosia

1 c. fresh pineapple chunks **1 c. coconut**
2 c. orange sections

Combine and chill at least an hour. Serves 6.

Stuffed Dates

Stuff dates with peanut butter and walnuts. Arrange on plate with dried apricots, pears, peaches, and figs.

Chilled Desserts

Banana Pudding

1 c. nonfat dry milk **1/4 c. sugar**
2 c. skim milk **1 t. lemon juice**
3 T. cornstarch **3 slices wholewheat zwieback, crushed**
3 fully ripe bananas **1/4 t. salt**

Scald 1½ c. Skim milk. Mix dry ingredients and ½ c. Cold skim milk. Slowly stir in scalded milk. Cook, stirring until smooth and thickened. Cool. Add lemon juice. Cover and chill until serving time. Line a 9" cake or pie pan with crushed zwieback. Add sliced bananas and cover with pudding. Serves 6.

Prune Puff

1/3 c. ice-cold water **2 T. sugar**
1/2 c. instant nonfat dry milk **1/8 t. salt**
2 T. lemon juice **1/2 c. finely cut, cooked prunes**

Put water and nonfat dry milk into a cold quart bowl. Beat with rotary or electric beater at high speed until mixture stands in soft peaks. Gradually beat in lemon juice, sugar, and salt until mixture is stiff. Fold in prunes. Spoon into dessert dishes. Garnish with additional pieces of prune or coconut. Chill about 30 minutes before serving. Makes 4 servings.

Prune Whip Freeze

3/4 c. milk **3 T. orange juice**
1 egg **3 T. lemon juice**
1/4 c. sugar **1/8 t. salt**
3/4 c. pureed cooked prunes (unsweetened) **1/3 c. of ice-cold water**
1/3 c. orange sections

Scald milk in a double boiler. Combine egg and sugar and add scalded milk slowly to mixture. Return to heat and cook only until custard coats a silver spoon. Blend remaining ingredients and add to custard. Freeze in refrigerator tray until firm.

Strawberry Cool

1 c. sour cream **2 c. fresh strawberries**
2 T. sugar

Combine sour cream and sugar. Crush berries lightly and fold into sour cream. Freeze until firm. Serves 4-6.

Sunny Orange Sherbet

1 can (6 oz.) frozen orange juice undiluted, unsweetened
3 T. sugar
Pinch of salt
1 c. evaporated milk

Chill evaporated milk in an ice cube tray in freezing compartment until ice crystals begin to form. Turn into a cold bowl and beat rapidly until it is stiff and will hold a peak. Mix thawed orange juice with sugar and salt and add gradually, whipping after each addition and until mixture is very stiff. Turn into freezer tray of refrigerator. Freeze until firm.

Pineapple juice concentrate or grape juice concentrate or an equal amount of crushed pineapple may be substituted for orange juice.

Cookies

Cinnarunes

2 c. whole wheat pastry flour
3 t. baking powder (low residue)
1/2 t. salt
1 t. cinnamon
1/2 c. firmly packed brown sugar
1/2 c. margarine
1 unbeaten egg
1/4 c. light molasses
1 c. shredded or flaked coconut
1 lb. large prunes, tenderized and pitted

Sift together flour, baking powder, salt, and cinnamon; set aside. Cream margarine and brown sugar well. Blend in unbeaten egg and molasses and beat well. Add dry ingredients gradually, mixing thoroughly. Stir in coconut. Chill dough before shaping. Flatten a rounded teaspoonful of dough for each cookie. Place a prune in the center, shaping dough around prune. Bake on ungreased baking sheet at 370° for 12-15 minutes until light brown. Makes 4 dozen cookies (1/2 t. sugar per cookie).

Coconut Balls

1 c. peanut butter
1/2 c. honey
3/4 c. nonfat dry milk
1 t. nonalcoholic vanilla

Shape in balls the size of a walnut. Roll in fresh ground coconut.

Coconut Stix

2-1/2 c. whole wheat pastry flour
1 t. baking powder (low residue)
1 t. salt
2/3 c. oil
2/3 c. firmly packed brown sugar
2 eggs
1/2 t. lemon extract
2 c. coconut

Combine oil and brown sugar. Add eggs and lemon extract. Beat well. Sift in dry ingredients and stir well. Add coconut and combine thoroughly. Using about two tablespoons of dough, roll into stick. Place on lightly greased baking sheet. Bake at 350° about 15 minutes until light brown. Makes 30 stix (1 t. sugar per stick).

Cottage Cheese Icebox Cookies

1/2 c. margarine
1/4 c. cottage cheese
1-1/4 c. whole wheat pastry flour
1-1/4 c. wheat germ
2 t. baking powder (low residue)
1/3 c. sugar
1/2 t. salt
3 T. orange juice
2 T. grated orange rind
1/2 c. chopped nuts

Cream sugar and margarine until light. Add cottage cheese, salt, orange juice, and grated orange rind. Sift together flour and baking powder and add to creamed mixture, blending well. Add wheat germ and mix well. Drop by teaspoonfuls onto greased cookie sheet. Bake 12-15 minutes at 350°.

Molasses Cookies

3/4 c. molasses
1/2 c. (cubes) margarine
2 eggs
2-1/4 c. sifted whole wheat pastry flour
1/2 t. salt
2 t. baking powder (low residue)
1-1/2 t. cinnamon
1/2 c. milk
1 c. seedless raisins, dark or light
1 c. chopped walnuts

Gradually beat molasses into margarine. Add eggs; beat well. Sift together dry ingredients and add alternately with milk. Stir in raisins and nuts. Drop by rounded teaspoonfuls 2 inches apart on greased cookie sheet. Top each with walnut half. Bake at 425° for 6-8 minutes or until done. Remove from pan immediately. Makes about 5 dozen cookies.

Oat Waffles

4 c. quick cook oatmeal
3 c. hot water
1 t. salt
1/3 c. oil
1/3 T. Soyagen powder

Mix all ingredients except flour. Heat heavy waffle iron and oil well for the first waffle. Bake until brown, about 10 minutes. Remove from waffle iron and put in slow oven (250°) to crisp, but not to brown. Will get very crisp. May be made ahead and put in the refrigerator or deep freeze and crisped up just before serving.

Peanut Butter Cookies

1/2 c. peanut butter
1/4 c. honey
1/4 t. salt
1-1/4 c. whole wheat pastry flour
1/4 c. oil
1/4 c. raw sugar
1 t. vanilla

Combine all ingredients except flour. Stir until well mixed. Add flour, mix until blended. Form into balls the size of a walnut. Place on ungreased cookie sheet, flatten with fork. Bake at 375°. Makes 18 cookies (1¼ t. sugar per cookie).

Peanut Butter Dandies

1/2 c. peanut butter
1/2 c. honey
3/4 c. nonfat dry milk
3/4 c. wheat germ

Blend peanut butter and honey. Add nonfat dry milk and wheat germ. Mix well. Shape into balls approximately the size of a walnut. Roll in additional wheat germ or finely ground coconut. Makes 24 balls.

Prune Confections

1/2 c. softened margarine
1/2 c. sugar
1/4 t. salt
1-1/4 c. sifted whole wheat pastry flour
1 T. cornstarch
1 T. prune water
1-1/2 c. chopped, soaked prunes
2 T. lemon juice
1 t. grated lemon rind
1 egg
1 T. oil
1 c. coconut

Combine margarine, ¼ c. sugar, salt, and flour. Mix until crumbs are formed. Press firmly into pan (about 9" x 9" x 2"), covering bottom and ¼ inch up sides. Prick with fork. Bake at 350° for 20 minutes. Add cornstarch to prune water and stir until blended. Combine with prunes, lemon juice, and rind. Bring to boiling point. Simmer until thickened, stirring occasionally. Cool. Spread prune mixture over pastry in pan. Beat egg, add remaining ¼ c. sugar and oil. Add coconut; mix well. Place coconut mixture evenly over prune filling. Bake at 350° for 30 minutes. Cool. Cut in squares. Makes 16 squares (2 t. sugar per square).

Prune Poppins

1/4 c. oil
2 c. sifted whole wheat pastry flour
3 t. baking powder (low residue)
1/2 t. salt
1/2 c. sugar
1 egg, beaten
1 c. milk
1-1/4 c. dried prunes, washed and cut into ¼ inch pieces

Sift together dry ingredients. Add 1 c. prune pieces. Combine oil, egg, and milk. Add to dry ingredients and mix until just blended. Fill greased muffin pans full of dough. Top with remaining ¼ c. prune pieces.

TOPPING:

1/4 c. oil
1/2 c. whole wheat pastry flour
1/4 t. cinnamon
1/4 c. brown sugar

Mix flour, cinnamon, brown sugar for topping. Add oil and blend. Sprinkle this mixture over the poppins. Bake at 375° for 30 minutes. Serve warm. Makes 18 poppins (2 t. sugar per serving).

Whole Wheat Crackers

3/4 c. oil
1-1/4 c. milk
1 t. salt
1 c. wheat germ
2 T. raw sugar
4 c. whole wheat flour

Mix ingredients thoroughly. Knead and roll thin. Cut into desired shapes and prick with fork. Bake at 300° until brown.

Whole Wheat Oat Sticks

2 c. whole wheat flour
2 c. date halves

2 c. oat flour or ground rolled oats
2/3 c. ground nut meats
1 t. salt
1/3 c. coconut
2/3 c.oil
3 T. honey
2/3 to 1 c. water
1/2 c. sesame seed

Combine dry ingredients and dates in a bowl. Emulsify oil with water and honey by whipping together with a fork. Add to dry ingredients and mix into a stiff dough. Add more water if necessary. Knead only enough to form dough ball. Divide dough and roll out on greased cookie sheet to 1/8 inch in thickness. Prick with a fork and cut into strips about ¾ x 3 inches. Bake at 400° until brown on top and bottom. Turn if necessary. Watch the sticks on the edges of the pan, as they brown first. Remove these as they bake, if necessary.

Cakes

Apple Cup Cakes

1/2 c. margarine
2/3 c. sugar
1 egg
2 c. whole wheat pastry flour
3 t. baking powder (low residue)
1/2 t. salt
1-1/2 t. cinnamon
1 c. applesauce
1/2 c. seedless raisins

Cream margarine and sugar. Add egg and beat well. Sift together flour, baking powder, salt, and cinnamon. Add alternately with applesauce to cream mixture. Add raisins. Pour into greased cupcake pans. Bake at 375° for 15-20 minutes. Cool 3-5 minutes. Remove from pan and cool on wire rack. Makes 15 cup cakes (¼ t. sugar per cake).

Apricot Nut Loaf

1 c. dried apricots
3 c. whole wheat pastry flour
3/4 c. sugar
4 t. baking powder (low residue)
1-1/2 t. salt
1 c. chopped walnuts
1 egg
1-1/2 c. milk
1/4 c. oil
2 T. grated orange rind

Rinse apricots, cover with water, and boil 15 minutes, or until barely tender. Cool, drain, and chop. Sift together flour, sugar, baking powder, and salt. Stir in walnuts. Beat egg lightly and add milk, oil, and rind. Stir liquid mixture and apricots into dry ingredients. Turn into greased loaf pan (about 9" x 4" x 3") and allow to stand for 15 minutes. Bake in moderate oven (350°) for 1 to 1½ hours. Remove from pan and cool on wire rack. Makes 15-18 slices (2 t. sugar per serving).

Apricot Scallop

2 c. dried apricots
1/4 c. firmly packed brown sugar
2 T. whole wheat pastry flour
6 T. nonfat dry milk
1/2 t. cinnamon
3 T. margarine
2 T. water

Cook apricots. Drain and cool. Combine brown sugar, flour, nonfat dry milk, and cinnamon. Add margarine; cut in with pastry blender to make crumbs. Alternate layers of apricots with layers of crumbs (finishing with crumbs) in a one-quart casserole. Sprinkle the 2 T.

water over top. Bake at 350° until lightly browned. About 30 minutes. Serve plain or with whipped topping. Makes 6 servings (2 t. sugar per serving).

Banana Loaf

1-3/4 c. sifted whole wheat pastry flour
2-3/4 t. baking powder (low residue)
1/2 t. salt
1/3 c. margarine
2 eggs
1 c. mashed ripe bananas (3-4)

Sift together flour, baking powder, and salt. Place margarine in mixing bowl and beat until creamy. Gradually add sugar, beating until light and fluffy. Add slightly beaten eggs and beat mixture until thick and pale lemon incolor. Add flour mixture and bananas alternately, blending thoroughly. Turn into greased and floured loaf pan. Bake at 350° for 60-70 minutes. Let cool 10 minutes in pan. Remove to rack and cool thoroughly. Makes 15-18 slices (2 t. sugar per serving).

Carrot Cake

1-1/2 c. water
1 c. seedless raisins
1/4 c. brown sugar
1 c. finely grated carrots
3 t. baking powder (low residue)
1/3 c. oil
1 t. cinnamon
1/2 t. salt
1 egg
2 c. sifted whole wheat pastry flour

Heat together water, raisins, sugar, carrots, oil, cinnamon, and salt. Cool. Add slightly beaten egg. Add flour and baking powder sifted together. Stir smooth. Pour into greased loaf pan. Bake about 45 minutes at 325°. Cool. Makes 15-18 slices (2/3 t. sugar per serving).

Date-Applesauce Cake

2 c. whole wheat pastry flour
2/3 c. brown sugar
1/2 c. margarine
2 eggs
1-1/2 c. applesauce
3 t. baking powder (low residue)
1-1/2 t. salt
1 t. cinnamon
1 c. chopped dates
1/2 c. nuts

Cream margarine and sugar thoroughly. Add well beaten eggs and applesauce. Sift all dry ingredients together and add to mixture. Blend thoroughly. Add dates and nuts. Bake in loaf pan 1 to 1 ¼ hours at 375°. Makes 15-18 slices (2 t. sugar per serving).

Pecan and Date Loaf Cake

1 lb. pitted dates
1 lb. pecans or walnuts
1 t. vanilla
1/2 c. honey or raw sugar
1 c. whole wheat pastry flour
1/2 t. salt
4 eggs

Place dates and nuts in bowl. Cover with flour and salt sifted together. Mix thoroughly. Stir in honey or raw sugar and vanilla. Whip egg yolks thiks. Fold in flour-fruit mixture. Beat egg whites stiff. Fold into other ingredients. Bake at 350° for 45 minutes in one large loaf pan, or 30-35 minutes in two small loaf pans (lined with waxed paper).

Prune-Orange Nut Cake

1 small orange
1/2 c. pitted soaked prunes
1/2 c. applesauce
2 c. whole wheat pastry flour
3 t. baking powder (low residue)
1/2 c. brown sugar
1/2 t. salt
1/2 c. chopped nut meats
2 eggs
2 T. oil

Cut orange in quarters and put through food chopper with prunes. (Chop prunes if too soft to put through food chopper.) Add applesauce. Sift dry ingredients together. Add nuts; mix. Combine slightly beaten eggs, oil, and fruit mixture. Stir moist ingredients into dry, only until well blended. Pour in well-greased loaf pans. Bake at 350° for 1 hour or until done. Turn on rack to cool. Place in plastic or tin and cover tightly. Chill in refrigerator overnight before slicing. Makes 15-18 slices (1½ t. sugar per serving).

Prune Soufflé

4 eggs
3 T. oil
3 T. whole wheat pastry flour
1/4 t. salt
1 c. milk
1 c. prune pulp
1/4 c. sugar
2 T. grated lemon rind
2 T. lemon juice

Heat oil; blend in flour and salt. Gradually add milk. Cook, stirring constantly, until thickened. Beat egg yolks and add milk mixture, stirring constantly. Add prune pulp, sugar, lemon rind, and juice; mix well. Beat egg whites stiff; fold into mixture. Pour into buttered casserole; set in pan of hot water 1 inch deep. Bake at 350° for 1½ hours. Serve immediately. Makes 6-8 servings (2 t. sugar per serving). Can serve with lemon juice.

Song of the Islands Cake

1 c. mashed sweet potatoes
1/2 c. mashed banana
1/4 c. sugar
1/2 t. salt
1 t. grated orange rind
2 eggs
1 c. milk
2 T. flaked or shredded coconut

Combine sweet potatoes and banana. Add sugar, salt, orange rind, and beaten eggs. Blend. Stir in milk. Pour into well-greased one-quart casserole. Sprinkle coconut over top. Bake at 300° for 1 hour, or until set. Chill. Garnish with whipped cream and banana slices. Serves 8 (1½ t. sugar per serving).

Low Calorie Whip Topping

1/3 c. ice water
1/3 c. nonfat dry milk
2 T. lemon juice
2 T. sugar
1 t. vanilla

Tarts and Pies

Apple Date Tarts

12 slices whole wheat bread
4 T. softened margarine
2 c. applesauce
1/4 c. chopped dates

3 T. sugar **1/4 c. chopped almonds**
1-1/2 t. cinnamon **Low-fat topping**

Remove crusts from thin slices of large bread. Spread with softened margarine. Mix sugar and cinnamon; sprinkle over bread slices. Fit slices into well-buttered muffin cups. Bake at 375° for 10-15 minutes or until delicate brown. Combine applesauce, dates, and chopped almonds. Chill. Spoon applesauce mixture into each bread cup. Top with puff of low-fat topping. Makes 12 servings (2 t. sugar per serving).

Banana Cream Pie

PIE CRUST:

1 c. whole wheat pastry flour, sifted **4 T. oil**
pinch of salt **2 T. boiling water**

Mix flour and salt. In a separate bowl, mix boiling water and oil with fork; add to flour. Mix to form a soft ball. Place at once into a warm pie plate. Press with fingers to cover plate to rim. This makes a thin, crisp crust. Prick with fork and bake at 400° until brown.

Dough can be cut into small balls and pressed into muffin tins to make tarts.

CREAM FILLING:

1/2 c. raw cashews **Pinch of salt**
12 pitted dates **1 t. vanilla**
2 c. water

Whip ingredients in liquefier, using 1 cup of water at a time. Place in pan and cook 15-20 minutes, stirring constantly until thickened. Cool. Refrigerate until ready to use.

To make pie, place a layer of the cream filling, then a layer of sliced bananas, then another layer of cream filling. Top with ground coconut or with fresh strawberry or cherry.

To make tarts, place slices of **bananas** in tart shell, cover with cream filling, and top with **coconut, strawberry,** or **cherry.**

Finger Pies

6 c. whole wheat pastry flour **1/2 c. seedless raisins**
2-1/4 t. salt **1/3 c. sugar**
1 to 1-1/2 c. water **1 t. grated lemon rind**
2 c. applesauce **1/2 c. nuts, coarsely chopped**

Mix all ingredients together and chill thoroughly. Just before serving, spoon into baked, cooled pie shell. Cover top with sweetened whipped cream (½ c. whipping cream, plus 1 T. confectioners sugar).

APPENDIX B

DR. RALPH STEINMAN

Loma Linda University School of Dentistry
Co-founder and Research Pioneer
(From personal interview, Jan 26, 2003)
1910-2007

Dr. Ralph Steinman graduated with honors from Emory University School of Dentistry and was selected for membership in the OKU honor dental society.

He seemed to be a born visionary, but at the same time a strong realist. He could readily sense when information was correct or if it lacked accuracy. Ralph just seemed to have a penchant for uncovering 'the rest of the story.'

He served in the United States Army where he developed appreciation not only for military efficiency but also for the short hairstyle that since has almost become a part of his persona—along with his distinctive bolo ties! The crew cut was simple enough that he taught himself to do it, which saved money during harder economic times and was a practice he continued into his later years.

Ralph had the conviction that his wife, Emily, should not have to find outside employment. If personal finances ever required that, he vowed he'd rather return to regular dental practice than to have her working outside the home. Times were not always easy. After 93 years of life, he looked back with satisfaction that Emily never had to seek employment even in those lean years when he was developing a position for dental research on the Loma Linda University campus.

His son, Douglas, practices medicine and both his daughters graduated from college. His always-cheerful wife Emily has ardently supported him, and he personally owed much to her intelligent care and concern over the years.

Before being called in 1951 to be one of the three originators of the Loma Linda University School of Dentistry, Dr. Steinman practiced dentistry near Asheville, North Carolina. Certain local air-borne allergens apparently caused him to have asthmatic attacks. These occurred with increasing frequency and severity to the extent that he found himself unable to sleep at night, desperately wondering if he'd even be able to breathe on his own until morning.

Fortunately, aminophylline injections brought great relief, at least at first. Less fortunately, the effectiveness of this medication soon faded, leaving him back almost where he started. This produced weeks and months when he could not schedule patients, and consequently lost income. In desperation, the young dentist took his family to coastal North Carolina to escape the high inland pollen counts. This gave him respiratory relief along with time to read and reflect.

He became impressed with the observations of writer Ellen G. White, mostly from *Counsels on Diet and Foods* and *The Ministry of Healing*. It was soon apparent that when he changed his lifestyle to include adequate rest, fresh air, regular exercise, and sound diet, advocated from these writings, that his condition improved. He discovered that as the rest of his body approached complete health, his asthmatic symptoms improved.

He pursued this further and eliminated as many refined foods made with white flour and sugar as possible. The recovery was remarkable. At first he tentatively returned to practice, advising his secretary not to book patients any further than two weeks in advance because of lingering uncertainty whether the asthma might return. Successful weeks stretched into months, and finally he was able to go the whole rest of the summer without allergic symptoms.

The more he pondered this experience, the more the realization stuck that the body takes care of itself from following simple eating and exercise practices. He felt stronger and healthier when he eliminated so many of the rich sweet, candies, pies, cakes, and pastries that he had grown up enjoying so much. Challenging his body's system with improper nutrients had weakened the proper balance and set him up for reduced resistance to a number of ailments.

As he became a stronger believer and advocate of eating overly refined foods, his family changed away from nearly all refined sweets in favor of more wholesome alternatives such as fresh fruits.

This wholistic emphasis was remarkable concept in itself, but later influenced Dr. Steinman's perceptions about how a healthfully functioning body might actually provide systemic resistance to dental decay.

As one of the three founding fathers, so to speak, Ralph was active in the early formation of the Loma Linda University School of Dentistry. There were serious decisions to be made. This was to be no ordinary dental school or else it wouldn't be worth the effort. It was to be a model institution reflective of the highest principles of the Seventh-day Adventist church and appropriately reflecting glory to God.

Dr. Webster Prince had asked several promising dentists who had graduated near the top of their class to join with him in starting this new dental school. He stipulated that no one would be considered for faculty appointment with less than a master's degree level education. At first, all but two turned him down. Dr. Ross Stromberg from Atlanta, Georgia and Dr. Ralph Steinman from Asheville, North Carolina, both went on for appropriate graduate training. Ralph attended the University of Michigan. This education enabled him to be the first instructor of Prosthodontics at the new school.

Those early days were successful despite some rather primitive conditions. The first class was accepted in 1953 before there was even a clinic. There were no basic science teachers so those classes were taken right along with medical students in what was then known as CME—the College of Medical Evangelists. Actual dental classes were taught in a building behind the Loma Linda Sanitarium up on "The Hill" where the School of Public Health is presently located.

The first dental class did not require actual clinical provisions until the third or junior year, which was around 1956. A small clinic was then set up with 10 dental chairs in the basement of Evans Hall (the old Microbiology building, now housing the Campus Center for Health Promotions offices). This arrangement existed in cramped spaces amidst steam pipes, low ceilings, and concrete floors, but served the purpose well enough until larger, more appropriate quarters could be obtained.

Dr. Steinman recalled back in the 1960s when some of the faculty were arguing fairly convincingly for moving the school out to Los Angeles in the Boyle Heights area. Their main point of concern was whether there could continue to be a ready source of patients in a location as remote as Loma Linda. After the decision was finally made to remain located in Loma Linda, the school not only proved to have sufficient patients to keep their schedule filled but would stand out from among other dental schools as uniquely self-supporting--largely from money generated by its own clinic income.

Around that time, Dean Prince recognized that a position needed to be created and funded for a dental researcher. It would need to be someone with a religious and philosophical background compatible with the school. Not only would the search task be difficult, but how much pay should the dean offer someone in this capacity? One morning he called Ralph to his office to consult about it. It was there that it dawned on Ralph that he personally could fill that need and save the school significant funds. He told Dr. Prince to look no further, that he would assume responsibility for that position himself. It was not an easy decision but after a long afternoon of fairly intense discussion, the dean agreed to it.

Ralph Steinman became the only dental research scientist that the dental school had for many years. It was not an easy start. Ralph describes himself as relatively untrained and uneducated when it came to performing original research. Fortunately, at that time the school of medicine had just acquired several young PhDs on their faculty. Ralph recalls finding ready acceptance by them. He had to go back and spend time studying his physiology and biochemistry books with renewed dedication to become sufficiently knowledgeable and conversant. He relished the wholesome interchange of ideas and knowledgeable opinions these specially trained individuals had to contribute. Dr. Steinman thrived on open-ended search for new information. Research became his favorite part of dentistry, and from that point he never looked back.

Projects were conducted in connection with the departments of Microbiology, Biochemistry, and Physiology. Interested dental students were invited to help. One of the first experiments was to measure relative failure of white blood cells' ability to phagocytize or engulf foreign blood particles when challenged with high levels of sugar. It was a simple, direct, and effective study which, after publication, was frequently referenced in the literature by other scientific writers.

This was an extension of Ralph's growing conviction that the body's defenses are influenced, if not sometimes controlled, by dietary intake. Such conviction went back to his own experience of changing his diet away from refined food products in order to overcome serious asthmatic symptoms. It was this cause-and-effect concept that remained paramount in Ralph's mind as he designed his experiments and interpreted their results.

When he started out, he observed other university's research facilities. He was impressed by the hundreds of white rats seen in cages at Harvard University's dental research center. He also visited the research center at the University of Michigan and recalls discussing the then-current *Lactobacillus*-caries theory with Dr. Phil Jay. It wasn't a theory Ralph necessarily agreed with (and has subsequently been disproven) but it was the best there was at the time. Coming back armed with new information, ideas, and enthusiasm he set up a rat experiment laboratory with the help of Dr. Mervyn Hardinge, PhD/PhD.

Dr. Steinman was frequently seen around the dental school wearing his white lab coat, wafting in characteristic aromas from the rat laboratory. Students couldn't help noticing, and soon affectionately referred to him as the "rat man," which Ralph seemed to enjoy in hia characteristically good-naturedly way.

He was ever innovative, approachable, confident, and upbeat. He always seemed to know exactly what he was doing, or at least trying to do, and glad to explain to anyone about it. It was refreshing for students to talk with such a knowledgeable and independent thinker.

Government research grants of $25,000 per year for at least a couple years kept things going along well. Inauspiciously, however, around 1981 a NIH grant was refused because the NIH site investigator somehow took the opinion that such research was not in line with any known accepted theories. Ironically, part of what true research is all about is the discovery and development of new theories. Ralph had been dependent on these important outside sources of research funding because the dental school budget did not include it. He showed the visiting scientist everything he could to explain its value to dentistry and the medical sciences, but unfortunately that grant assessor's mind had already been made up. After that, it became very difficult to find further financial research support.

Based on information from the dental literature on a possible dentinal fluid flow mechanism and his own observations, Dr. Steinman became convinced that physiological mechanism(s) might be involved in maintaining dental health. This innovative concept was based on his observation that the movement of a fluorescent dye through the dentin could be significantly inhibited by feeding a cariogenic diet to rats compared to the movement observed in rats fed a noncariogenic diet. Such an innovative concept was anathema to those who embraced the acidogenic theory as the primary causal factor for cariogenesis to occur. It was at this point that Dr. Steinman felt his physiological background was not sufficient to identify the possible physiological mechanism(s) and consulted with Dr. Leonora. Dr. Leonora suggested that in all probability hormonal mechanism(s) were involved. It was from this discussion that their research collaboration began, leading to discovery of a new endocrine system--the hypothalamic parotid gland endocrine axis (HPEA)--which regulates/stimulates dentinal fluid flow.

Dr. Steinman retired to Sunny Valley, Oregon in 1997. He was 94 years old at the time of this interview. Unfortunately progressive macular degeneration had severely affected his ability to read. Despite this handicap, his mind remained active and he continued offering thoughtful new insights and approaches for further research in his correspondence until his passing at age 97 in 2007. His wife Emily passed away a year later, also at the age of 97.--two long and very dedicated lives.

--Clyde Roggenkamp, DDS
Fall, 2004

DR. JOHN LEONORA

Professor of Physiology and Endocrinology
Lecturer and Researcher
Loma Linda University School of Medicine
(Information submitted to Wikipedia from family)
1928-2006

John Leonora was born in Milwaukee, Wisconsin, soon after his parents arrived as immigrants from Sicily. Upon the death of his father in 1942, John's mother found employment stitching leather by hand in an Italian shoe factory. He became an errand boy for various businesses throughout Milwaukee. Meanwhile, he excelled in school and became proficient with the piano. He accompanied and played at jazz combos. John was an active member of the Italian club at Lincoln High School. Because of excellent grades he was awarded a one-year scholarship at the University of Wisconsin, Milwaukee, WI.

Upon receiving his B.S. degree at the University of Wisconsin, Madison, WI, he took an interim position as a laboratory assistant in chemistry and obtained teaching credentials at what is now Andrews University, Berrien Springs, MI. John returned to Madison and the University of Wisconsin. There he and his wife lived as he completed his education with a PhD in endocrine physiology, obtained a federal fellowship and embarked on his career as an endocrinologist.

Dr. Leonora was active in his chosen field of medical physiology for nearly 40 years. He received over one million dollars in research grant awards from such entities as the National Institutes of Health, the Walter E. Macpherson Society, the Don Baxter Foundation, the Pediatric Research Endowment Fund and the Basic Science Research Fund.

He served as Professor and Co-Chairman, Department of Physiology and Pharmacology, Loma Linda University, from 1970 to 2002. Dr. Leonora not only mentored numerous graduate students, but provided leadership for research conducted in his own laboratory. In his research he demonstrated remarkable surgical skills whether with a pig weighing 200 pounds or a mouse weighing only a few ounces. He also delighted in teaching. His lectures were remembered by students for their clarity and quiet humor.

Gonadotropic Hormones. Based on his doctoral studies and subsequent research fellowship, John Leonora initially intended to devote his career to the investigation of gonadotropic hormones.

Dentinal Fluid Transport. One day he received a telephone call from Dr. Ralph R. Steinman, a dental colleague, who had been studying the flow of dentinal fluid in the teeth of rats from the odontoblasts in the dental pulp through the dentin using an intraperitoneal injection of the fluorescent dye, acriflavine hydrochloride. Steinman found that in the teeth of rats fed a cariogenic diet the flow of dentinal fluid, as an indigenous means of caries protection within the tooth, was markedly reduced. He wondered if some systemic mechanism might be involved in this impairment and so decided to contact Dr. John Leonora as an endocrinologist.

The Hypothalamus. This was the beginning of a fascinating, decades-long collaborative journey. John Leonora first suggested that none of the recognized hormones were plausible candidates for regulating dentinal fluid transport (DFT), but that the hypothalamus might well be an alternative hormonal source. Quickly they found that infusing rats with a crude extract from rabbit hypothalami triggered increased DFT activity. This, however, raised the question whether the hypothalamic factor had a direct effect on the teeth or rather had an indirect effect characteristic of other hypothalamic hormones.

The Parotid Hormone. Assuming that the hypothalamic factor was mediated through one of the major salivary glands, John Leonora, along with co-investigators Ralph Steinman and Jean-Marc Tièche, found that this factor was biologically active when administered to rats with intact parotid glands but was wholly ineffective in rats that had the parotid glands removed. There was no involvement of the other salivary glands. Direct regulation of dentinal fluid flow was found to be by the parotid glands and this endocrine function was controlled by the hypothalamus.

Neural Stimuli of the Hypothalamus. The next question was what physiological factors normally stimulate the secretion of the parotid hormone? Feeding pigs a standard pig chow proved to effectively stimulate parotid hormone secretion along with a copious secretion of saliva. Surprisingly, pigs fed nonnutritive substances and exposed to auditory, olfactory and visual cues salivated profusely but these cues did not change the fasting level of the parotid hormone. The endocrine and exocrine functions of the parotid glands, therefore, occur concurrently but they must be controlled by different mechanisms. Apparently nutritive substrates activate neural stimuli going to the hypothalamus, which in turn activates the hypothalamic-parotid gland endocrine axis that then stimulates the dentinal fluid transport mechanism.

The Formation of Dentin. At this critical juncture a group of investigators at the University of Oulu Dental School, Oulu, Finland [Tjäderhane, L. et al] discovered that the parotid hormone not only regulates the flow of dentinal fluid but also is involved in the formation of dentin—dentinogenesis. They also found that a high sucrose diet in young rats suppressed primary dentinogenesis. The injection of carbamyl phosphate significantly reversed the effect of sucrose—but only in intact rats. Furthermore, carbamyl phosphate prevented the atrophy of the parotid glands associated with the ingestion of sucrose.

The Synthesis of the Parotid Hormone. Subsequent research successfully cloned the porcine cDNAs that code for the parotid hormone gene. The amino acids encoded by these cDNAs agreed with the amino acid sequence of the hormone isolated from the porcine parotid glands. In addition, a commercially available synthetic parotid hormone was found to have an activity indistinguishable from the isolated parotid hormone or the gene-expressed hormone.

The Acinar Cell Source of the Parotid Hormone. Meanwhile, it was discovered that the acinar cells of the parotid glands are apparently the source of the parotid hormone.

The Regulation of Insulin Secretion. Preliminary research suggested the parotid hormone not only regulates dental structures but also influences insulin secretion by the pancreas.

Other Tissues/Organs. These systemic effects have yet to be followed up but may well include other glandular and/or avascular tissues. As Dr. Leonora stated in an undated letter, "I anticipate finding receptors [for the Parotid Hormone] in the odontoblasts in teeth, osteocytes in bone matrix, [and] Islets of Langerhans…."

Dr. Leonora, with what may be considered irrefutable evidence, introduced the controlling role played by Parotid Hormone in dental health and its interaction with insulin and other systemic metabolic chemical factors. He was instrumental in recognizing that the parotid gland possesses dual functions. Besides excreting saliva into the oral cavity, it produces a hormone that activates fluid from the dental pulp to be expressed outwardly through the radiating tubular structure of the dentin and microscopic pores of the enamel. If the dentinal fluid transport theory is correct, this maintains and protects teeth particularly during eating. The Parotid Hormone is also to have interaction with insulin and other systemic metabolic factors but this aspect deserves further investigation. John's life ended before he could pursue this research and it would be a tribute to his eager investigative spirit if medicine, dentistry and basic science would collaboratively continue this quest. Important new facets of discovery important to our knowledge and treatment of health are undoubtedly waiting to be found in this very rewarding and promising area.

APPENDIX C

PERSONAL TRIBUTES TO DR. STEINMAN
(Presented in alphabetical order)

Tribute to Dr.Steinman

It was with some degree of interest that I first listened to the lectures of Dr. Steinman on dental decay. As a beginning dental student, the thought of why or how caries exists was of much less importance than the treatment. Fillings, crowns, partials, dentures and surgery had specific requirements for graduation and represented the difference between financial failure and success in private practice. Thirty years later the emphasis of dental education and practice has not appreciably changed--"Show me the money!" still rules.

Disease epidemiology, etiology and progression leading to concepts of prevention still take a distant back seat to treatment in most areas of medicine and dentistry. The loudest cries for help come from those who already have the disease, not from those who may or may not get it. This is seen most lately in AIDS where money has poured in to expensive therapies that most of the world cannot afford even if access to care were available. This is also obvious in cardiovascular disease, cancer and most infectious diseases including dental decay which is perhaps the most wide-spread infectious disease.

Politics within caries research has also strongly impacted this struggling arena. Forceful opinions within groups of scientists have, as frequently happens, sidelined the concepts of other researchers, which stalled overall progress in the field. One of the most eloquent papers in this regard has been recently penned by Dr. Larmas in the *Journal of Dental Research* 82(4):253-256, 2003 where he uncovers a 35-year history of rejected manuscripts and concepts because strong, well positioned researchers only believed in the acid theory of tooth decay. A strong appeal is then made to study the pathobiology of the caries process involving odontoblasts and dentin-pulp physiology in a similar manner in which bone physiologists evaluate osteoblasts and osteoporosis. It's beginning to look a lot like Ralph.

It is in this context that the work of Dr.Steinman regarding the physiologic relationships of fluid movement in teeth, sugar, and a possible hypothalamic-parotid endocrine axis stands fairly isolated from both the monied aspects of dentistry and the small world of dental caries research. Yet the problem of dental caries has not lessened, and years after those dental school lectures I still find myself treating rampant decay in many children and adults who live within a few miles of Loma Linda University. The dental disease of these patients is as bad, many times worse than that which I have seen in any of my third world mission trips, and these patients do have access to tooth brushes, fluoride and dental care. It is clear that both our knowledge and methods are deficient as we are not winning this war. This perplexing enigma causes me to cherish the larger concepts of dental health and disease espoused by Dr. Steinman in the classroom, and in our private discussions at the dental school and in his home.

This compilation of the prodigious work of Dr. Steinman is a tribute to a fine researcher who worked against great odds nationally, worldwide but especially locally. His research presents an extremely important perspective of a monstrous worldwide disease. It is time to carefully consider the broader picture of this painful and debilitating disease, which we will never be able to conquer with surgical methods alone.

We applaud this wonderful friend, gentleman and scientist.

--Stanton S. Appleton DDS, MPH, MSD
Professor and Section Chief
Oral Medicine, Orofacial Pain
LLU School of Dentistry

Dr. Ralph Steinman was my teacher, mentor, and friend. As my professor of Prosthodontics he constantly asked the question, "Why?" --Why should we have this problem of tooth decay?

Teeth are a living part of a living organism, ingeniously created to last. What has gone wrong? Why do some people have this disease and some do not? He believed that with the proper understanding of human physiology and biochemistry that this problem, which has plagued a large part of humanity, could be solved and prevented.

His tenacity and sheer willpower together with his work ethic, his wisdom, and his faith led this man to accomplish what very few could.

Though his research involved working with nutritionists, physiologists, biochemists, pharmacologists and many others, it was his personal drive, determination and total dedication to the task that was the key to his accomplishments.

This summary of his work has been compiled by another of his students and friends, Dr. Clyde Roggenkamp. May someone of Dr. Steinman's courage, ability, and undaunted spirit build on this storehouse of information and continue with this pertinent work.

--Dr. James Crawford, DDS, MPH
Former Dean, LLU School of Public Health

As one of the initial faculty members present when Loma Linda University School of Dentistry opened in 1953, Dr. Ralph Steinman deserves special recognition. Additionally, he deserves accolades for his contributions to the history of outstanding research at Loma Linda that has improved the quality of life for countless patients.

Without question, the research thrust of the School of Dentistry was initiated through the early work of Dr.Steinman. He set a standard of excellence that was unique to that time in history. We owe much to his efforts and he is rightfully recognized as the "Father of Research" at Loma Linda University School of Dentistry.

--Charles Goodacre, DDS
Dean, LLU School of Dentistry

Dental health remains a major public health concern with millions of edentulous adults and countless children needing extensive dental care in spite of the well-documented benefits of fluoridation. The research of Dr. Ralph Steinman presented a primary prevention approach that if implemented could have a significant impact on decreasing the burden of dental disease. Dr. Steinman understood the concept of dietary effects being mediated systemically and not just in an external local sense. Such an understanding belies a simplistic approach and is in keeping with the understanding of our bodies as complex interrelated physiologic systems that if given proper support through diet, as well as exercise, will function optimally. Public health salutes a forward- thinking man, a careful researcher and a committed Christian.

--Patricia Johnston, DrPH, MS, RD
Dean, LLU School of Public Health

Remembering the past...

During my junior and senior years (1957-1958) as a dental student, I had the opportunity to work for Dr. Steinman in research. In his work with various sugars he proposed to feed mice from birth to the time they would be weaned with a variety of formulas. A task I was assigned to perform was to be a stand-in for the mother mouse.

I was impressed with the innovative thinking of Dr. Steinman as we designed and assembled an array of glass pipes, plastic tubing, and an assortment of glass containers terminating with a row of nipples. Part of the assembly was located in refrigeration where formulae were kept fresh, then transported through this maze and delivered to its destination at room temperature. Experiencing repeated setbacks with this approach, we were impressed with the uniqueness of the mother mouse and sought a more simplified approach. We found that miniature milk bottles used by children as they simulate the feeding of their baby doll would simplify the concept of automated feeding. This proved to be the system of choice, even though this was work-intensive, since feeding these little ones by hand occurred every 4 hours around the clock.

As a dental student with lessons to be learned and little exposure to research, I observed in Dr. Steinman the vision, the tenacity, and the ability to regroup when faced with odds.

I have been enriched in knowing this man as an instructor, colleague, friend, and scientist.

--Robert L. Kinzer, DDS
Professor of Restorative Dentistry
LLU School of Dentistry

Dr. Steinman has been a stalwart leadership figure in dental research at the LLU School of Dentistry from the earliest period of his faculty service. After his graduation from Atlanta Southern Dental College (subsequently Emory University School of Dentistry) in 1943, he has applied his considerable energy toward realizing high standards of clinical dentistry, and to areas of research that support this quest. In his early years of practice in the Asheville, North Carolina area, he began to focus on the possibility of systemic factors that influence general health, and this led to his concern that these systemic factors might also influence a patient's susceptibility to dental disease.

When an opportunity came to join the faculty at the newly developing dental school in Loma Linda, California in 1952, he accepted the new Dean's invitation somewhat as a mandate to pursue the research that occupied most of his subsequent professional career.

In my long acquaintance with Dr. Steinman, one of my earliest memories was observing him present a table clinic to the American Dental Association on the shrinkage effect of solder joints in fixed prostheses, emphasizing the distortion to the prosthesis such shrinkage could produce. This bit of research in the arena of dental materials was at a very practical level, relating to then-common techniques in restorative dentistry.

A much larger allocation of Ralph's time and effort developed as he pursued a better understanding of the causes of dental caries, and our understanding of caries as a disease process, rather than merely as a collection of dental defects to be repaired mechanically, with "fillings", inlays or crowns.

His interest in learning the cause(s) of dental decay with the hope of preventing this widespread health problem may not, at that time, have been in the most popular field of dental research activity. Investigators studying the physical properties of various dental materials, particularly those used in restorative and prosthetic dentistry, were more commonly found in the mainstream; those relating to the causes and prevention of dental disease were mainly devoted to concepts resulting from acids etching enamel, and the subsequent need to mechanically repair or replace the missing tooth structure.

The School of Dentistry realized numerous tangible benefits from the inspiration and diligence Dr. Steinman applied to his research efforts. Among the School's early faculty, whose efforts (because of minimal staffing) were stretched over the entire dental curriculum, he was virtually alone in his chosen interest in caries etiology. He was a model of diligence in the use of his time and effort, and well-disciplined in seeking to broaden his knowledge of basic sciences as they applied to his research interests. His basic science colleagues, notably Dr. John Leonora, were constant in their support of his study and research efforts. Over the entire period of Dr. Steinman's faculty service he inspired many younger faculty colleagues and dental alumni in the pursuit of his research goals.

--Judson Klooster, DDS
Dean Emeritus
LLU School of Dentistry

In the history of Loma Linda University School of Dentistry are found giants. As a school dedicated to the compassionate care of patients, it is built on the shoulders of those who set examples as to what that means. Among those is included the name of Dr. Ralph Steinman. Dr. Steinman was a scholar who, because of his philosophical belief that the maintenance of oral health is more effectively achieved through application of health principles and the prevention of disease than through the symptomatic treatment of disease sequelae, followed lines of research leading to prevention of dental caries, the preponderant dental disease affecting all societies.

His seminal work on the role of diet, the systemic foundation of dental health and the importance of implementing effective oral health practices are just beginning to be recognized today, some forty years after he propounded those ideas. The mechanisms by which sugar weakens the system and promotes dental caries are only beginning to be understood outside of this institution.

Thank you Dr. Steinman for setting the stage for the next generation of oral health management and giving those of us who follow in your footsteps encouragement to persevere in a traditionalist environment.

--**George Lessard, PhD**
Director of Research Activities
LLU School of Dentistry

In my senior year (1967) at LLUSD, I had an amazing experience in a lecture given by Dr Ralph Steinman. It was a slide view demonstration of dentinal fluid being transported through the dentin and enamel. That picture has remained with me over the past 35 years of dental practice.

During that year I spent significant time and study with Ralph exploring his concepts and became convinced that the teeth do have an immune response to the initial stages of caries, and that the teeth do possess a physiology just as bone and soft tissue.

Through the years, these principles have been used as the primary approach to prevention in my practice and has served me well with great satisfaction with the results for my patients.

I visited Ralph regularly to keep pace with his progress over the years and update my practice approach to prevention. In 1988, I met with Dr John Leonora, Ralph's long time associate in their research in the medical center laboratory to discuss the status of their work and found all their notebooks, some 15 or so lying on a lower shelf gathering dust. Somewhat shocked, I ask John if these were the only records of their work. They were, so I asked his permission to use them to organize, outline and index them. Over the next five years, I spent many hours in the library looking up his references, duplicating all his documenting references, reading, outlining and building an index. I now have over 400 research papers from various authors collaborating his work along with over 50 of his own articles. They are organized, indexed and outlined.

Ralph was retired then and living in Yucaipa, but still doing literature research for John on Wednesday morning at the library. Each Wednesday I spent some time discussing his research to guide me in my work. At this time, I gained a great respect for his tremendous intellect, memory, and dedication to this research.

Ralph has made a major discovery and contribution to an important cause and treatment of caries. It has taken, and will yet take many years before the full impact of this will reach the daily practice of dentistry.

As one of the four original faculty of Loma Linda university school of dentistry, founder of the dental research department, researcher extraordinaire and person of great stature and humility, he should receive a place of true honor and respect at the school of dentistry.

--**Lin Martin, DDS**
Assistant professor
LLU School of Dentistry

My first encounter with Dr. Steinman was when I was a second year dental student at Loma Linda University (then the College of Medical Evangelists) in 1957. Dr. Steinman, to say the least, was significantly different than other faculty at that time. He was an independent thinker that was not afraid to face the dental establishment at the time and to stimulate their thinking in the area of the etiology of dental caries. That the etiology of dental caries was in any way connected to a systemic effect mediated by the individual's diet and the intake of carbohydrates was equivalent to thinking that people traveled between Mars and Earth and back again. His willingness to pursue a conviction, regardless of its acceptance by the establishment and his critical thinking and inquisitive mind were like a magnet attracting me to him.

I volunteered to work with Dr. Steinman on his research in the hope that some of his intelligence and critical thinking would be transferred, by some act of magic, to me. The major project, on which I worked with him as a student, was evaluating the effect of the intake of different carbohydrates in the diet on the status of the odontoblastic processes within the dentinal tubules of rat's teeth. He was anxious to examine the odontoblastic process under the electron microscope. Up to this time, however, it was necessary to decalcify the dentin in order to section it thin enough to view under transmission electron microscopy. The harsh tissue preparation process for decalcification greatly altered the integrity of the odontoblastic process. We were successful in developing a mechanism by which it was possible to section non-decalcified dentin for viewing under transmission electron microscopy. This allowed us to identify a significant difference in the odontoblastic processes of littermate laboratory rats with the controlled variable being the amount and type of carbohydrate ingested in their diet.

These early experiences in critical thinking and the exploration of the unknown in science eventually led me to become involved in teaching and scientific investigation. I owe a great deal to Dr. Steinman for the example he set in having the courage to follow his convictions even when they are not consistent with commonly held beliefs.

--**Steven Morrow, DDS**
Assoc. Professor
Clinical Administrator
LLU School of Dentistry

SPECIAL TRIBUTE FROM THE LLU CENTER FOR DENTAL RESEARCH

The Center for Dental Research is proud and honored to salute Dr. Ralph R. Steinman, one of Loma Linda University School of Dentistry's early pioneers in dental research. Dr. Steinman's published works span a period of over 4 decades from 1954 to 1994. During this time he produced a body of literature that has impacted other researchers as well as the dental profession. As you read through the pages of this book, you will see firsthand the contributions of Dr. Steinman's research on the etiology and prevention of dental caries.

To showcase Dr. Steinman's findings, this collection of publications has been produced with the help of many of his colleagues and former students. It is hoped that future generations of dentists and dental hygienists may enjoy the fruits of his labor.

Let me add that this entire undertaking would not have been possible without the initiative and commitment of Dr. Clyde Roggenkamp. Dr. Roggenkamp was the driving force behind this project. So, on behalf of the Center for Dental Research, I am pleased to extend my thanks and congratulations to him for his outstanding effort in collecting this scientific information. I also want to recognize and thank those who included individual tributes to Dr. Steinman. You'll find their personal comments further highlight the value of Dr. Steinman's research and the impact he had in their professional development.

These collected works will also appear in the 2004 edition of *Committed to Research* in CD-ROM format. Copies can be obtained through Continuing Education.

Please join us in saluting Dr. Steinman.

--Carlos A. Muñoz-Viveros, DDS, MSD
Director, Biomaterials Research
LLU School of Dentistry

A fluid transport system and the prevention of tooth decay

In 1971, discoveries by Ralph R. Steinman, DDS, MS, professor of oral medicine, School of Dentistry, and John Leonora, PhD, professor of physiology and biophysics, School of Medicine, demonstrated a change in fluid dynamics within teeth: a transport system flowing from the pulp through the dentinal tubules.

Dr. Steinman had studied the dental literature back to the 1880s and had discovered an interesting minority view based on research indicating that teeth might possess a defensive mechanism against cavities. This information motivated Dr. Steinman to explore this theory. He developed a rapid technique to visualize dentinal fluid flow using a fluorescent dye as a marker. By tracking the dye, Dr. Steinman was able to document an astounding observation: that the teeth are internally active. In the absence of sugar, the dentinal fluid flowed within the tooth from the dentin-pulp interface through the dentin. In contrast, no significant flow occurred in the presence of a high sugar intake. The fact that sugar in the diet could affect an internal process in teeth had not been documented before.

The discovery had important implications regarding the eventual prevention of dental decay. The significance of the outward dentinal fluid flow is: (1) It prevents the penetration of bacterial acids into the tooth structure, and (2) It neutralizes the bacterial acids on the surface of the teeth.

To answer the question of how this mechanism was controlled, Dr. Steinman consulted with Dr. Leonora who suggested that a hormonal mechanism would be most appropriate controlling dentinal fluid flow. Their collaborative studies led to the discovery of a new endocrine system: the hypothalamic-parotid gland endocrine axis.

They isolated the parotid hormone in a pure form, and showed that it stimulates dentinal fluid flow. They demonstrated that a high sugar diet suppresses the function of this endocrine axis and consequently dentinal fluid flow. They went on to demonstrate in rats that they could physiologically prevent the suppressive effect of the high sugar diet on dentinal fluid flow and prevent dental decay 80 to 100 percent of the time.

Subsequent research by others has concluded that dentinal fluid flow also exists in human teeth. As in rats, dentinal fluid flow may be an important defensive mechanism for preventing dental decay in humans.

--Richard A. Schaefer
LLU Historian
(Written in collaboration with Dr. John Leonora,
for the *LLU Observer*, April 1971)

As a dental hygiene student at Loma Linda University School of Dentistry in the mid-1960s, I had the privilege of having Dr. Ralph Steinman as the course director for my Nutrition and Dental Caries class.

He impressed upon us students the importance of diet in the control of dental caries. He cited his wife and himself as examples whose personal dental histories were replete with restorations; and yet his own children had no history of carious lesions--therefore espousing his philosophy that there was more than genetics at work.

He was a 20th century pioneer (in his research with mice) into the relationship and interaction between the body and the oral cavity. In this modern age, the medical/dental community has come to increasingly support this very important relationship.

--Karen A. Simpson, MPH, RDH
Associate Professor, Dental Hygiene

I came across Dr. Steinman's Research projects in my freshman year of Dental School in 1979. I had to do an errand on the 4th floor, where dental research was located at the time, and happened to run into Ralph in his lab. I was asking for directions to a different department at the time, but Dr. Steinman seemed to take a liking to me and handed me a folder of all the papers he had published and written up to that point. I had looked them over and promptly went back into student mode in order to graduate on time. Sometime later after I had finished school and was out on my own, in my own business did I come across his papers and begin to reread them. Stimulated by the content, I looked Ralph up and found he had recently retired from the Dental School / Research program and was still living in Yucaipa. He consented to having me drop by and we discussed the overall sum of his findings. From there we decided to meet with Dr. Leonora, Dr. Tièche, Dr. Beltz and have lunch on a once a month basis to stimulate interest on the topic of "Dentinal Fluid Transport." Soon after we began to meet, Ralph moved up to Oregon where he and his wife have retired. The monthly get-togethers continued until May of 2002, when

I stopped teaching in the Dental School. I still keep in touch with Dr. Steinman from time to time and converse with Dr. Leonora, although more infrequently now.

It was always a mystery for me why the pulp has such a large blood supply, nervous innervation, and lymphatic supply, just to let you know when you had a tooth ache! The information given to me from instructors was always found wanting. In fact, it was apparent that no one knew the answer to my question. But, when I read Ralph's papers on the proposed function of the dental pulp, odontoblasts in particular, I was convinced he was on to something. The fact that the pulp changes into a hydrodynamic pump under the direction of a hormone produced by the Parotid Gland not only supplies a quantitative answer, it also makes perfect sense! The teeth have a natural defense mechanism after all! Now we could counsel patients how to avoid getting cavities in a way that makes a difference. . . . in the diet, and avoiding sugar before meals!

I wish there had been time for me to be involved with Ralph's research (still ongoing). But, fate has determined that I just be acquainted with the body of knowledge instead. I am very gratified that I met Dr. Steinman and became knowledgeable of his quest for understanding about diet and dental disease interaction. I am confident the skeptics will come around to the scientific table in time.

--Herbert Woodward III, DDS
General Dentist, Carlsbad, CA

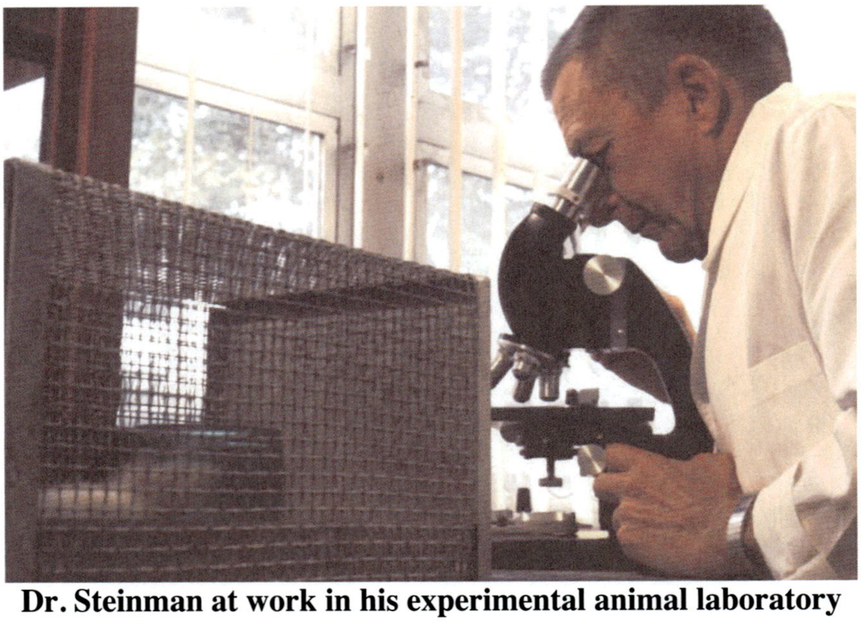

Dr. Steinman at work in his experimental animal laboratory

FIGURES

TABLES

INDEX

Subjects are listed by page numbers; *T* indicates Table(s) and **Bold printed numbers** indicate Figure(s).

E

F

Dentinal Fluid Transport

GLOSSARY OF ABBREVIATIONS AND TERMS

↑	Increases, increased
↓	Decreases, decreased
½ round bur	½ mm-diameter round-shaped dental rotating bur
μg	Microgram
AA	Amino acid(s)
ADP	Adenosine diphosphate
Aliquot	A portion or sample of a liquid used to test the composition of the whole
AMP	Adenosine monophosphate
ATP	Adenosine triphosphate
BSL	Blood sugar level
CAA	Carbamyl aspartic acid; an IDDP-stimulating compound
CAP	Carbamyl phosphate
C	Carbon
cDNA	Cloned DNA
C	Centigrade degrees
CHO	Carbohydrate
Cr	Chromium
DEJ	Dentinoenamel junction
DFM	Dentinal fluid movement (used interchangeably with DFT, dentinal fluid transport)
DFT	Dentinal fluid transport (used interchangeably with DFM, dentinal fluid movement)
Diamox	Trademark for preparations of acetazolamide, a carbonic anhydride inhibitor (used sometimes as a urinary alkalizer)
Diuril	A chlorothiazide diuretic
DNA	Deoxyribonucleic acid
DNP	Dinitrophenol
DOCA	Desoxycorticosterone trimethylacetate
ELISA	Enzyme linked immunoadsorbent assay
F	Fluoride
FM	Fluid movement
FMR	Fluid movement ratio
GI	Gastrointestinal
GTT	Glucose tolerance test
H, h	Hour
HE	Hypothalamic extract
HPEA	Hypothalamic-parotid endocrine axis
HSD	High sucrose diet
IDDP	Intradentinal dye penetration
iPH	Immunoreactive parotid hormone
i.p., I.P.	Intraperitoneal (within the abdominal space)
i.v., I.V.	Intravenous
KCN	Potassium cyanide

mRNA	Messenger RNA
MAO	Monoamine oxidase(s), present in tissues probably for detoxification
Mbd	Molybdenum
Me	Methane gas or Methionine (a sulfur-containing amino acid)
Mersalyl	A mercurial diuretic administered intramuscularly or intravenously
Mg	Magnesium
Mo	Molybdenum
NaCl	Sodium chloride, table salt
NIH	National Institutes of Health, Washington, DC
Ninhydrin	Trademark for a preparation of triketohydrindene hydrate used as chemical test for the presence of protein
P	Phosphorus
Pg	Picogram
PH	Parotid hormone
pH	Negative logarithm of the hydrogen ion concentration; a measure of acidity or alkalinity
PHRF	Parotid hormone releasing factor, comes from the hypothalamus
Pi	Inorganic phosphorus
PRF	Parotin releasing factor
[ref]	Indicates references available in the original article
RIA	Radioimmunoassay
RNA	Ribonucleic acid
SD, SDase	Succinic dehydrogenase, an iron-containing flavoprotein found in the mitochondria, transfers H atoms or electrons from substrate to molecular oxygen
SH	Sulfhydryl (chemical group containing sulfur plus hydrogen)
SS	Disulfide
UV	Ultraviolet
TE	Trace elements
Zn	Zinc